Update on Robotic Gastrointestinal Surgery

Update on Robotic Gastrointestinal Surgery

Editors

Marco Milone
Paolo Pietro Bianchi

MDPI • Basel • Beijing • Wuhan • Barcelona • Belgrade • Manchester • Tokyo • Cluj • Tianjin

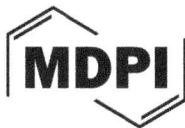

Editors
Marco Milone
Department of Clinical
Medicine and Surgery
University of Naples
"Federico II"
Naples
Italy

Paolo Pietro Bianchi
Department of Health Science
University of Milan
Milano
Italy

Editorial Office
MDPI
St. Alban-Anlage 66
4052 Basel, Switzerland

This is a reprint of articles from the Special Issue published online in the open access journal *Journal of Personalized Medicine* (ISSN 2075-4426) (available at: www.mdpi.com/journal/jpm/special_issues/Gastrointestinal_Surgery).

For citation purposes, cite each article independently as indicated on the article page online and as indicated below:

LastName, A.A.; LastName, B.B.; LastName, C.C. Article Title. *Journal Name* **Year**, *Volume Number*, Page Range.

ISBN 978-3-0365-7679-4 (Hbk)
ISBN 978-3-0365-7678-7 (PDF)

© 2023 by the authors. Articles in this book are Open Access and distributed under the Creative Commons Attribution (CC BY) license, which allows users to download, copy and build upon published articles, as long as the author and publisher are properly credited, which ensures maximum dissemination and a wider impact of our publications.
The book as a whole is distributed by MDPI under the terms and conditions of the Creative Commons license CC BY-NC-ND.

Contents

About the Editors vii

Preface to "Update on Robotic Gastrointestinal Surgery" ix

Marco Milone and Paolo Pietro Bianchi
Robotic Gastrointestinal Surgery: State of the Art and Future Perspectives
Reprinted from: *J. Pers. Med.* **2023**, *13*, 568, doi:10.3390/jpm13030568 1

Sara Vertaldi, Anna D'Amore, Michele Manigrasso, Pietro Anoldo, Alessia Chini and Francesco Maione et al.
Robotic Surgery and Functional Esophageal Disorders: A Systematic Review and Meta-Analysis
Reprinted from: *J. Pers. Med.* **2023**, *13*, 231, doi:10.3390/jpm13020231 3

Marco Milone, Michele Manigrasso, Pietro Anoldo, Anna D'Amore, Ugo Elmore and Mariano Cesare Giglio et al.
The Role of Robotic Visceral Surgery in Patients with Adhesions: A Systematic Review and Meta-Analysis
Reprinted from: *J. Pers. Med.* **2022**, *12*, 307, doi:10.3390/jpm12020307 19

Simona Giuratrabocchetta, Giampaolo Formisano, Adelona Salaj, Enrico Opocher, Luca Ferraro and Francesco Toti et al.
Update on Robotic Total Mesorectal Excision for Rectal Cancer
Reprinted from: *J. Pers. Med.* **2021**, *11*, 900, doi:10.3390/jpm11090900 45

Giampaolo Formisano, Luca Ferraro, Adelona Salaj, Simona Giuratrabocchetta, Andrea Pisani Ceretti and Enrico Opocher et al.
Update on Robotic Rectal Prolapse Treatment
Reprinted from: *J. Pers. Med.* **2021**, *11*, 706, doi:10.3390/jpm11080706 57

Giuseppe Giuliani, Francesco Guerra, Lorenzo De Franco, Lucia Salvischiani, Roberto Benigni and Andrea Coratti
Review on Perioperative and Oncological Outcomes of Robotic Gastrectomy for Cancer
Reprinted from: *J. Pers. Med.* **2021**, *11*, 638, doi:10.3390/jpm11070638 67

Michele Manigrasso, Sara Vertaldi, Alessandra Marello, Stavros Athanasios Antoniou, Nader Kamal Francis and Giovanni Domenico De Palma et al.
Robotic Esophagectomy. A Systematic Review with Meta-Analysis of Clinical Outcomes
Reprinted from: *J. Pers. Med.* **2021**, *11*, 640, doi:10.3390/jpm11070640 77

Michele Manigrasso, Sara Vertaldi, Pietro Anoldo, Anna D'Amore, Alessandra Marello and Carmen Sorrentino et al.
Robotic Colorectal Cancer Surgery. How to Reach Expertise? A Single Surgeon-Experience
Reprinted from: *J. Pers. Med.* **2021**, *11*, 621, doi:10.3390/jpm11070621 103

Fabio Rondelli, Alessandro Sanguinetti, Andrea Polistena, Stefano Avenia, Claudio Marcacci and Graziano Ceccarelli et al.
Robotic Transanal Total Mesorectal Excision (RTaTME): State of the Art
Reprinted from: *J. Pers. Med.* **2021**, *11*, 584, doi:10.3390/jpm11060584 115

Gianluca Rompianesi, Roberto Montalti, Luisa Ambrosio and Roberto Ivan Troisi
Robotic versus Laparoscopic Surgery for Spleen-Preserving Distal Pancreatectomies: Systematic Review and Meta-Analysis
Reprinted from: *J. Pers. Med.* **2021**, *11*, 552, doi:10.3390/jpm11060552 131

Wanda Petz, Simona Borin and Uberto Fumagalli Romario
Updates on Robotic CME for Right Colon Cancer: A Qualitative Systematic Review
Reprinted from: *J. Pers. Med.* **2021**, *11*, 550, doi:10.3390/jpm11060550 . . . . **143**

About the Editors

Marco Milone

Marco Milone was born in Naples, Italy. He is an Assistant Professor and Attending Surgeon at "Federico II" University of Naples, Italy. He received his undergraduate degree in Naples, Italy, and underwent postgraduate clinical and research training in Italy and in the United Kingdom. He holds a PhD in Surgical Science and Advanced Techniques. He has long been engaged in clinical and research work of the gastrointestinal surgery, especially in those of minimally invasive surgery. He has a track record of over 130 publications in peer-reviewed journals, with an h-index of 23 and a citation count of >1400.

He is member of the editorial board of numerous peer-reviewed journals. He is currently a member of the Executive Board of the Italian Society of Endoscopic Surgery (SICE).

Paolo Pietro Bianchi

Doctor Paolo Pietro Bianchi graduated from the University of Milano in 1989, with an early interest in minimally invasive surgery.

He developed his initial experience in Belgium at the European School of Laparoscopy and in France and Strasbourg at the IRCAD.

He was Chief of the Colorectal and Minimally Invasive Unit in 2004 at the Istituto Clinico Humanitas in Rozzano (Italy) and became the Director of the Minimally Invasive Unit at the European Institute of Oncology in Milano in 2008.

Doctor Bianchi's main interest is digestive surgery and especially colorectal surgery, and he is an expert of sentinel lymphnode detection in colon cancer anda pioneer of laparoscopic ultrasound.

In recent years, he worked on the development of robotic surgery and its application to oncological digestive diseases.

Doctor Bianchi is a Professor of Surgical Technique at the Postgraduate School of General Surgery at the University of Milano, a director of the live courses of laparoscopic surgery in colon cancer, and a founding member of the School of Robotic Surgery at the European Institute of Oncology In Milano.

He is an author and co-author of many peer-reviewed publications and a reviewer for some of the most important journals of minimally invasive surgery.

Preface to "Update on Robotic Gastrointestinal Surgery"

Since its inception, robotic surgery has made incredible progress and has undergone significant development in an extremely short period of time. In the field of minimally invasive surgery, robotic platforms could potentially be used to realize improvements for both the patient and the surgeon. Several barriers of laparoscopic surgery could be overcome through the introduction of 3D vision, stable and magnified images, EndoWrist instruments, physiologic tremor filtering, and motion scaling. Minimally invasive surgery is constantly evolving so as to allow surgeons to achieve essential goals in terms of survival and functionality; robotic platforms could play a key role in obtaining these goals. For this reason, it is necessary to evaluate the oncological and functional outcomes of robotic surgery.

Regarding surgical oncology, robotic surgery may offer several benefits through precise visualization and dissection along the embryological planes. One example of its advantageous application is rectal cancer surgery, especially in the case of male narrow pelvis and bulking tumors [1]. Even in esophageal cancer surgery, the robotic approach appears to be slightly superior to laparoscopic surgery, resulting in less postoperative pneumonia and higher numbers of harvested nodes [2].

If the results of robotic surgery, in oncological terms, are encouraging, the same can be said for gastrointestinal functional disorders. Even if, on the one hand, robotic surgery proved to be non-inferior to laparoscopic surgery in the treatment of functional esophageal disorders [3], on the other hand, it showed better postoperative outcomes in the treatment of pelvic floor disorders, such as lower complication rates and shorter lengths of hospital stay [4].

Robotic surgery has also begun to play an important role in endoluminal surgery with the evolution of systems for transanal surgery that allow for the execution of highly complex procedures, such as RTaTME, for low-lying rectal cancer [5].

Although, to date, there are no specific indications for the use of robotic surgery compared to laparoscopic surgery, the former's lower unplanned conversion rate has been amply demonstrated in the literature. Therefore, one of the targets of this surgery could be patients with known or suspected abdominal adhesions [6].

This Special Issue focuses on the application of robotic surgery in the context of gastrointestinal surgery and its safety and efficacy in the performance of various procedures, even those of high complexity. Increased costs, poor availability, and dedicated training are still barriers which prevent the widespread adoption of this system. In the near future, emerging robotic platforms will lead to major competition and consequent reductions in costs, encouraging the use of this platform and raising its potential as a standard surgery for many procedures.

Marco Milone and Paolo Pietro Bianchi
Editors

Editorial

Robotic Gastrointestinal Surgery: State of the Art and Future Perspectives

Marco Milone [1,*] and Paolo Pietro Bianchi [2]

1 Department of Clinical Medicine and Surgery, University of Naples "Federico II", 80131 Naples, Italy
2 Department of Health Science, University of Milan, 20142 Milano, Italy
* Correspondence: milone.marco.md@gmail.com

Since its inception, robotic surgery has made incredible progress and has undergone significant development in an extremely short period of time. In the field of minimally invasive surgery, robotic platforms could potentially be used to realize improvements for both the patient and surgeon. Several barriers of laparoscopic surgery could be overcome through the introduction of 3D vision, stable and magnified images, EndoWrist instruments, physiologic tremor filtering, and motion scaling. Minimally invasive surgery is constantly evolving so as to allow surgeons to achieve essential goals in terms of survival and functionality; robotic platforms could play a key role in obtaining these goals. For this reason, it is necessary to evaluate the oncological and functional outcomes of robotic surgery.

Regarding surgical oncology, robotic surgery may offer several benefits through precise visualization and dissection along the embryological planes. One example of its advantageous application is rectal cancer surgery, especially in the case of male narrow pelvis and bulking tumors [1]. Even in esophageal cancer surgery, the robotic approach appears to be slightly superior to laparoscopic surgery, resulting in less postoperative pneumonia and higher numbers of harvested nodes [2].

If the results of robotic surgery, in oncological terms, are encouraging, the same can be said for gastrointestinal functional disorders. Even if, on the one hand, robotic surgery proved to be non-inferior to laparoscopic surgery in the treatment of functional esophageal disorders [3], on the other hand, it showed better postoperative outcomes in the treatment of pelvic floor disorders, such as lower complication rates and shorter lengths of hospital stay [4].

Robotic surgery has also begun to play an important role in endoluminal surgery with the evolution of systems for transanal surgery that allow for the execution of highly complex procedures, such as RTaTME, for low-lying rectal cancer [5].

Although, to date, there are no specific indications for the use of robotic surgery compared to laparoscopic surgery, the former's lower unplanned conversion rate has been amply demonstrated in the literature. Therefore, one of the targets of this surgery could be patients with known or suspected abdominal adhesions [6].

This Special Issue concerns the application of robotic surgery in the context of gastrointestinal surgery and its safety and efficacy in the performance of various procedures, even those of high complexity. Increased costs, poor availability and dedicated training are still barriers which prevent the widespread adoption of this system. In the near future, emerging robotic platforms will lead to major competition and consequent reductions in costs, encouraging the use of this platform and raising its potential as a standard surgery for many procedures.

Conflicts of Interest: There are no conflict of interest to declare.

References

1. Giuratrabocchetta, S.; Formisano, G.; Salaj, A.; Opocher, E.; Ferraro, L.; Toti, F.; Bianchi, P.P. Update on Robotic Total Mesorectal Excision for Rectal Cancer. *J. Pers. Med.* **2021**, *11*, 900. [CrossRef] [PubMed]
2. Manigrasso, M.; Vertaldi, S.; Marello, A.; Antoniou, S.A.; Francis, N.K.; De Palma, G.D.; Milone, M. Robotic Esophagectomy. A Systematic Review with Meta-Analysis of Clinical Outcomes. *J. Pers. Med.* **2021**, *11*, 640. [CrossRef] [PubMed]
3. Vertaldi, S.; D'Amore, A.; Manigrasso, M.; Anoldo, P.; Chini, A.; Maione, F.; Pesce, M.; Sarnelli, G.; De Palma, G.D.; Milone, M. Robotic Surgery and Functional Esophageal Disorders: A Systematic Review and Meta-Analysis. *J. Pers. Med.* **2023**, *13*, 231. [CrossRef]
4. Formisano, G.; Ferraro, L.; Salaj, A.; Giuratrabocchetta, S.; Pisani Ceretti, A.; Opocher, E.; Bianchi, P.P. Update on Robotic Rectal Prolapse Treatment. *J. Pers. Med.* **2021**, *11*, 706. [CrossRef]
5. Rondelli, F.; Sanguinetti, A.; Polistena, A.; Avenia, S.; Marcacci, C.; Ceccarelli, G.; Bugiantella, W.; De Rosa, M. Robotic Transanal Total Mesorectal Excision (RTaTME): State of the Art. *J. Pers. Med.* **2021**, *11*, 584. [CrossRef] [PubMed]
6. Milone, M.; Manigrasso, M.; Anoldo, P.; D'Amore, A.; Elmore, U.; Giglio, M.C.; Rompianesi, G.; Vertaldi, S.; Troisi, R.I.; Francis, N.K.; et al. The Role of Robotic Visceral Surgery in Patients with Adhesions: A Systematic Review and Meta-Analysis. *J. Pers. Med.* **2022**, *12*, 307. [CrossRef] [PubMed]

Disclaimer/Publisher's Note: The statements, opinions and data contained in all publications are solely those of the individual author(s) and contributor(s) and not of MDPI and/or the editor(s). MDPI and/or the editor(s) disclaim responsibility for any injury to people or property resulting from any ideas, methods, instructions or products referred to in the content.

Systematic Review

Robotic Surgery and Functional Esophageal Disorders: A Systematic Review and Meta-Analysis

Sara Vertaldi [1,*], Anna D'Amore [1], Michele Manigrasso [2], Pietro Anoldo [2], Alessia Chini [1], Francesco Maione [1], Marcella Pesce [1], Giovanni Sarnelli [1], Giovanni Domenico De Palma [1] and Marco Milone [1]

1. Department of Clinical Medicine and Surgery, University of Naples "Federico II", 80131 Naples, Italy
2. Department of Advanced Biomedical Sciences, University of Naples "Federico II", 80131 Naples, Italy
* Correspondence: vertaldisara@gmail.com; Tel.: +39-340-86-03-360

Abstract: The functional disease of the esophago-gastric junction (EGJ) is one of the most common health problems. It often happens that patients suffering from GERD need surgical management. The laparoscopic fundoplication has been considered the gold standard surgical treatment for functional diseases of the EGJ. The aim of our meta-analysis is to investigate functional outcomes after robotic fundoplication compared with conventional laparoscopic fundoplication. A prospective search of online databases was performed by two independent reviewers using the search string "robotic and laparoscopic fundoplication", including all the articles from 1996 to December 2021. The risk of bias within each study was assessed with the Cochrane ROBINS-I and RoB 2.0 tools. Statistical analysis was performed using Review Manager version 5.4. In addition, sixteen studies were included in the final analysis, involving only four RCTs. The primary endpoints were functional outcomes after laparoscopic (LF) and robotic fundoplication (RF). No significant differences between the two groups were found in 30-day readmission rates ($p = 0.73$), persistence of symptomatology at follow-up ($p = 0.60$), recurrence ($p = 0.36$), and reoperation ($p = 0.81$). The laparoscopic fundoplication represents the gold standard treatment for the functional disease of the EGJ. According to our results, the robotic approach seems to be safe and feasible as well. Further randomized controlled studies are required to better evaluate the advantages of robotic fundoplication.

Keywords: robotic fundoplication; laparoscopic fundoplication; reflux; hiatal hernia; functional outcomes

1. Introduction

The functional disease of the esophago-gastric junction (EGJ) is one of the most common health problems, affecting more than 50% of the world's population and resulting in a serious deterioration of quality of life with important economic implications [1]. Medical treatment with a proton pump inhibitor (PPI) can help control reflux symptoms, but on the other hand, it implies cost-effective, long-lasting medicine-based treatment. It often happens that GERD patients do not achieve complete control of the symptoms, needing surgical management [2].

The laparoscopic fundoplication has been performed with patient satisfaction since its introduction during the twentieth century, becoming the gold standard for the surgical treatment of functional disease of the EGJ [3,4].

Additionally, after the first robotic-assisted Nissen fundoplication (RALF) reported by Cadiere in 1999 [5], it has been debated if the robotic approach could improve surgical outcomes due to the three-dimensional view and the enhanced manipulation of instruments [6] compared with the conventional laparoscopic fundoplication (CLF). Several previous studies have demonstrated the safety and feasibility of a robot-assisted approach in this setting [7–10].

The aim of our meta-analysis is to investigate the functional outcomes after minimally invasive surgery, both laparoscopic and robotic, for the treatment of functional disease of the EGJ.

2. Materials and Methods

2.1. Literature Search and Eligibility Criteria

This systematic review complied with PRISMA (preferred reporting items for systematic reviews and meta-analyses) reporting standards [11] and was developed in line with MOOSE (meta-analysis of observational studies in epidemiology) guidelines [12].

A prospective search of Embase, PubMed, SCOPUS, and Web of Science was performed using the search string "robotic and laparoscopic fundoplication".

The analysis included all the articles from 1996 to December 2021. The last search was performed in January 2022.

Case reports, case series without a control group, indexed abstracts of posters and podium presentations at international meetings, and non-English articles were excluded. Systematic reviews and meta-analyses were only consulted to identify additional studies of interest. In addition, the reference lists of the retrieved studies were manually reviewed. In cases of overlapping series in different studies, only the most recent article was included. Publications with no data about functional results after minimally invasive fundoplication were also excluded.

The research question was structured using the PICO (problem/population, intervention, comparison, and outcome) framework. The populations of interest included patients affected by functional esophageal disease (GERD, hiatal hernia, or paraesophageal hernia). The intervention was robotic fundoplication, and the comparator was laparoscopic fundoplication. The functional outcomes after surgery were analyzed: 30-day readmission; persistent symptomatology at follow-up, including delayed gastric emptying; postoperative pyrosis or dysphagia; disease recurrence; need for reintervention.

The literature search and study selection were performed independently by two reviewers (S.V. and A.D.), showing a high level of inter-reader agreement ($\kappa = 1$). In case of disagreement, a third investigator (Mi.Ma.) was consulted, and an agreement was reached by consensus.

2.2. Data Extraction and Assessment of Risk of Bias in Included Studies

The titles and abstracts were screened and reviewed independently by S.V. and A.D., followed by full-text reading. In addition, ineligible studies were excluded after full-text reading. The data extraction was conducted independently and in duplicate by the two reviewers. Further, the data extraction form was created in accordance with the guidelines in the Cochrane Handbook for systematic reviews of interventions by the consensus of both reviewers.

The following data were extracted from each included study: first author, year of publication, study design, period of study, surgical indication, sample size, number of patients in each surgical group, gender, mean age, mean BMI, type of intervention (Nissen, Dor, Toupet, or no fundoplication), redo surgery, operative time, 30 days readmission, mean follow-up, persistence of symptomatology at follow-up, complaining of delayed gastric emptying, pyrosis, or dysphagia, needing of reintervention. The data extracted from studies were then separated into the following sections: study characteristics, population characteristics, intervention characteristics, and functional outcomes.

Additionally, after data extraction was completed, the risk of bias within each study was assessed.

The Cochrane ROBINS-I (Risk of Bias in Non-randomized Studies of Interventions) tool [13], which is a risk of bias tool to assess the quality of non-randomized studies of interventions, was adopted to evaluate the methodological quality of each cohort-type study. The scoring system encompasses seven domains. The first two domains, covering confounding and selection of participants into the study, address issues before the start of the interventions that are to be compared ("baseline"). The third domain addresses the classification of the interventions themselves. The other four domains address issues after the start of interventions: biases due to deviations from intended interventions, missing data, measurement of outcomes, and selection of the reported result. The categories for risk of bias judgments are "low risk", "moderate risk", "serious risk", "critical risk", and "no information" when insufficient data are reported to permit a judgment.

In cases of randomized controlled trials (RCTs), the risk of bias was evaluated using the revised Cochrane Risk of Bias tool (RoB 2.0) [14]. According to this scoring system, seven domains were evaluated as "low risk of bias", "high risk of bias", or "unclear" according to the reporting on sequence generation, allocation concealment, blinding of participants, blinding of outcome assessment, incomplete outcome data, selective outcome reporting, and other potential threats to validity.

2.3. Statistical Analysis

The statistical analysis was performed using Review Manager (RevMan Version 5.4, Copenhagen, Denmark: The Nordic Cochrane Centre, The Cochrane Collaboration, 2020).

The primary outcomes of this study were the functional results after robotic fundoplication in patients suffering from GERD, hiatal hernia, or paraesophageal hernia compared to a laparoscopic approach. In addition, the differences among cases and controls were expressed as risk difference (RD) with pertinent 95% CI for dichotomous variables, to maintain analytic consistency and include all available data, according to Messori et al. [15]; the differences among cases and controls were expressed as mean difference (MD) with pertinent 95% confidence intervals (95% CI) for continuous variables. The risk difference represents the difference between the observed risks (proportions of individuals with the outcome of interest) in the two groups. If studies reported only the median, range, and size of the trial, the means and standard deviations were calculated according to Luo et al. and Wan et al. [16,17]. When studies reported only means for continuous variables and the sample size of the trial, a standard deviation was imputed, according to Furukawa et al. [18].

The overall effect was tested using Z scores, and significance was set at $p < 0.05$. Statistical heterogeneity between studies was tested by the Q statistic and quantified by the I^2 statistic, a measurement of the inconsistency across study results and a description of the proportion of total variation in study estimates, that is due to heterogeneity rather than sampling error. In detail, an I^2 value of 0% indicates no heterogeneity, 25% low, 25–50% moderate, and >50% high heterogeneity [19].

According to DerSimonian and Laird [20], the random-effects model was used for all analyses to account for the heterogeneity among included studies.

The presence of publication bias was investigated through a funnel plot, where the summary estimate of each study (Risk Difference) was plotted against a measure of study precision (Standard Error). In addition to visual inspection and the funnel plot, symmetry was tested using Egger's linear regression method. [21] p values < 0.05 were considered statistically significant.

3. Results

3.1. Study Selection

A total of 339 articles were identified from electronic databases. After the removal of duplicate studies, 287 publications were screened according to the PRISMA flowchart (Figure 1).

Of the 72 articles that were selected for the title and abstract, 51 studies were excluded because they did not meet the inclusion criteria. Furthermore, the online full version of five articles was not available, and it was not possible to extract data from the abstract. The remaining 16 studies [22–37] were selected as they met the eligibility criteria and were included in the final analysis.

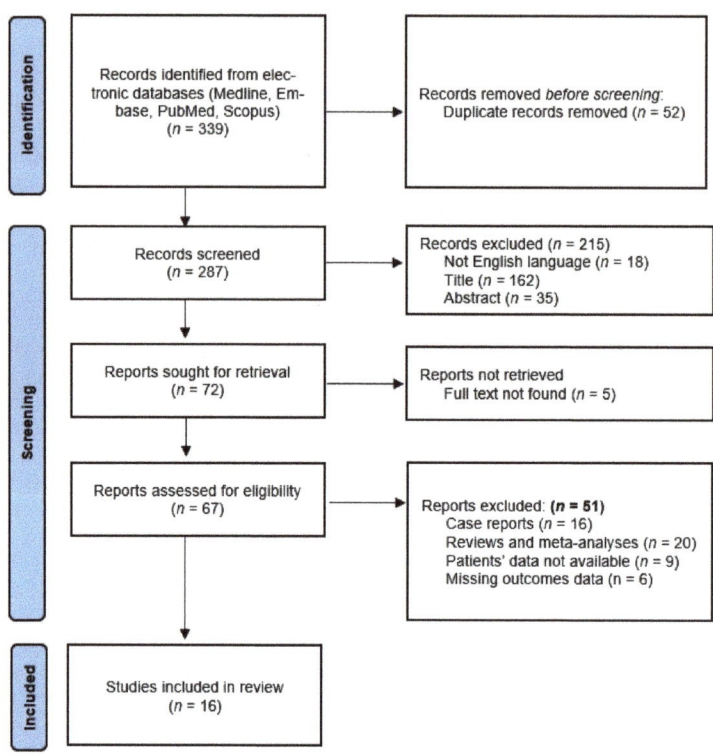

Figure 1. PRISMA 2020 flow diagram.

3.2. Baseline Characteristics of the Included Studies

This meta-analysis included 16 monocentric studies published between 2002 and 2021, involving 1064 patients suffering from GERD, hiatal hernia, or paraesophageal hernia, whereof 618 underwent laparoscopic and 445 robotic fundoplication, respectively. There were 4 RCT [27,32–34], 10 retrospective [22–26,28–30,35,36], and 2 prospective [31,37] trials. The number of patients ranged between 12 and 687, the mean age was between 3.8 and 72.5 years, and the mean BMI varied from 10.1 kg/m^2 to 37.0 kg/m^2.

Major characteristics of the studies are shown in Table 1.

Intervention characteristics are described in detail in Table 2. Nissen fundoplication (360°) was performed in fourteen studies [22,24–28,30–37], Toupet fundoplication (270°) was reported in seven papers [23,25,29,31,35–37], Dor fundoplication (180°) was described in two articles [29,36], while in only one study [35] Watson partial anterior fundoplication was performed. Only two studies [22,36] included redo fundoplications.

Table 1. Baseline characteristics of the included studies.

Study	Study Design	Study Period	Patients (n)			Male/Female (n)		Age (years) (SD)		BMI (kg/m²) (SD)		Diagnosis
			Total	Lap	Rob	Lap	Rob	Lap	Rob	Lap	Rob	
Albassam AA et al., 2009 [22]	Retrospective	Jan. 2005–Jul. 2008	50	25	25	9/16	11/14	3.8 (3.25)	5.4 (3.42)	10.9 (4.65)	10.1 (3.14)	GERD
Benedix F et al., 2021 [23]	Retrospective	Jan. 2016–Jul. 2020	140	85	55	29/56	18/37	62.9 (11.6)	63.5 (12.3)	29.3 (3.8)	29.5 (4.4)	Hiatal hernia and GERD
Ceccarelli G et al., 2009 [24]	Retrospective	Oct. 1992–Sep. 2007	183	137	45	-	-	52.5 (8.3)	55.0 (11.75)	27.0 (2.0)	28.0 (3.0)	GERD
Ceccarelli G et al., 2020 [25]	Retrospective	Dec. 2009–Dec. 2019	5	2	3	2/0	3/0	72.5 (13.5)	68.3 (14.2)	30.0 (2.6)	29.1 (5.6)	Giant Hiatal hernia
Copeland DR et al., 2008 [26]	Retrospective	1994–2005	100	50	50	-	-	8.9 (5.9)	9.75 (5.3)	33.0 (24.0)	37.0 (23.0)	-
Draaisma WA et al., 2006 [27]	RCT	Jan. 2003–Oct. 2005	50	25	25	17/8	16/9	50.5 (12.7)	39.0 (0.5)	31.0 (7.0)	27.0 (4.5)	GERD
Gehrig T et al., 2013 [28]	Retrospective	2003–2007	29	17	12	12/5	3/9	60.2 (11.8)	68.1 (7.9)	26.6 (4.4)	25.4 (2.6)	Paraesophageal hernia
Hartmann J et al., 2009 [29]	Retrospective	Jan. 2003–Dec. 2003	80	62	18	30/33	9/9	53.0 (14.0)	57.0 (13.0)	30.0 (4.7)	27.2 (4.3)	GERD
Jensen JS et al., 2017 [30]	Retrospective	Apr. 2013–Apr. 2015	103	64	39	23/41	18/21	49.4 (15.4)	52.0 (14.6)	26.9 (3.4)	26.5 (3.1)	GERD
Melvin WS et al., 2002 [31]	Prospective	-	40	20	20	7/13	13/7	49.6 (0.5)	42.9 (0.5)	-	-	GERD
Morino M et al., 2006 [32]	RCT	-	50	25	25	18/7	19/6	46.3 (11.3)	43.0 (12.8)	26.1 (2.3)	25.5 (2.9)	GERD
Muller-Stich BP et al., 2009 [33]	RCT	Aug. 2004–Dec. 2005	40	20	20	12/8	10/10	50.5 (12.4)	49.6 (12.0)	26.2 (3.4)	29.2 (5.83)	GERD

Table 1. Cont.

Study	Study Design	Study Period	Patients (n)			Male/Female (n)		Age (years) (SD)		BMI (kg/m²) (SD)		Diagnosis
			Total	Lap	Rob	Lap	Rob	Lap	Rob	Lap	Rob	
Nakadi IE et al., 2006 [34]	RCT	-	20	11	9	8/3	6/3	48.0 (4.0)	44.0 (4.0)	24.8 (0.7)	25.3 (1.2)	GERD
Samar AM et al., 2020 [35]	Retrospective	Jan. 2014–Jun. 2016	44	26	18	13/13	9/9	55.7 (8.2)	49.2 (7.75)	-	-	-
Tolboom RC et al., 2016 [36]	Retrospective	Jan. 2008–Dec. 2013	75	30	45	11/19	12/33	57.2 (2.2)	56.0 (2.2)	-	-	Hiatal hernia and GERD
Wilhelm A et al., 2021 [37]	Prospective	July 2015–June 2019	55	19	36	5/14	13/23	71.7 (13.5)	69.0 (11.5)	29.0 (6.5)	30.0 (3.5)	Hiatal hernia

Table 2. Intervention characteristics.

Study	De Novo Surgery		Redo Surgery		Nissen Fundoplication		Dor Fundoplication		Toupet Fundoplication		No Fundoplication		Operative Time (min)	
	Lap	Rob	Lap	Rob	Lap	Rob	Lap	Rob	Lap	Rob	Lap	Rob	Lap	Rob
Albassam AA et al., 2009 [22]	24	24	1	1	25	25	0	0	0	0	0	0	193.12 (26.6)	186.04 (21.1)
Benedix F et al., 2021 [23]	-	-	-	-	0	0	0	0	85	55	0	0	125.0 (35.5)	149.0 (42.1)
Ceccarelli G et al., 2009 [24]	-	-	-	-	137	45	0	0	0	0	0	0	86.2 (14.2)	65.0 (10.8)
Ceccarelli G et al., 2020 [25]	2	3	0	0	1	1	0	0	1	1	0	1	165.0 (5.0)	203.3 (17.8)
Copeland DR et al., 2008 [26]	50	50	0	0	50	50	0	0	0	0	0	0	107.0 (31.0)	160.0 (61.0)
Draaisma WA et al., 2006 [27]	25	25	0	-	25	25	0	0	0	0	0	0	115.0 (37.5)	125.0 (25.0)
Gehrig T et al., 2013 [28]	17	12	0	0	9	6	0	0	0	0	8	6	168.0 (42.0)	172.0 (31.0)

Table 2. Cont.

Study	De Novo Surgery		Redo Surgery		Nissen Fundoplication		Dor Fundoplication		Toupet Fundoplication		No Fundoplication		Operative Time (min)	
	Lap	Rob	Lap	Rob	Lap	Rob	Lap	Rob	Lap	Rob	Lap	Rob	Lap	Rob
Hartmann J et al., 2009 [29]	62	18	0	0	0	0	62	18	0	0	0	0	116.0 (63.0)	207.0 (45.0)
Jensen JS et al., 2017 [30]	64	39	0	0	49	15	0	0	15	24	0	0	86.0 (19.0)	135.0 (27.0)
Melvin WS et al., 2002 [31]	20	20	0	0	17	17	0	0	3	3	0	0	101.7 (30.7)	160.2 (45.7)
Morino M et al., 2006 [32]	25	25	0	0	25	25	0	0	0	0	0	0	91.1 (10.6)	131.6 (18.3)
Muller-Stich BP et al., 2009 [33]	20	20	0	0	20	20	0	0	0	0	0	0	102.0 (19.0)	88.0 (18.0)
Nakadi IE et al., 2006 [34]	11	9	0	0	11	9	0	0	0	0	0	0	96.0 (5.0)	137.0 (12.0)
Samar AM et al., 2020 [35]	-	-	-	-	15	3	7 *	2 *	4	13	0	0	164.0 (43.0)	129.0 (22.0)
Tolboom RC et al., 2016 [36]	0	0	30	45	6	4	2	12	20	27	1	2	98.7 (6.2)	120.0 (2.5)
Wilhelm A et al., 2021 [37]	-	-	-	-	4	0	0	0	15	29	0	7	179.5 (42.0)	182.2 (6.9)

* Watson partial anterior fundoplication (120°).

3.3. Risk of Bias

The Cochrane RoB 2.0 and ROBINS-I tools were used to assess the quality of the included papers.

Additionally, regarding the four randomized controlled trials, only one study [33] reported a low risk of bias. The other three studies [27,32,34] showed a high risk of bias, with the major bias due to deviations from the intended interventions, i.e., conversions to an open approach. Two conversions from laparoscopy were described by Draaisma et al. [27], and two conversions from the robotic approach were reported by Morino et al. and Nakadi et al. [32,34].

Due to the nature of the surgical interventions, blinding was impossible, but the results are unlikely to be affected by the lack of blinding.

All non-randomized studies reported a risk of bias due to baseline confounding. Only three [22,26,31] authors with a consequent moderate risk of bias performed propensity score matching, while the other nine [23–25,28–30,35–37] had a severe risk of bias due to insufficient adjustment for confounding domains.

The results of the RoB 2.0 and ROBINS-I quality assessments are reported in Figures 2a,b and 3a,b, which were created with Robvis (Risk-of-Bias VISualization), a web app that facilitates rapid production of publication-quality risk-of-bias assessment figures.

3.4. Primary Outcomes

The functional outcomes after laparoscopic (LF) and robotic fundoplication (RF) were analysed during a mean follow up period of 1-93.6 months, as described in Table 3.

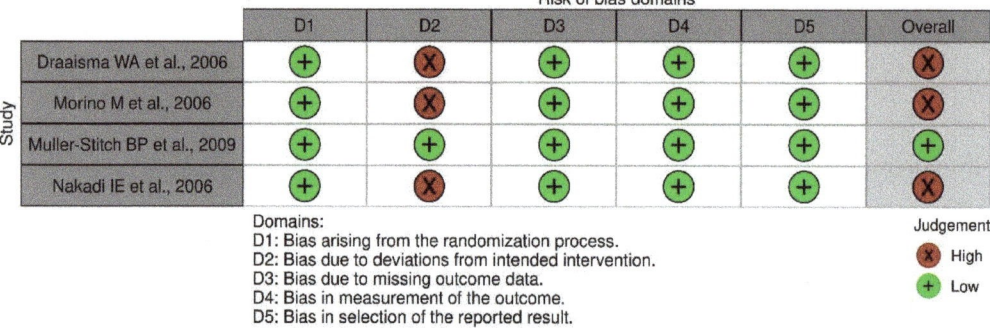

(a)

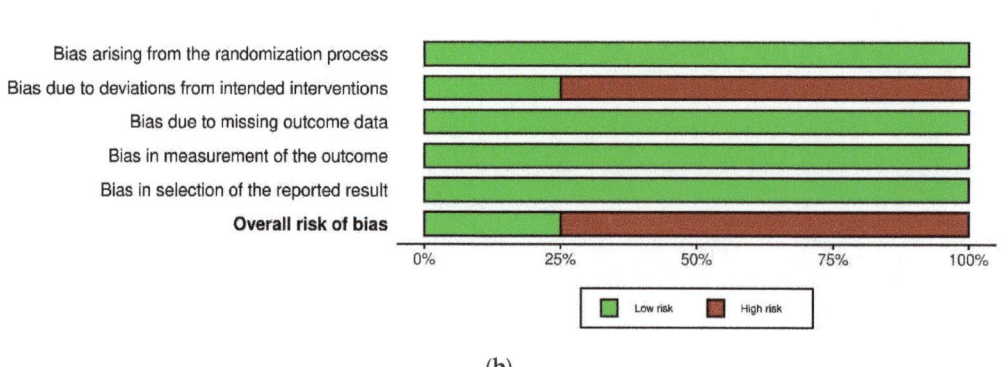

(b)

Figure 2. Summary of risk of bias for RCT studies [27,32–34].

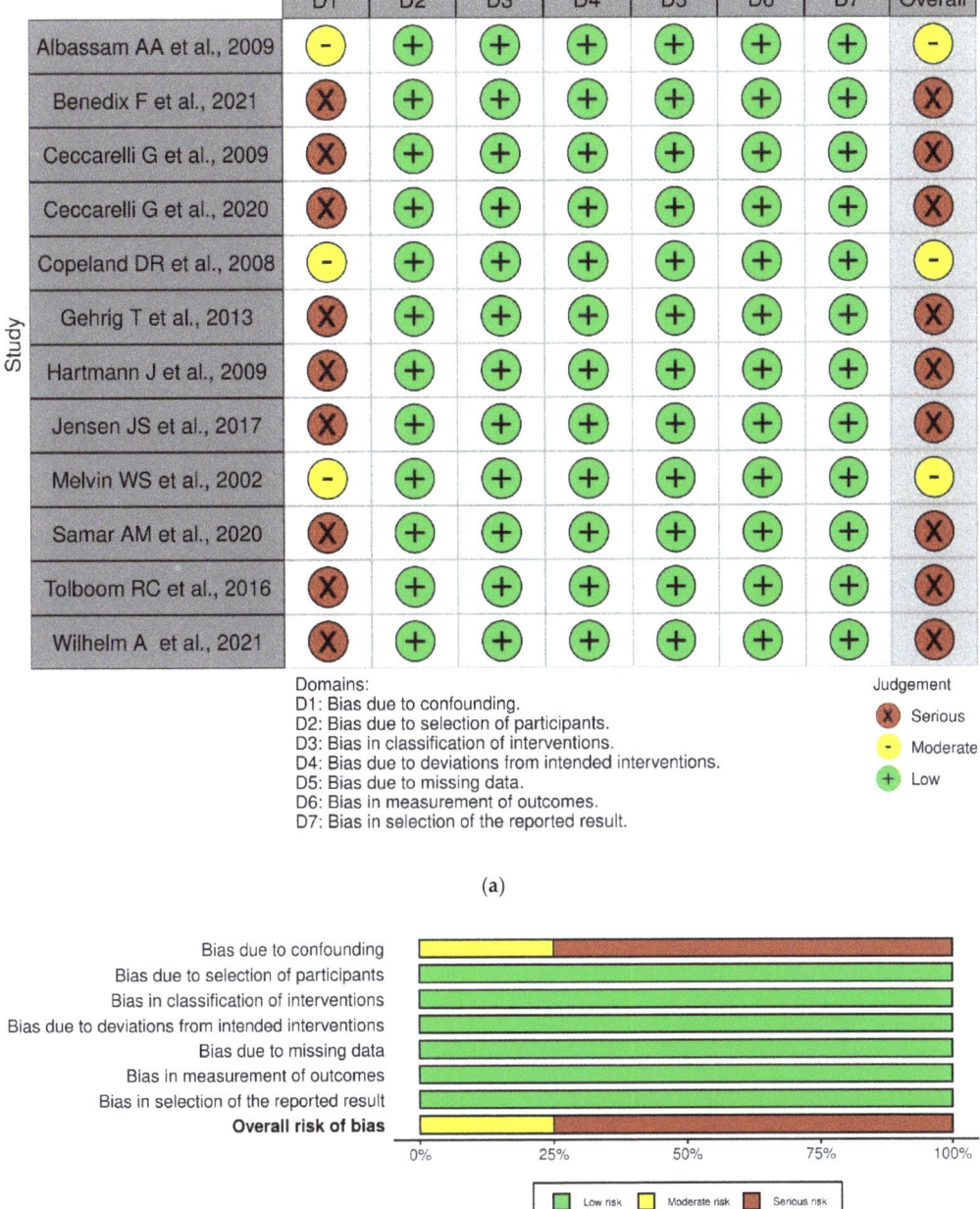

Figure 3. Summary of risk of bias for non-RCT studies [22–26,28–31,35–37].

Table 3. Functional outcomes.

Study	Mean Follow-Up (months)		30-days Readmission (n)		Persistence of Symptoms (n)		Delayed Gastric Emptying (n)		Pyrosis (n)		Dysphagia (n)		Recurrence (n)		Reoperation (n)	
	Lap	Rob	Lap	Rob	Lap	Rob	Lap	Rob	Lap	Rob	Lap	Rob	Lap	Rob	Lap	Rob
Albassam AA et al., 2009 [22]	19.25	19.25	0	0	10	9	1	2	-	-	1	0	0	0	0	0
Benedix F et al., 2021 [23]	3	3	2	3	-	-	-	0	-	-	8	5	-	-	1	1
Ceccarelli G et al., 2009 [24]	93.6	43.2	-	-	15	5	-	-	-	-	3	1	5	2	-	-
Ceccarelli G et al., 2020 [25]	6	6	0	0	0	0	0	0	-	-	-	-	0	0	0	0
Copeland DR et al., 2008 [26]	1	1	0	0	-	-	-	-	-	-	14	15	-	-	-	-
Draaisma WA et al., 2006 [27]	6	6	-	-	1	2	-	-	-	-	2	1	3	1	2	2
Gehrig T et al., 2013 [28]	-	-	-	-	-	-	2	0	-	-	-	-	-	-	0	1
Hartmann J et al., 2009 [29]	-	-	-	-	18	5	-	0	-	-	-	-	-	-	-	-
Jensen JS et al., 2017 [30]	22.5	26	-	-	-	-	0	0	-	-	4	2	1	0	5	2
Melvin WS et al., 2002 [31]	10.5	6.7	-	-	18	13	-	0	4	3	5	3	6	0	1	0
Morino M et al., 2006 [32]	12	12	-	-	-	-	-	-	0	0	0	0	-	-	-	-
Muller-Stich BP et al., 2009 [33]	12	12	0	0	5	5	-	-	-	-	0	1	2	0	0	1
Nakadi IE et al., 2006 [34]	12	12	-	-	2	1	-	-	0	0	0	0	0	0	0	1
Samar AM et al., 2020 [35]	1	1	-	-	11	5	-	-	2	2	4	2	-	-	-	-
Tolboom RC et al., 2016 [36]	11.7	3	-	-	16	23	3	3	9	6	3	6	-	-	4	4
Wilhelm A et al., 2021 [37]	28.7	31	0	0	0	0	0	1	-	-	1	1	0	2	0	0

3.4.1. 30-Days Readmission Rates

Only seven authors [22,23,25,26,33,35,37] reported 30-day readmission rates including 434 patients (207 RF and 227 LF) with no significant differences between the two groups [$p = 0.73$, RD = 0.00, 95% CI (−0.02, 0.03)]. No heterogeneity among the studies [$Tau^2 = 0.00$; $Chi^2 = 0.85$; df = 6 ($p = 0.99$); $I^2 = 0\%$] was reported (Figure 4).

Study or Subgroup	Robotic Events	Robotic Total	Laparoscopic Events	Laparoscopic Total	Weight	Risk Difference M-H, Random, 95% CI
Albassam AA et al. 2009	0	25	0	25	12.0%	0.00 [-0.07, 0.07]
Benedix F et al. 2021	3	55	2	85	14.4%	0.03 [-0.04, 0.10]
Ceccarelli G et al. 2020	0	3	0	2	0.2%	0.00 [-0.53, 0.53]
Copeland DR et al. 2008	0	50	0	50	45.8%	0.00 [-0.04, 0.04]
Muller-Stich BP et al. 2009	0	20	0	20	7.9%	0.00 [-0.09, 0.09]
Samar AM et al. 2020	0	18	0	26	8.6%	0.00 [-0.09, 0.09]
Wilhelm A et al. 2021	0	36	0	19	11.0%	0.00 [-0.08, 0.08]
Total (95% CI)		**207**		**227**	**100.0%**	**0.00 [-0.02, 0.03]**
Total events	3		2			

Heterogeneity: Tau² = 0.00; Chi² = 0.85, df = 6 (P = 0.99); I² = 0%
Test for overall effect: Z = 0.34 (P = 0.73)

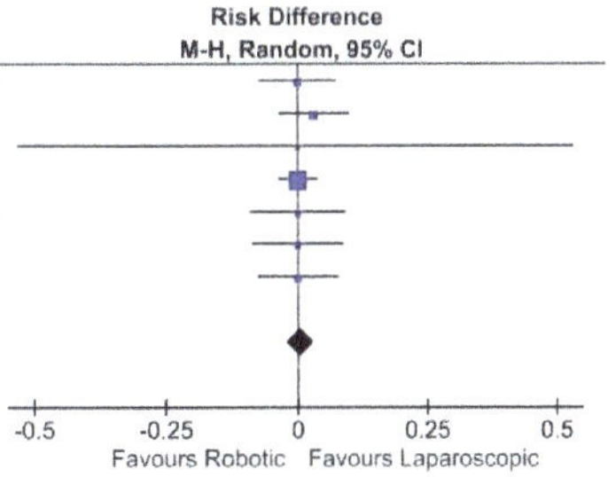

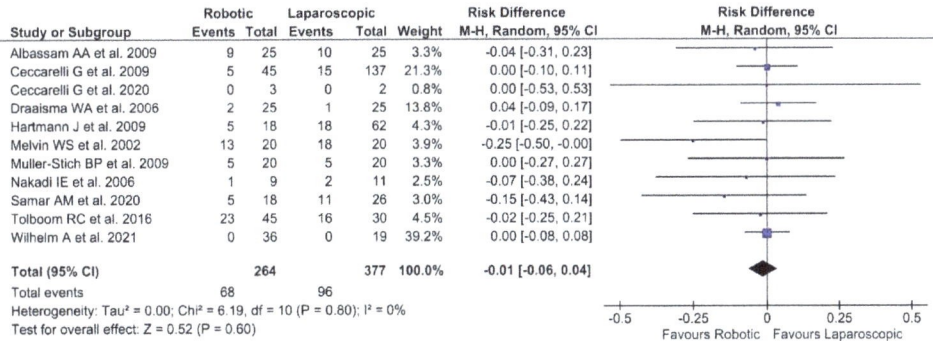

Figure 4. Forest plot of laparoscopic vs. robotic 30day readmission rates [22,23,25,26,33,35,37].

3.4.2. Persistence of Symptoms

Eleven studies [22,24,25,27,29,31,33–37] investigated the persistence of symptomatology after almost 1 month of follow-up. In addition, apart from two studies [25,37], which reported no ongoing symptoms, in the other nine [22,24,27,29,31,33–36], a total of 164 of the 641 patients referred reported lasting symptomatology without statistically significant differences between robotic and laparoscopic procedures ($p = 0.60$). Neither heterogeneity among the studies [$Tau^2 = 0.00$; $Chi^2 = 6.19$; df = 10 ($p = 0.80$); $I^2 = 0\%$] was described (Figure 5).

Study or Subgroup	Robotic Events	Robotic Total	Laparoscopic Events	Laparoscopic Total	Weight	Risk Difference M-H, Random, 95% CI
Albassam AA et al. 2009	9	25	10	25	3.3%	-0.04 [-0.31, 0.23]
Ceccarelli G et al. 2009	5	45	15	137	21.3%	0.00 [-0.10, 0.11]
Ceccarelli G et al. 2020	0	3	0	2	0.8%	0.00 [-0.53, 0.53]
Draaisma WA et al. 2006	2	25	1	25	13.8%	0.04 [-0.09, 0.17]
Hartmann J et al. 2009	5	18	18	62	4.3%	-0.01 [-0.25, 0.22]
Melvin WS et al. 2002	13	20	18	20	3.9%	-0.25 [-0.50, -0.00]
Muller-Stich BP et al. 2009	5	20	5	20	3.3%	0.00 [-0.27, 0.27]
Nakadi IE et al. 2006	1	9	2	11	2.5%	-0.07 [-0.38, 0.24]
Samar AM et al. 2020	5	18	11	26	3.0%	-0.15 [-0.43, 0.14]
Tolboom RC et al. 2016	23	45	16	30	4.5%	-0.02 [-0.25, 0.21]
Wilhelm A et al. 2021	0	36	0	19	39.2%	0.00 [-0.08, 0.08]
Total (95% CI)		**264**		**377**	**100.0%**	**-0.01 [-0.06, 0.04]**
Total events	68		96			

Heterogeneity: Tau² = 0.00; Chi² = 6.19, df = 10 (P = 0.80); I² = 0%
Test for overall effect: Z = 0.52 (P = 0.60)

Figure 5. Forest plot of laparoscopic vs. robotic persistence of symptomatology [22,24,25,27,29,31,33–37].

In particular, thirteen studies [22–24,26,27,30–37] reported the presence of postoperative dysphagia without significant differences between the two groups [39/387 RF and 47/529 LF, $p = 0.77$, RD = 0.00, 95% CI (−0.03, 0.02)]. Supplementary Materials: Figure S1.

Seven authors [22,23,25,28,30,36,37] reported data regarding delayed gastric emptying: a total of 6 patients in each group had gastric paresis at follow-up, with no statistically significant differences between the two groups [6/215 RF vs. 6/242 LF; $p = 0.99$, RD = 0.00, 95% CI (−0.02, 0.02)]. Supplementary Materials: Figure S2.

Only five articles [31,32,34–36] described the presence of postoperative pyrosis in 11 of 117 patients for the robotic group and 15 of 122 patients for the laparoscopic group, with no statistically significant differences between the two groups [$p = 0.58$, RD = −0.02, 95% CI (−0.09, 0.05)]. Supplementary Materials: Figure S3.

3.4.3. Recurrence

In nine studies [22,24,25,27,30,31,33,34,37], recurrence of symptoms of reflux was described in 22 patients (5 RF and 17 LF), with no significant differences between the two groups [$p = 0.36$, RD = -0.02, 95% CI (-0.07, 0.03)]. The moderate heterogeneity among the studies [Tau^2 = 0.00; Chi^2 = 13.42; df = 8 ($p = 0.10$); I^2 = 40%] was reported (Figure 6).

Study or Subgroup	Robotic Events	Total	Laparoscopic Events	Total	Weight	Risk Difference M-H, Random, 95% CI
Albassam AA et al. 2009	0	25	0	25	18.0%	0.00 [-0.07, 0.07]
Ceccarelli G et al. 2009	2	45	5	137	19.5%	0.01 [-0.06, 0.08]
Ceccarelli G et al. 2020	0	3	0	2	0.8%	0.00 [-0.53, 0.53]
Draaisma WA et al. 2006	1	25	3	25	7.7%	-0.08 [-0.23, 0.07]
Jensen JS et al. 2017	0	39	1	64	23.8%	-0.02 [-0.07, 0.03]
Melvin WS et al. 2002	0	20	6	20	4.5%	-0.30 [-0.51, -0.09]
Muller-Stich BP et al. 2009	0	20	2	20	7.4%	-0.10 [-0.25, 0.05]
Nakadi IE et al. 2006	0	9	0	11	5.9%	0.00 [-0.18, 0.18]
Wilhelm A et al. 2021	2	36	0	19	12.4%	0.06 [-0.05, 0.16]
Total (95% CI)		**222**		**323**	**100.0%**	**-0.02 [-0.07, 0.03]**
Total events	5		17			

Heterogeneity: Tau² = 0.00; Chi² = 13.42, df = 8 (P = 0.10); I² = 40%
Test for overall effect: Z = 0.92 (P = 0.36)

Figure 6. Forest plot of laparoscopic vs. robotic recurrence of reflux symptoms [22,24,25,27,30,31,33,34,37].

3.4.4. Reoperation

A total of nine studies [22,25,27,30,31,33,34,36,37] reported reintervention during follow-up involving 22 patients with no significant differences between the two groups [$p = 0.81$, RD = 0.00, 95% CI (-0.04, 0.03)]. In addition, ten patients underwent reintervention after an initially successful robotic fundoplication: five experienced troublesome dysphagia [27,30,33,36], three had persistent GERD symptoms [36], one had an incisional hernia at the umbilicus [27], and another patient with a gastric torsion underwent a laparoscopic procedure with reduction of the torsion and fixation of the anterior gastric wall to the abdominal wall [34]. In the laparoscopic group, twelve patients were subject to reoperation during follow-up for persistent symptoms: six presented recurrent GERD symptoms [30,31,36] and six had severe dysphagia [27,30]. No heterogeneity among the studies [Tau^2 = 0.00; Chi^2 = 2.58; df = 8 ($p = 0.96$); I^2 = 0%] was reported (Figure 7).

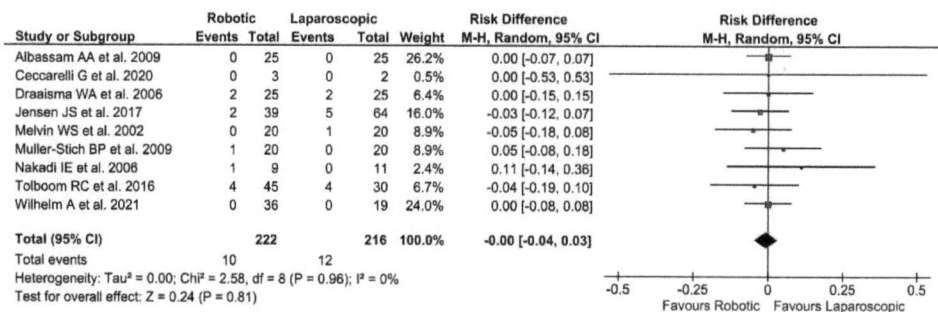

Figure 7. Forest plot of laparoscopic vs. robotic reoperation rates [22,25,27,30,33,34,36,37].

3.5. Publication Bias

It is recognized that publication bias can affect the results of meta-analyses; thus, we attempted to assess this potential bias using funnel plot analysis performed with Comprehensive Meta-analysis Software (CMA v.2). In evaluating all the analysed outcomes, we observed a symmetrical distribution of the studies without any publication bias by the Egger's linear regression method (30-day readmission $p = 0.84$; recurrence $p = 0.23$; reoperation $p = 0.60$; persistence of symptomatology $p = 0.12$) (Supplementary Materials: Figures S4–S7).

4. Discussion

The functional disease of the esophago-gastric junction (EGJ) is a common health problem that often causes a serious deterioration of quality of life. Sometimes GERD patients do not achieve complete control of the symptoms with medical treatment with a proton pump inhibitor (PPI), needing surgical management.

Up until now, laparoscopic fundoplication has been considered the gold standard for the surgical treatment of functional disease of the EGJ [3,4].

Additionally, after the first robotic-assisted Nissen fundoplication (RALF) [5], it has been debated if the robotic approach could improve surgical outcomes compared with the conventional laparoscopic fundoplication (CLF) [6], considering the documented safety and feasibility of the robot-assisted approach in this setting [7–10].

It could be rational to hypothesize advantages of robotic surgery to improve functional results; limitations of laparoscopic procedures due to lack of dexterity, lack of tactile sense, magnification of natural tremors, and two-dimensional visualization could be overcome.

However, the robotic technique presents an important limitation that is related to the high functional costs, as shown by Hartmann et al. [29], Morino et al. [32], and Albassam et al. [22], due to the instrumentation and reusable materials, the nursing costs, the investment costs, and the maintenance costs [34].

According to current literature, there is no clear evidence as to which minimally invasive surgical approach is superior for the treatment of functional diseases of the EGJ. In addition, to the best of our knowledge, this is the first meta-analysis reported on the comparative efficacy of available interventions in the management of functional diseases of the EGJ.

Several limitations must be considered in our study: first, because of the novelty of this topic, few studies are present in the literature. In fact, only 16 studies [22–37] published between 2002 and 2021 could be included in this meta-analysis, with a narrow sample size of 1064 patients suffering from GERD, hiatal hernia, or paraesophageal hernia.

Then, only four studies were RCTs [27,32–34] and two were prospective trials [31,37]. All the other ten included studies were retrospective [22–26,28–30,35,36]; the observed results in each study could be affected by many factors, such as standards in patients' selection, the surgeon's experience, or technical details.

It is important to highlight that no one study had functional results as its primary outcome.

According to our results, both robotic and laparoscopic fundoplication are effective as well, reporting no significant differences between the two groups in terms of 30-day readmission rates ($p = 0.73$), lasting of symptomatology at almost 1 month of follow-up ($p = 0.60$), recurrence of symptoms of reflux ($p = 0.36$), and needing for reintervention during follow-up ($p = 0.81$). Moreover, two conversions from laparoscopy were described by Draaisma et al. [27], and two conversions from the robotic approach were reported by Morino et al. and Nakadi et al. [32,34]. Although nowadays the risk of conversion to open surgery has decreased due to higher surgeon expertise, it is important to underline that the conversion rate from robotic surgery is lower than that from laparoscopy, according to current literature [38–40].

Furthermore, regarding the persistence of symptomatology after 1 month from the intervention, no differences were found in postoperative dysphagia ($p = 0.77$), gastric paresis ($p = 0.99$) and postoperative pyrosis ($p = 0.58$). It is fair to specify that both persistence of symptomatology and recurrence could appear even after years with a treatment failure rate of 40%, as shown by Spechler SJ [41]. However, there is a lack of data concerning a follow-up longer than five years for both the medical and surgical approaches.

Even if, on the basis of our results, we can state that the robotic approach was effective and feasible for the surgical treatment of the functional disease of EGJ, we cannot declare any advantage on the basis of the functional analysis results. Both laparoscopic and robotic approaches could be selected to perform a Nissen fundoplication. On the other hand, the current literature presents a lack of ad hoc papers evaluating some important features, such as:

- the functional outcomes obtained by a laparoscopic versus robotic approach.
- data concerning a follow-up longer than 5 years for both medical and surgical approach.
- indications and parameters for GERD-surgery.

The rationale is that robotic surgery should improve functional outcomes due to the magnified view and endowrist technology. However, it required making a call for future well-designed multicentre high-quality randomized controlled studies to evaluate the functional outcomes after robotic surgery for the treatment of functional disease of the EGJ, indications and parameters for GERD-surgery, and the long-term follow-up longer than 5 years.

Funding: This research received no external funding.

Supplementary Materials: The following supporting information can be downloaded at: https://www.mdpi.com/article/10.3390/jpm13020231/s1. Figure S1: Forest plot of laparoscopic vs. robotic persistence of postoperative dysphagia [22–24,26,27,30–37]; Figure S2: Forest plot of laparoscopic vs. robotic presence of gastric paresis [22,23,25,28,30,36,37]; Figure S3: Forest plot of laparoscopic vs. robotic presence of postoperative pyrosis [31,32,34–36]. Figure S4: Funnel plot of 30-day readmission rates; Figure S5: Funnel plot of recurrence of reflux symptoms; Figure S6: Funnel plot of reoperation; Figure S7: Funnel plot of persistence of symptomatology.

Institutional Review Board Statement: The study was conducted according to the guidelines of the Declaration of Helsinki. This study involved a systematic review and meta-analysis; as such, ethical review and approval were waived.

Informed Consent Statement: Informed consent was obtained from all subjects involved in the study.

Data Availability Statement: The data presented in this study are available on request from the corresponding author.

Conflicts of Interest: The authors declare no conflict of interest.

References

1. Darling, G.; Deschamps, C. Technical Controversies in Fundoplication Surgery. *Thorac. Surg. Clin.* **2005**, *15*, 437–444. [CrossRef] [PubMed]
2. Dallemagne, B.; Weerts, J.M.; Jehaes, C.; Markiewicz, S.; Lombard, R. Laparoscopic Nissen fundoplication: Preliminary report. *Surg. Laparosc. Endosc.* **1991**, *1*, 138–143. [PubMed]
3. Wright, A.S.; Gould, J.C.; Melvin, W.S. Computer-assisted robotic antireflux surgery. *Minerva Gastroenterol. E Dietol.* **2004**, *50*, 253–260.
4. Lunca, S.; Bouras, G.; Stanescu, A.C. Gastrointestinal robot-assisted surgery. A current perspective. *Rom. J. Gastroenterol.* **2005**, *14*, 385–391. [PubMed]
5. Cadière, G.B.; Himpens, J.; Vertruyen, M.; Bruyns, J.; Fourtanier, G. Fundoplicature Selon Nissen Réalisée à Distance Du Pa-tient Par Robotique [Nissen Fundoplication Done by Remotely Controlled Robotic Technique]. *Ann. Chir.* **1999**, *53*, 137–141.
6. Ruurda, J.P.; Draaisma, W.A.; van Hillegersberg, R.; Rinkes, I.H.B.; Gooszen, H.G.; Janssen, L.W.; Simmermacher, R.K.; Broeders, I.A. Robot-Assisted Endoscopic Surgery: A Four-Year Single-Center Experience. *Dig. Surg.* **2005**, *22*, 313–320. [CrossRef]
7. Brenkman, H.J.; Parry, K.; van Hillegersberg, R.; Ruurda, J.P. Robot-Assisted Laparoscopic Hiatal Hernia Repair: Promising Anatomical and Functional Results. *J. Laparoendosc. Adv. Surg. Tech.* **2016**, *26*, 465–469. [CrossRef]
8. Falkenback, D.; Lehane, C.W.; Lord, R.V.N. Robot-assisted oesophageal and gastric surgery for benign disease: Antireflux operations and Heller's myotomy. *ANZ J. Surg.* **2014**, *85*, 113–120. [CrossRef]
9. Kastenmeier, A.; Gonzales, H.; Gould, J.C. Robotic Applications in the Treatment of Diseases of the Esophagus. *Surg. Laparosc. Endosc. Percutaneous Tech.* **2012**, *22*, 304–309. [CrossRef]
10. Mi, J.; Kang, Y.; Chen, X.; Wang, B.; Wang, Z. Whether robot-assisted laparoscopic fundoplication is better for gastroesophageal reflux disease in adults: A systematic review and meta-analysis. *Surg. Endosc.* **2010**, *24*, 1803–1814. [CrossRef]
11. Page, M.J.; McKenzie, J.E.; Bossuyt, P.M.; Boutron, I.; Hoffmann, T.C.; Mulrow, C.D.; Shamseer, L.; Tetzlaff, J.M.; Akl, E.A.; Brennan, S.E.; et al. The PRISMA 2020 Statement: An Updated Guideline for Reporting Systematic Reviews. *BMJ* **2021**, *372*, n71. [CrossRef] [PubMed]
12. Brooke, B.S.; Schwartz, T.A.; Pawlik, T.M. MOOSE Reporting Guidelines for Meta-analyses of Observational Studies. *JAMA Surg.* **2021**. [CrossRef] [PubMed]
13. Sterne, J.A.C.; Hernán, M.A.; Reeves, B.C.; Savović, J.; Berkman, N.D.; Viswanathan, M.; Henry, D.; Altman, D.G.; Ansari, M.T.; Boutron, I.; et al. ROBINS-I: A tool for assessing risk of bias in non-randomised studies of interventions. *BMJ* **2016**, *355*, i4919. [CrossRef] [PubMed]

14. Higgins, J.P.T.; Altman, D.G.; Gøtzsche, P.C.; Jüni, P.; Moher, D.; Oxman, A.D.; Savović, J.; Schulz, K.F.; Weeks, L.; Sterne, J.A.C.; et al. The Cochrane Collaboration's tool for assessing risk of bias in randomised trials. *BMJ* **2011**, *343*, d5928. [CrossRef] [PubMed]
15. Messori, A.; Maratea, D.; Fadda, V.; Trippoli, S. Using risk difference as opposed to odds-ratio in meta-analysis. *Int. J. Cardiol.* **2013**, *164*, 127. [CrossRef]
16. Luo, D.; Wan, X.; Liu, J.; Tong, T. Optimally estimating the sample mean from the sample size, median, mid-range, and/or mid-quartile range. *Stat. Methods Med Res.* **2018**, *27*, 1785–1805. [CrossRef]
17. Wan, X.; Wang, W.; Liu, J.; Tong, T. Estimating the sample mean and standard deviation from the sample size, median, range and/or interquartile range. *BMC Med Res. Methodol.* **2014**, *14*, 1–13. [CrossRef]
18. Furukawa, T.A.; Barbui, C.; Cipriani, A.; Brambilla, P.; Watanabe, N. Imputing missing standard deviations in meta-analyses can provide accurate results. *J. Clin. Epidemiol.* **2006**, *59*, 7–10. [CrossRef]
19. Barili, F.; Parolari, A.; Kappetein, P.; Freemantle, N. Statistical Primer: Heterogeneity, random- or fixed-effects model analyses? *Interact. Cardiovasc. Thorac. Surg.* **2018**, *27*, 317–321. [CrossRef]
20. DerSimonian, R.; Laird, N. Meta-analysis in clinical trials. *Control Clin. Trials* **1986**, *7*, 177–188. [CrossRef]
21. Egger, M.; Smith, G.D.; Schneider, M.; Minder, C. Papers Bias in Meta-Analysis Detected by a Simple, Graphical Test. *BMJ* **1997**, *315*, 629–631. [CrossRef] [PubMed]
22. Albassam, A.A.; Mallick, M.S.; Gado, A.; Shoukry, M. Nissen Fundoplication, Robotic-assisted Versus Laparoscopic Procedure: A Comparative Study in Children. *Eur. J. Pediatr. Surg.* **2009**, *19*, 316–319. [CrossRef] [PubMed]
23. Benedix, F.; Adolf, D.; Peglow, S.; Gstettenbauer, L.M.; Croner, R. Short-term outcome after robot-assisted hiatal hernia and anti-reflux surgery—Is there a benefit for the patient? *Langenbeck's Arch. Surg.* **2021**, *406*, 1387–1395. [CrossRef] [PubMed]
24. Ceccarelli, G.; Patriti, A.; Biancafarina, A.; Spaziani, A.; Bartoli, A.; Bellochi, R.; Casciola, L. Intraoperative and Postoperative Outcome of Robot-Assisted and Traditional Laparoscopic Nissen Fundoplication. *Eur. Surg. Res.* **2009**, *43*, 198–203. [CrossRef] [PubMed]
25. Ceccarelli, G.; Pasculli, A.; Bugiantella, W.; De Rosa, M.; Catena, F.; Rondelli, F.; Costa, G.; Rocca, A.; Longaroni, M.; Testini, M. Minimally invasive laparoscopic and robot-assisted emergency treatment of strangulated giant hiatal hernias: Report of five cases and literature review. *World J. Emerg. Surg.* **2020**, *15*, 1–12. [CrossRef]
26. Copeland, D.R.; Boneti, C.; Kokoska, E.R.; Jackson, R.J.; Smith, S.D. Evaluation of Initial Experience and Comparison of the da Vinci Surgical System With Established Laparoscopic and Open Pediatric Nissen Fundoplication Surgery. *JSLS J. Soc. Laparosc. Robot. Surg.* **2008**, *12*, 238–240.
27. Draaisma, W.A.; Ruurda, J.P.; Scheffer, R.C.H.; Simmermacher, R.K.J.; Gooszen, H.G.; Jong, H.G.R.; Buskens, E.; Broeders, I.A.M.J. Randomized clinical trial of standard laparoscopic *versus* robot-assisted laparoscopic Nissen fundoplication for gastro-oesophageal reflux disease. *Br. J. Surg.* **2006**, *93*, 1351–1359. [CrossRef]
28. Gehrig, T.; Mehrabi, A.; Fischer, L.; Kenngott, H.; Hinz, U.; Gutt, C.N.; Müller-Stich, B.P. Robotic-assisted paraesophageal hernia repair—A case-control study. *Langenbeck's Arch. Surg.* **2012**, *398*, 691–696. [CrossRef]
29. Hartmann, J.; Menenakos, C.; Ordemann, J.; Nocon, M.; Raue, W.; Braumann, C. Long-term results of quality of life after standard laparoscopic vs. robot-assisted laparoscopic fundoplications for gastro-oesophageal reflux disease. A comparative clinical trial. *Int. J. Med Robot. Comput. Assist. Surg.* **2009**, *5*, 32–37. [CrossRef]
30. Jensen, J.S.; Antonsen, H.K.; Durup, J. Two years of experience with robot-assisted anti-reflux surgery: A retrospective cohort study. *Int. J. Surg.* **2017**, *39*, 260–266. [CrossRef]
31. Melvin, W. Computer-Enhanced vs. Standard Laparoscopic Antireflux Surgery. *J. Gastrointest. Surg.* **2002**, *6*, 11–16. [CrossRef] [PubMed]
32. Morino, M.; Pellegrino, L.; Giaccone, C.; Garrone, C.; Rebecchi, F. Randomized clinical trial of robot-assisted *versus* laparoscopic Nissen fundoplication. *Br. J. Surg.* **2006**, *93*, 553–558. [CrossRef] [PubMed]
33. Müller-Stich, B.P.; Reiter, M.A.; Wente, M.N.; Fischer, L.; Köninger, J.; Gutt, C.N. No relevant difference in quality of life and functional outcome at 12 months' follow-up—A randomised controlled trial comparing robot-assisted versus conventional laparoscopic Nissen fundoplication. *Langenbeck's Arch. Surg.* **2009**, *394*, 441–446. [CrossRef]
34. El Nakadi, I.; Mélot, C.; Closset, J.; De Moor, V.; Bétroune, K.; Feron, P.; Lingier, P.; Gelin, M. Evaluation of da Vinci Nissen Fundoplication Clinical Results and Cost Minimization. *World J. Surg.* **2006**, *30*, 1050–1054. [CrossRef]
35. Samar, A.M.; Bond, A.; Ranaboldo, C. Comparison of FreeHand® robot-assisted with human-assisted laparoscopic fundoplication. *Minim. Invasive Ther. Allied Technol.* **2020**, *31*, 24–27. [CrossRef]
36. Tolboom, R.C.; Draaisma, W.A.; Broeders, I.A.M.J. Evaluation of conventional laparoscopic versus robot-assisted laparoscopic redo hiatal hernia and antireflux surgery: A cohort study. *J. Robot. Surg.* **2016**, *10*, 33–39. [CrossRef] [PubMed]
37. Wilhelm, A.; Nocera, F.; Schneider, R.; Koechlin, L.; Daume, D.L.; Fourie, L.; Steinemann, D.; von Flüe, M.; Peterli, R.; Angehrn, F.V.; et al. Robot-assisted vs. laparoscopic repair of complete upside-down stomach hiatal hernia (the RATHER-study): A prospective comparative single center study. *Surg. Endosc.* **2021**, 1–9. [CrossRef]
38. Jayne, D.; Pigazzi, A.; Marshall, H.; Croft, J.; Corrigan, N.; Copeland, J.; Quirke, P.; West, N.; Rautio, T.; Thomassen, N.; et al. Effect of Robotic-Assisted vs Conventional Laparoscopic Surgery on Risk of Conversion to Open Laparotomy Among Patients Undergoing Resection for Rectal Cancer: The ROLARR Randomized Clinical Trial. *JAMA* **2017**, *318*, 1569–1580. [CrossRef] [PubMed]

39. Milone, M.; de'Angelis, N.; Beghdadi, N.; Brunetti, F.; Manigrasso, M.; De Simone, G.; Servillo, G.; Vertaldi, S.; De Palma, G.D. Conversions related to adhesions in abdominal surgery. Robotic versus laparoscopic approach: A multicentre experience. *Int. J. Med Robot. Comput. Assist. Surg.* **2020**, *17*, e2186. [CrossRef]
40. Milone, M.; Manigrasso, M.; Anoldo, P.; D'Amore, A.; Elmore, U.; Giglio, M.C.; Rompianesi, G.; Vertaldi, S.; Troisi, R.I.; Francis, N.K.; et al. The Role of Robotic Visceral Surgery in Patients with Adhesions: A Systematic Review and Meta-Analysis. *J. Pers. Med.* **2022**, *12*, 307. [CrossRef]
41. Spechler, S.J. Evaluation and Treatment of Patients with Persistent Reflux Symptoms Despite Proton Pump Inhibitor Treatment. *Gastroenterol. Clin. N. Am.* **2020**, *49*, 437–450. [CrossRef] [PubMed]

Disclaimer/Publisher's Note: The statements, opinions and data contained in all publications are solely those of the individual author(s) and contributor(s) and not of MDPI and/or the editor(s). MDPI and/or the editor(s) disclaim responsibility for any injury to people or property resulting from any ideas, methods, instructions or products referred to in the content.

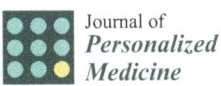

Systematic Review

The Role of Robotic Visceral Surgery in Patients with Adhesions: A Systematic Review and Meta-Analysis

Marco Milone [1,*], Michele Manigrasso [2], Pietro Anoldo [2], Anna D'Amore [1], Ugo Elmore [3], Mariano Cesare Giglio [1], Gianluca Rompianesi [1], Sara Vertaldi [1], Roberto Ivan Troisi [1], Nader K. Francis [4] and Giovanni Domenico De Palma [1]

1. Department of Clinical Medicine and Surgery, University of Naples "Federico II", 80131 Naples, Italy; anna.damore1993@libero.it (A.D.); mariano.giglio@hotmail.it (M.C.G.); gianluca.rompianesi@unina.it (G.R.); vertaldisara@gmail.com (S.V.); roberto.troisi@unina.it (R.I.T.); giovanni.depalma@unina.it (G.D.D.P.)
2. Department of Advanced Biomedical Sciences, University of Naples "Federico II", 80131 Naples, Italy; michele.manigrasso@unina.it (M.M.); pietro.anoldo@gmail.com (P.A.)
3. Department of Surgery, San Raffaele Hospital and San Raffaele Vita-Salute University, 20132 Milan, Italy; elmore.ugo@hsr.it
4. Yeovil District Hospital, Somerset BA21 4AT, UK; nader.francis@ydh.nhs.uk
* Correspondence: milone.marco.md@gmail.com; Tel.: +39-333-299-3637

Abstract: Abdominal adhesions are a risk factor for conversion to open surgery. An advantage of robotic surgery is the lower rate of unplanned conversions. A systematic review was conducted using the terms "laparoscopic" and "robotic". Inclusion criteria were: comparative studies evaluating patients undergoing laparoscopic and robotic surgery; reporting data on conversion to open surgery for each group due to adhesions and studies including at least five patients in each group. The main outcomes were the conversion rates due to adhesions and surgeons' expertise (novice vs. expert). The meta-analysis included 70 studies from different surgical specialities with 14,329 procedures (6472 robotic and 7857 laparoscopic). The robotic approach was associated with a reduced risk of conversion (OR 1.53, 95% CI 1.12–2.10, $p = 0.007$). The analysis of the procedures performed by "expert surgeons" showed a statistically significant difference in favour of robotic surgery (OR 1.48, 95% CI 1.03–2.12, $p = 0.03$). A reduced conversion rate due to adhesions with the robotic approach was observed in patients undergoing colorectal cancer surgery (OR 2.62, 95% CI 1.20–5.72, $p = 0.02$). The robotic approach could be a valid option in patients with abdominal adhesions, especially in the subgroup of those undergoing colorectal cancer resection performed by expert surgeons.

Keywords: conversion; abdominal adhesions; laparoscopic surgery; robotic surgery

1. Introduction

Robotic surgery was introduced in the early 2000s to overcome some technical limitations of conventional laparoscopic surgery. However, even if some benefits of the robotic approach over laparoscopy have been described [1–5], it is currently considered the gold standard treatment only for radical prostatectomy [6].

Specific interventions that could benefit from the robotic approach are yet to be identified. It is worth mentioning that one of the most extensively reported advantages of robotic surgery is the lower rate of unplanned open conversions [7–14]. Conversion to open surgery can be multifactorial, and when all causes of conversion were examined in ROLARR Randomized Controlled Clinical Trial (RCT), no difference was found between robotic and laparoscopic techniques during rectal cancer surgery [15].

Intra-abdominal adhesions due to prior abdominal surgery are a common and well-recognised risk factor for conversion [16–18], and it is not known whether the robotic approach could allow a lower conversion rate than laparoscopy in patients with adhesions. The rationale lies in the potential technical advantages of robotic surgery—magnified 3D

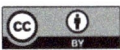

vision with a more stable operative field, preservation of natural eye-hand-instrument alignment, precisely controlled EndoWrist instruments with better ergonomics and reduced physiologic tremor—heightened in case of distortion of the normal abdominal anatomy related to adhesions, which makes the visualisation more difficult and increases the difficulty of surgical procedure.

Since the indications for the robotic technique outside prostatectomy are far from being established by high levels of evidence, a meta-analysis of the available literature addressing pertinent questions related to the possible benefits of the robotic approach over laparoscopy is required to guide the expansion of the application of the robotic techniques. The aim of this study was to systematically review the literature and pool the evidence in order to evaluate and compare the adhesion-related conversions to open surgery are in patients undergoing robotic and laparoscopic surgery across all specialities.

2. Materials and Methods

2.1. Literature Search and Study Selection

To identify all available studies, an electronic search of Cochrane Library (including the Cochrane Central Register of Controlled Trials), EMBASE, PubMed, SCOPUS and Web of Science was conducted according to PRISMA (Preferred Reporting Items for Systematic reviews and Meta-Analyses) guidelines [19]. This systematic review was performed following the meta-analysis of observational studies epidemiology (MOOSE) guidelines [20].

The search terms "laparoscopic" and "robotic" were used. The search was limited to studies regarding humans and published in English between June 1993 and March 2020.

Inclusion criteria were as follows: (1) comparative studies evaluating patients undergoing laparoscopic and robotic surgery; (2) studies reporting data on conversion to open surgery for each group due to adhesions; and (3) studies including at least 5 patients in each group, to minimise the imprecision associated with very small populations. Indexed abstracts of posters and podium presentations at international meetings were not included. Systematic reviews and meta-analyses were consulted to find additional studies of interest. Reference lists of the selected studies were screened to find additional studies of interest. If the same author or institution published overlapping series in different articles, only the most recent study was included. Two reviewers (Mi.Ma. and S.V.) independently assessed the reports for eligibility at the title and abstract level. In case of discrepancies, a third author (M.M.) was consulted, and an agreement was reached by consensus.

2.2. Data Extraction and Quality Assessment of Included Studies

The following data were extracted from each included study: first author, year of publication, study design, propensity score analysis, surgical field, diagnosis, type of intervention, total number of patients, number of patients undergoing laparoscopic and robotic surgery, and number of conversions related to intraoperative adhesions. Although widely reported by surgical studies, the definition of conversion within the literature varies [21]; therefore, we searched for this information in all the included studies. Surgeons' expertise (classified as novice vs. expert) has been described in many of the included studies, even if only a few studies reported the number of procedures performed by the surgeons. None of the studies provided an exact definition of the various steps of the surgical procedure. Thus, the criteria to define expertise remains heterogeneous.

Furthermore, attempts to examine the quality assurance of surgical techniques of the studies according to Foster JD et al. [22] was performed for the assessment of surgeon-dependent performance bias.

The following patients' characteristics were extracted and registered: gender, mean age, mean BMI, American Society of Anesthesiologists (ASA) score and previous abdominal surgery.

Study quality assessment for non-randomised clinical trial was performed using the Newcastle Ottawa Scale (NOS) [23]. This scoring system encompasses three major domains (selection, comparability and exposure), with a resulting score that varies between 0 (low quality) and 9 (high quality). In the case of randomised controlled trial (RCTs), the risk of bias was evaluated according to the Cochrane Collaboration Tool for assessing the risk of bias [24]. According to this scoring system, seven domains were evaluated as "Low risk of bias" or "High risk of bias" or "Unclear" according to reporting on sequence generation, allocation concealment, blinding of participants, blinding of outcome assessment, incomplete outcome data, selective outcome reporting and other potential threats to validity. The results of the quality assessment are reported in Table 1.

Table 1. NOS quality assessment of the included non-randomised trials.

Study	Selection				Comparability	Outcome			Total
	Representativeness of Exposed Cohort	Selection of the Non-Exposed Cohort	Ascertainment of Exposure	Outcome Not Present at the Start of the Study		Assessment of Outcome	Length of Follow-Up	Adequacy of Follow-Up	
Albassam A.A. et al., 2009 [25]		*	*	*	*	*	*	*	*******
Alfieri S. et al., 2019 [26]	*	*	*	*	**	*	*	*	*********
Alhossaini R.M. et al., 2019 [27]	*	*	*	*	*	*	*	*	********
Alimi Q. et al., 2018 [28]		*	*	*	*	*	*	*	*******
Ayloo S. et al., 2011 [29]		*	*	*	*	*	*	*	*******
Beak J. et al., 2010 [30]	*	*	*	*	**	*	*	*	*********
Benizri E.I. et al., 2013 [31]		*	*	*	*	*	*	*	*******
Benway B.M. et al., 2009 [32]		*	*	*	*	*	*	*	*******
Bilgin I.A. et al., 2019 [33]		*	*	*	**	*	*	*	********
Boggess J.F. et al., 2008 [34]		*	*	*	*	*	*	*	*******
Buchs N.C. et al., 2014 [35]		*	*	*	**	*	*	*	********
Butturini G. et al., 2014 [36]	*	*	*	*	**	*	*	*	*********
Cassini D. et al., 2018 [37]	*	*	*	*	**	*	*	*	*********
Chiu L.H. et al., 2015 [38]	*	*	*	*	*	*	*	*	********
Coronado P.J. et al., 2012 [39]		*	*	*	**	*	*	*	********

Table 1. Cont.

Study	Selection				Comparability	Outcome		Total
	Representativeness of Exposed Cohort	Selection of the Non-Exposed Cohort	Ascertainment of Exposure	Outcome Not Present at the Start of the Study	Assessment of Outcome	Length of Follow-Up	Adequacy of Follow-Up	
Corrado G. et al., 2018 [40]		*	*	*	*	*	*	*******
Crippa J. et al., 2019 [41]		*	*	*	**	*	*	********
Cuendis-Velazquez A. et al., 2018 [42]	*	*	*	*	*	*	*	********
Elliott P.A. et al., 2015 [43]	*	*	*	*	**	*	*	*********
Escobar F. et al., 2011 [44]		*	*	*	*	*	*	*******
Esen E. et al., 2018 [45]	*	*	*	*	**	*	*	*********
Feroci F. et al., 2016 [46]		*	*	*	**	*	*	********
Gallotta V. et al., 2018 [47]	*	*	*	*	*	*	*	********
Gangemi A. et al., 2017 [48]		*	*	*	**	*	*	********
Gao Y. et al., 2018 [49]	*	*	*	*	**	*	*	*********
Goçmen A. et al., 2012 [50]	*	*	*	*	*	*	*	********
Goh B.K.P. et al., 2016 [13]	*	*	*	*	**	*	*	*********
Golcoechea J.C. et al., 2010 [51]	*	*	*	*	*	*	*	********
Gorgun E. et al., 2016 [52]	*	*	*	*	**	*	*	*********
Gray K.D. et al., 2018 [53]	*	*	*	*	**	*	*	*********
Guillotrean et al., 2012 [54]		*	*	*	**	*	*	********
Hoekstra A.V. et al., 2009 [55]		*	*	*	**	*	*	********
Holz D.O. et al., 2010 [56]		*	*	*	*	*	*	*******
Ielpo B. et al., 2014 [57]		*	*	*	**	*	*	********
Johnson L. et al., 2016 [58]	*	*	*	*	**	*	*	*********
Karabulut K.K. et al., 2012 [59]	*	*	*	*	*	*	*	********

Table 1. *Cont.*

Study	Selection				Comparability	Outcome			Total
	Representativeness of Exposed Cohort	Selection of the Non-Exposed Cohort	Ascertainment of Exposure	Outcome Not Present at the Start of the Study	Assessment of Outcome	Length of Follow-Up	Adequacy of Follow-Up		
Kilic G. et al., 2011 [60]	*	*	*	*	*	*	*		********
Kim J.C. et al., 2018 [61]	*	*	*	*	**	*	*		*********
Kim Y.W. et al., 2015 [62]	*	*	*	*	*	*	*		********
Kong Y. et al., 2019 [63]	*	*	*	*	**	*	*		*********
Krucharoen U. et al., 2019 [64]		*	*	*	**	*	*		********
Law W.L. et al., 2016 [65]	*	*	*	*	**	*	*		*********
Lee S.Y. et al., 2014 [66]		*	*	*	**	*	*		********
Leitao M.M. et al., 2012 [67]		*	*	*	*	*	*		*******
Lim P.C. et al., 2010 [68]		*	*	*	*	*	*		*******
Liu et al., 2016 [69]		*	*	*	*	*	*		*******
Maenpaa M.M. et al., 2016 [70]	*	*	*	*	*	*	*		********
Mantoo S. et al., 2013 [71]		*	*	*	**	*	*		********
Mehmood R.K. et al., 2014 [72]	*	*	*	*	*	*	*		********
Montalti R. et al., 2014 [73]		*	*	*	**	*	*		********
Morelli L. et al., 2016 [74]		*	*	*	*	*	*		*******
Najafi N. et al., 2020 [75]	*	*	*	*	**	*	*		*********
Nezhat F.R. et al., 2014 [76]	*	*	*	*	*	*	*		********
Niglio A. et al., 2019 [77]		*	*	*	**	*	*		********
Ozben V. et al., 2019 [78]	*	*	*	*	**	*	*		*********
Park J.Y. et al., 2015 [79]		*	*	*	*	*	*		*******

Table 1. Cont.

Study	Selection				Comparability	Outcome			Total
	Representativeness of Exposed Cohort	Selection of the Non-Exposed Cohort	Ascertainment of Exposure	Outcome Not Present at the Start of the Study	Assessment of Outcome	Length of Follow-Up	Adequacy of Follow-Up		
Ramji K.M. et al., 2015 [80]	*	*	*	*	*	*	*		*******
Rencuzogullari A. et al., 2016 [81]		*	*	*	**	*	*	*	*******
Seror J. et al., 2016 [82]	*	*	*	*	**	*	*	*	********
Smith A.L. 2012 [83]	*	*	*	*	*	*	*	*	*******
Spinoglio G. et al., 2018 [84]	*	*	*	*	**	*	*	*	********
Troisi R.I. et al., 2013 [85]	*	*	*	*		*	*	*	******
Turunen H. et al., 2013 [86]		*	*	*	**	*	*	*	*******
Vasilescu C. et al., 2012 [87]		*	*	*	*	*	*	*	******
Wang A.J. et al., 2009 [88]		*	*	*	**	*	*	*	*******
Wang Z.Z. et al., 2019 [89]	*	*	*	*	**	*	*	*	********
Warren J.A. et al., 2016 [90]	*	*	*	*	**	*	*	*	********
Wong M.T.C. et al., 2011 [91]		*	*	*	*	*	*	*	******
Yamaguchi T. et al., 2015 [92]	*	*	*	*	**	*	*	*	********
Zhao X. et al., 2018 [93]		*	*	*	*	*	*	*	******

2.3. Statistical Analysis

Statistical analysis was performed using RevMan (Version 5.4, Copenhagen: The Nordic Cochrane Centre, The Cochrane Collaboration, 2020).

The primary outcome of this study was the open conversion rate to open surgery due to adhesions. The odds ratio (OR) along with 95% confidence interval (CI) was used as an effect estimate for dichotomous outcomes, with OR values < 1 indicating fewer events in the robotic group. In the case of zero events, a 0.5 correction was added to incorporate all available data in the meta-analysis and to maintain analytic consistency [94]. When studies provided only means for continuous variables and sample size of the trial, a standard deviation was imputed, according to Furukawa et al. [95]. The summary estimate was computed according to the random effect model described by DerSimonian and Laird [96]. A conservative random effect model was chosen a priori in consideration of foreseen heterogeneity among the studies, which were from different surgical fields. The heterogeneity among studies was tested by Q statistic and quantified by I^2 statistic, with I^2 values < 25%, between 25 and 50%, and >50% indicating respectively low, moderate, and high heterogeneity [97].

With the aim to assess if that differences among included studies may be affected by demographic (gender, age and BMI) and clinical variables (ASA Score and previous abdominal surgery), we planned to perform meta-regression analyses in case of the significance of the meta-analysis after implementing a regression model with incidence of the main outcome as dependent variable (y) and the above-mentioned covariates as independent variables (x). Meta-regression analyses were performed with Comprehensive Meta-analysis (Version 2.2, Biostat Inc., Englewood, NJ, USA, 2005), provided by Biostat Inc. [98].

The presence of publication bias was investigated through a funnel plot where the summary estimate of each study (OR) was plotted against a measure of study precision (standard error). In addition to visual inspection, funnel plot symmetry was tested using Egger's linear regression method [99]. p values < 0.05 were considered statistically significant.

Furthermore, different subgroups analyses, including studies about each surgical field (colorectal, oesophagogastric, hepatobiliary, pancreatic, endocrine, urologic and gynaecologic surgery) and the surgeons' expertise (novice and expert) were performed. Furthermore, in case of a statistically significant difference in any of the above-mentioned surgical fields, further analyses were performed to understand if the significance was present in the case of benign and or malignant disease.

3. Results

3.1. Study Selection

The electronic search provided a total of 49,891 results. After the removal of duplicates, 10,489 studies underwent screening on the basis of title. Of the 4050 full-text articles assessed for eligibility, 3978 studies were excluded for several reasons: 431 were not published in the English language, 444 were case reports, 2179 were reviews, 535 were off-topic after scanning abstract, and for 391, data were not available. At the end of the selection process, 70 studies were included in the meta-analysis [13,25–93].

3.2. Study Characteristics

The selected studies included a total of 14,329 patients, of whom 6472 underwent robotic surgery and 7857 laparoscopic surgery. Fifty-one studies were retrospective [13,25–27,32,33,37, 39–49,51–53,56–58,63–69,71,73–90,92,93], eighteen were prospective [28–31,34–36,38,50,54,55, 59–62,65,72,91], and there was only one randomised controlled trial [70]. Studies were from different fields of surgery, including colorectal (n = 19), oesophagogastric (n = 10), hepatobiliary (n = 5), pancreatic (n = 6), gynaecologic (n = 19), urologic (n = 5), endocrine (n = 3) vascular (n = 1), abdominal wall (n = 1) and splenic surgery (n = 1). In six studies, robotic surgery was performed by early surgeons, and by expert surgeons in other 47 studies. The other 17 studies did not provide these data. The characteristics of the included studies are reported in Table 2.

Table 2. Characteristics of the included studies.

Study	Design	Patients		Surgical Field	Pathology	Procedure	Expertise
		Lap	Rob				
Albassam A.A., 2009 [25]	Retrospective	25	25	Oesophago-gastric	GERD	Nissen fundoplication	Expert
Alfieri S. et al., 2019 [26]	Retrospective	85	96	Pancreatic	pNETs	Distal pancreatectomy	Expert
Alhossaini R.M. et al., 2019 [27]	Retrospective	30	25	Oesophago-gastric	Remnant gastric cancer	Completion total gastrectomy	NR
Alimi Q. et al., 2018 [28]	Prospective	50	50	Urologic	Renal tumour	Partial nephrectomy	Expert
Ayloo S. et al., 2011 [29]	Prospective	39	30	Oesophago-gastric	Morbid obesity	Sleeve gastrectomy	NR
Beak J. et al., 2010 [30]	Prospective	41	41	Colorectal	Rectal cancer	Rectal resection with TME	Early
Benizri E.I. et al., 2013 [31]	Prospective	100	100	Oesophago-gastric	Morbid obesity	Roux-en-Y gastric bypass	Expert

Table 2. Cont.

Study	Design	Patients		Surgical Field	Pathology	Procedure	Expertise
		Lap	Rob				
Benway B.M. [32]	Retrospective	118	129	Urologic	Renal tumour	Partial nephrectomy	Expert
Bilgin I.A. et al., 2019 [33]	Retrospective	22	20	Colorectal	Diverticular disease	Sigmoidectomy	Expert
Boggess J.F. et al., 2008 [34]	Prospective	81	103	Gynaecologic	Endometrial cancer	Hysterectomy	Early
Buchs N.C. et al., 2014 [35]	Prospective	389	388	Oesophago-gastric	Morbid obesity	Roux-en-Y gastric bypass	Expert
Butturini G. et al., 2014 [36]	Prospective	21	22	Pancreatic	Pancreatic tumours	Distal pancreatectomy	Expert
Cassini D. et al., 2018 [37]	Retrospective	92	64	Colorectal	Diverticular disease	Sigmoidectomy	Expert
Chiu L.H. et al., 2015 [38]	Prospective	128	88	Gynaecologic	Benign pathology or carcinoma IS	Hysterectomy	NR
Coronado P.J. et al., 2012 [39]	Retrospective	84	71	Gynaecologic	Endometrial cancer	Hysterectomy with bilateral salpingo-oophorectomy	NR
Corrado G. et al., 2018 [40]	Retrospective	406	249	Gynaecologic	Low-grade endometrial carcinoma	Hysterectomy	Expert
Crippa J. et al., 2019 [41]	Retrospective	283	317	Colorectal	Rectal cancer	LAR or APR with TME	Expert
Cuendis-Velazquez A. et al., 2018 [42]	Retrospective	40	35	Hepatobiliary	Bile duct injury	Hepaticojejunostomy	NR
Elliott P.A. et al., 2015 [43]	Retrospective	20	11	Colorectal	Diverticulitis	Sigmoidectomy	Expert
Escobar P.F. et al., 2011 [44]	Retrospective	30	30	Gynaecologic	Endometrial cancer	Hysterectomy	Expert
Esen E. et al., 2018 [45]	Retrospective	78	100	Colorectal	Rectal cancer	Rectal resection with TME	Expert
Feroci F. et al., 2016 [46]	Retrospective	58	53	Colorectal	Rectal cancer	Rectal resection with TME	Expert
Gallotta V. et al., 2018 [47]	Retrospective	140	70	Gynaecologic	Early cervical cancer	Hysterectomy	Expert
Gangemi A. et al., 2017 [48]	Retrospective	289	676	Hepatobiliary	Cholelithiasis/cholecystitis	Cholecystectomy	Expert
Gao Y. et al., 2018 [49]	Retrospective	163	163	Oesophago-gastric	Gastric cancer	Partial and total gastrectomy	Expert
Goh B.K.P. et al., 2016 [13]	Retrospective	31	8	Pancreatic	Pancreatic tumours	Distal pancreatectomy	Early
Goioechea J.C. et al., 2010 [51]	Retrospective	173	102	Gynaecologic	Endometrial cancer	Hysterectomy	Expert
Gorgun E. et al., 2016 [52]	Retrospective	27	29	Colorectal	Rectal cancer in obese patients	LAR and APR	NR
Goçmen A. et al., 2012 [50]	Prospective	60	60	Gynaecologic	Benign gynaecologic disease	Hysterectomy	NR
Gray K.D. et al., 2018 [53]	Retrospective	66	18	Oesophago-gastric	Revision of bariatric surgery	AGB, VSG, RYGB, VBG	Expert
Guillotrean J. et al., 2012 [54]	Prospective	226	210	Urologic	Small renal mass	Partial nephrectomy	NR
Hoekstra A.V. et al., 2009 [55]	Prospective	7	32	Gynaecologic	Endometrial cancer	Hysterectomy with bilateral salpingo-oophorectomy	Expert
Holtz D.O. et al., 2019 [56]	Retrospective	20	13	Gynaecologic	Endometrial cancer	Hysterectomy with bilateral salpingo-oophorectomy	Expert
Ielpo B. et al., 2017 [57]	Retrospective	112	86	Colorectal	Rectal cancer	Rectal resection	Expert
Johnson L. et al., 2016 [58]	Retrospective	187	353	Gynaecologic	Endometrial cancer	Hysterectomy	NR
Karabulut K.K. et al., 2012 [59]	Prospective	50	50	Endocrine	Pheochromocytoma	Adrenalectomy	Expert

Table 2. *Cont.*

Study	Design	Patients		Surgical Field	Pathology	Procedure	Expertise
		Lap	Rob				
Kilic G.S. et al., 2011 [60]	Prospective	34	25	Gynaecologic	Benign gynaecologic disease	Hysterectomy	Expert
Kim J.C. et al., 2018 [61]	Prospective	53	20	Colorectal	Colon cancer	Left colectomy	NR
Kim Y.W. et al., 2015 [62]	Prospective	288	87	Oesophago-gastric	Gastric cancer	Distal gastrectomy	Expert
Kong Y. et al., 2019 [63]	Retrospective	532	266	Oesophago-gastric	Gastric cancer	Partial and total gastrectomy	Expert
Krucharoen U. et al., 2019 [64]	Retrospective	16	18	Vascular	Median arcuate ligament syndrome	MAL release	Expert
Law W.L. et al., 2016 [65]	Prospective	171	220	Colorectal	Rectal cancer	Hartmann procedure, LAR and APR	NR
Lee S.Y. et al., 2014 [66]	Retrospective	131	37	Pancreatic	Pancreatic tumours	Distal pancreatectomy	Expert
Leitao M.M. et al., 2012 [67]	Retrospective	302	347	Gynaecologic	Uterine cancer	Hysterectomy	Expert
Lim P.C. et al., 2019 [68]	Retrospective	122	122	Gynaecologic	Endometrial cancer	Hysterectomy	Expert
Liu et al., 2016 [69]	Retrospective	25	27	Pancreatic	Periampullary neoplasms	PD	Expert
Maenpaa M.M. et al., 2016 [70]	Rct	48	51	Gynaecologic	Low-grade endometrial carcinoma	Hysterectomy	Expert
Mantoo S. et al., 2013 [71]	Retrospective	74	44	Colorectal	Obstructed defecation	Ventral mesh rectopexy	NR
Mehmood R.K. et al., 2014 [72]	Prospective	34	17	Colorectal	Rectal prolapse	Ventral mesh rectopexy	NR
Montalti R. et al., 2015 [73]	Retrospective	72	36	Hepatobiliary	Liver diseases	Posterosuperior segments resection	Expert
Morelli L. et al., 2016 [74]	Retrospective	41	41	Endocrine	Benign or malignant adrenal tumour	Adrenalectomy	Expert
Najafi N. et al., 2020 [75]	Retrospective	40	35	Pancreatic	Benign and borderline tumours	Distal pancreatic resection and enucleation	NR
Nezhat F.R. et al., 2014 [76]	Retrospective	13	9	Gynaecologic	Early ovarian cancer	Salpingo-oophorectomy	NR
Niglio A. et al., 2019 [77]	Retrospective	64	40	Endocrine	Adrenal cancer	Adrenalectomy	NR
Ozben V. et al., 2019 [78]	Retrospective	56	26	Colorectal	Benign or malignant pathology	Subtotal or total colectomy	Expert
Park J.Y. et al., 2015 [79]	Retrospective	622	148	Oesophago-gastric	Early gastric cancer	Partial and total gastrectomy	Expert
Ramji K.M. et al., 2015 [80]	Retrospective	27	26	Colorectal	Rectal cancer	Rectal resection	Early
Rencuzogullari A. et al., 2016 [81]	Retrospective	21	21	Colorectal	IBD	Proctectomy	Early
Seror J et al., 2013 [82]	Retrospective	106	40	Gynaecologic	Endometrial cancer	Hysterectomy with bilateral salpingo-oophorectomy	Expert
Smith A.L. et al., 2012 [83]	Retrospective	106	116	Gynaecologic	Endometrial cancer	Hysterectomy	Early
Spinoglio G. et al., 2018 [84]	Retrospective	100	100	Colorectal	Right colon cancer	Right colectomy with CME	Expert
Troisi R.I. et al., 2013 [85]	Retrospective	223	40	Hepatobiliary	Liver diseases	Liver resection	Expert
Turunen H. et al., 2013 [86]	Retrospective	150	67	Gynaecologic	Endometrial cancer	Hysterectomy	Expert
Vasilescu C. et al., 2012 [87]	Retrospective	22	10	Splenic	Hereditary spherocytosis	Splenectomy	NR
Wang A.J. et al., 2009 [88]	Retrospective	62	40	Urologic	Renal cell carcinoma	Partial nephrectomy	Expert

Table 2. Cont.

Study	Design	Patients		Surgical Field	Pathology	Procedure	Expertise
		Lap	Rob				
Wang Z.Z. et al., 2019 [89]	Retrospective	48	92	Hepatobiliary	Benign or malignant hepatic lesions	Hemiepatectomy	Expert
Warren J.A. et al., 2016 [90]	Retrospective	103	53	Abdominal wall	Ventral hernia	Ventral hernia repair	NR
Wong M.T.C. et al., 2011 [91]	Prospective	40	23	Colorectal	Complex rectocele	Ventral mesh rectopexy	Expert
Yamaguchi T. et al., 2015 [92]	Retrospective	239	203	Colorectal	Rectal cancer	Rectal resection	Expert
Zhao X. et al., 2018 [93]	Retrospective	101	101	Urologic	Renal tumour	Simple enucleation with single layer renorrhaphy	Expert

GERD—gastroesophageal reflux disease; pNET—pancreatic neuroendocrine tumour; IS—in situ; IBD—intestinal bowel disease; TME—total mesorectal excision; LAR—low anterior resection; APR—abdominoperineal resection; AGB—adjustable gastric banding; VSG—vertical sleeve gastrectomy; RYGB—Roux-en-Y gastric bypass; VBG—vertical banded gastroplasty; MAL—median arcuate ligament; PD—pancreaticoduodenectomy; CME—complete mesocolic excision; NR—not reported.

3.3. Quality Assessment of Studies and Performance

All studies had NOS quality scores greater than 6, indicating that all these studies had a high methodological quality. Specifically, twenty-one studies had NOS quality score = 9; thirty studies had NOS quality score = 8; eighteen studies had NOS quality score = 7. The NOS quality score is shown in Table 1. The only randomised controlled trial (RCT) showed a low risk of bias.

Among the expert surgeons, none of the included studies reported on the quality assurance of surgical technique as described by Foster et al. [22]. Thus, it was not possible to perform further analyses on the quality of surgical performance among expert or early surgeons.

3.4. Conversion to Open Surgery Due to Adhesions

Seventy studies provided data about the conversion to open surgery due to anastomotic adhesions [13,25–93], even if only nine of them [13,35,41,43,45,46,50,78,84] reported the definition of conversion. The robotic approach was associated with a reduced risk of conversion (OR 1.53, 95% CI 1.12–2.10, $p = 0.007$, Figure 1), with consistent results across all the 70 studies since no heterogeneity was observed ($I^2 = 0\%$, $p = 0.95$).

Regarding surgeons' expertise, 47 studies classified surgeons as "expert" [25,26,28,31–33, 35–37,40,41,43–49,51,53,55–57,59,60,62–64,66–70,73,74,78,79,82,84–86,88,89,91–93] and 6 studies as "novice" [13,30,34,80,81,83]. The analysis of the procedures performed by expert surgeons involved 11,172 procedures, of which 6283 laparoscopic and 4889 robotic and showed a statistically significant difference in favour of robotic surgery (OR 1.48, 95% CI 1.03–2.12, $p = 0.03$), with no heterogeneity among the studies ($I^2 = 0\%$, $p = 0.71$). The analysis of the procedures performed by "novice" surgeons involved 622 procedures, of which 307 laparoscopic and 315 robotic and showed no significant difference between the two groups (OR 1.53, 95% CI 0.44–5.28, $p = 0.50$), without any heterogeneity among the studies ($I^2 = 0\%$, $p = 0.91$). Data on surgeons' expertise are shown in Figure 2.

Our meta-regression analysis showed that no demographic or clinical outcomes significantly impacted conversion, as shown in Table 3.

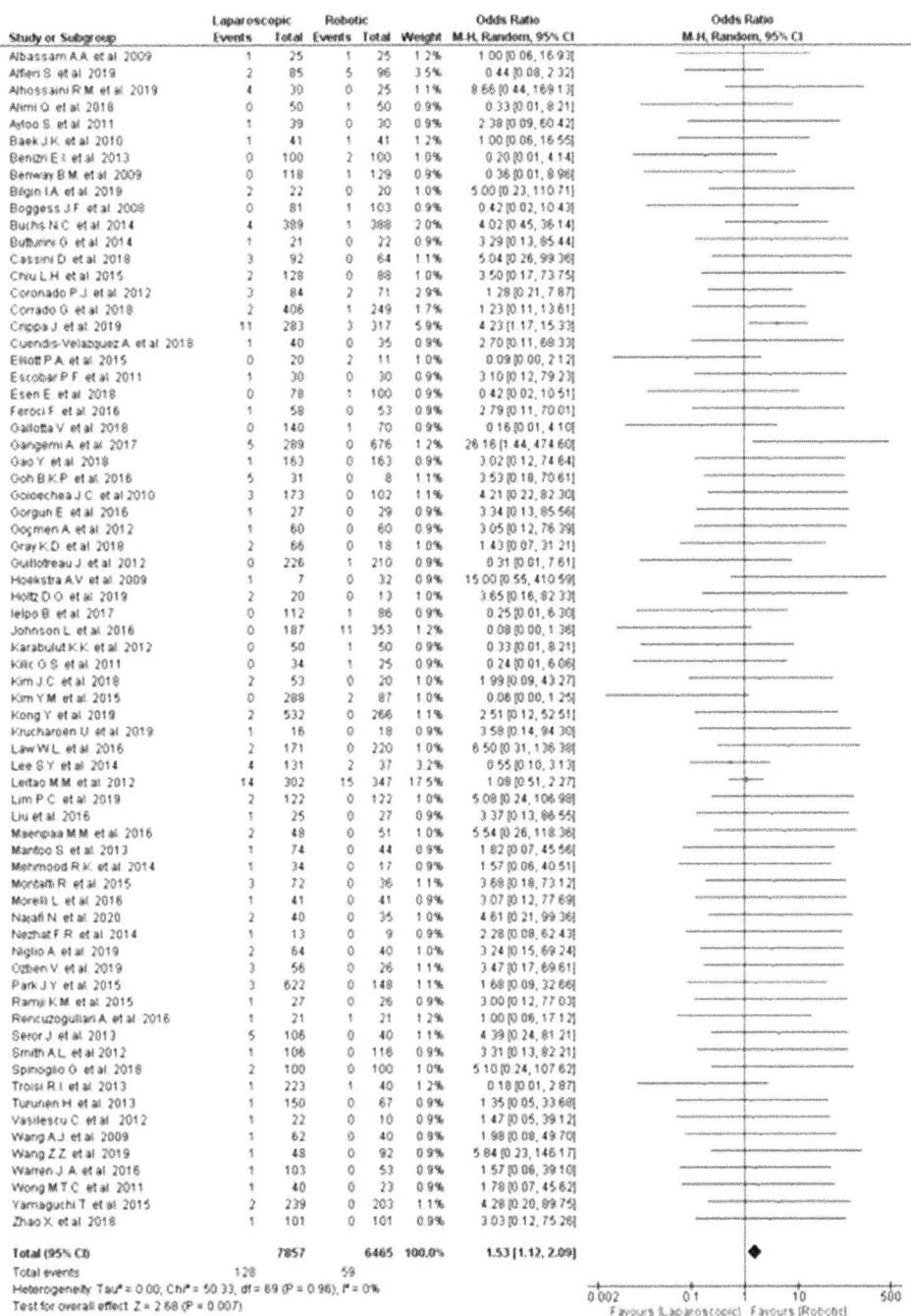

Figure 1. Meta-analysis of the included studies on conversion due to adhesions.

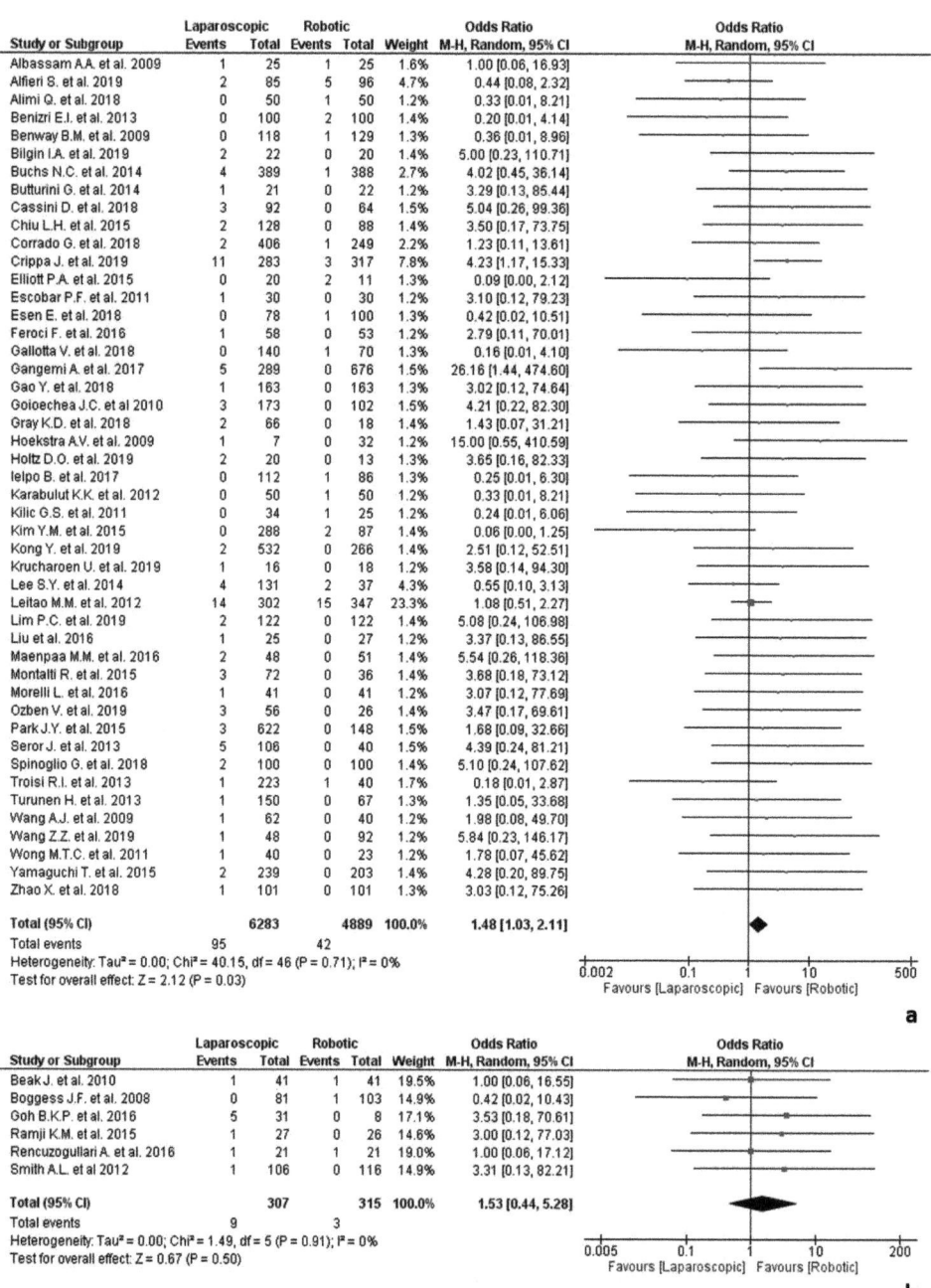

Figure 2. Conversions due to adhesions according to surgeons' expertise: (**a**) in procedures performed by expert surgeons; (**b**) in procedures performed by "early" surgeons.

Table 3. *p*-values of the meta-regression analysis.

Covariates	p Value
Mean age	0.67
Female gender	0.5
BMI	0.99
ASA Score I	0.44
ASA Score II	0.92
Tumour stage II	0.36
Tumour stage IV	0.22
Previous abdominal surgery	0.03

BMI—body mass index.

3.5. Subgroup Analysis

3.5.1. Colorectal Surgery

The results of the studies about colorectal surgery are shown in Figure 3. Nineteen studies [30,33,37,41,43,45,46,52,57,61,65,71,72,78,80,81,84,91,92] included in the final analysis were including colorectal surgery cases and involved 2969 procedures, of which 1548 laparoscopic and 1421 robotic. Of the included studies, eleven were on colorectal cancer [30,41,45,46,52,57,61,65,80,84,92], three on rectocele or rectal prolapse [71,72,91] and three on diverticular disease patients [33,37,43]. Ozben et al. [78] described surgical procedures related to both benign and malign diseases. Rencuzogullari et al. [81] was the only one to report surgical proctectomy performed for IBD, so it was excluded from the subgroup analysis.

In the overall colorectal surgery analysis, a significant difference in terms of conversion rate related to adhesions was observed between the two groups in favour of robotics (OR 2.22, 95% CI 1.18–4.19, $p = 0.01$), with no heterogeneity among the included studies ($I^2 = 0\%$, $p = 0.93$).

Meta-regression analysis showed that none of the demographic and clinical parameters (gender, age, BMI, ASA and tumoural stage) significantly impacted the conversion rate due to adhesions, with the exception of "previous abdominal surgery" ($p = 0.03$).

In a further analysis about colorectal cancer the significance was confirmed (OR 2.62, 95% CI 1.20–5.72, $p = 0.02$), with no heterogeneity among the included studies ($I^2 = 0\%$, $p = 0.89$). Even including only studies about rectal cancer [30,41,45,46,52,57,61,65,80,84,92], the significance was confirmed (OR 2.54, 95% CI 1.10–5.88, $p = 0.03$), with no heterogeneity among the included studies ($I^2 = 0\%$, $p = 0.79$).

Meta-regression analysis on colorectal cancer showed that none of the demographic or clinical parameters significantly impacted the analysed outcome.

No statistically significant differences in terms of conversion rate due to adhesions were observed between robotics and laparoscopy in the studies about rectocele/rectal prolapse [72,73,91] and diverticular disease [33,37,43] (OR 1.72, 95% CI 0.27–11.16, $p = 0.57$ and OR 1.36, 95% CI 0.10–18.02, $p = 0.81$, respectively), with no significant heterogeneity among the studies ($I^2 = 0\%$, $p = 1.00$ and $I^2 = 53\%$, $p = 0.12$, respectively).

Within the colorectal surgery studies, surgeons were classified as "expert" in eleven studies [33,37,41,43,45,46,57,78,84,91,92] and as "novice" in other three studies [30,80,81]. Five studies did not provide these data [52,61,65,71,72]. The analysis about expertise in colorectal surgeries showed that a significant difference in terms of conversion rate related to adhesions was found in colorectal surgery performed by expert surgeons in favour of robotic approach (OR 2.34, 95% CI 1.07–5.11, $p = 0.03$), while no statistically significant differences were observed among colorectal (OR 1.35, 95% CI 0.25–7.40, $p = 0.73$) "novice" surgeons.

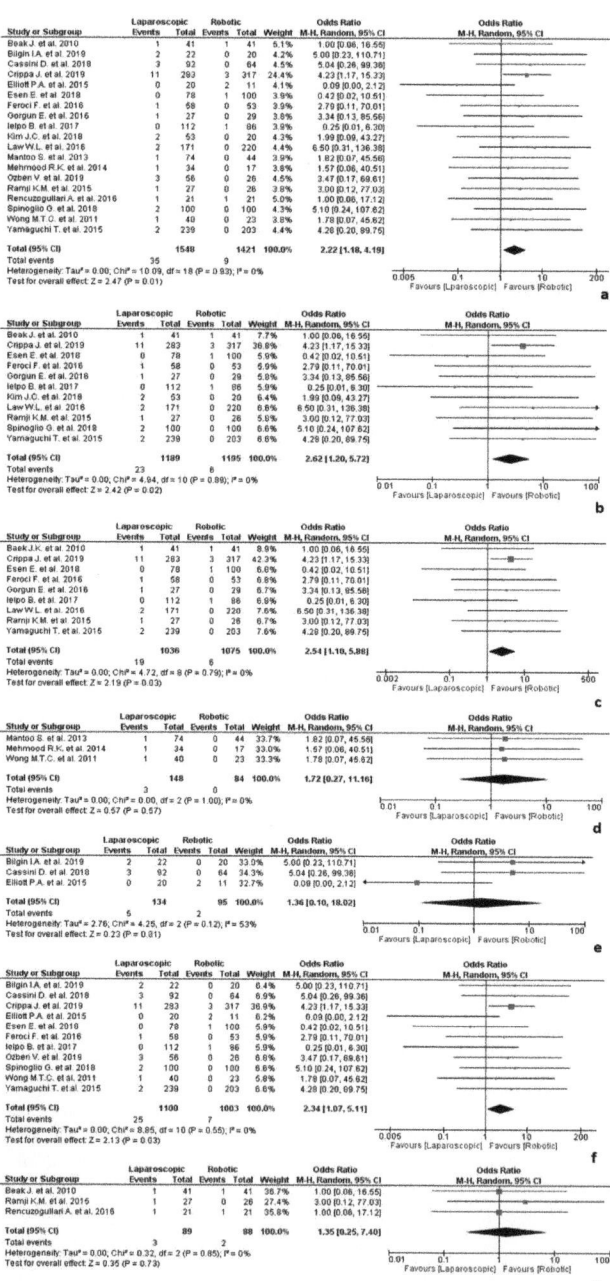

Figure 3. Results of the studies about colorectal surgery: (**a**) conversion due to adhesions in colorectal surgery; (**b**) conversion due to adhesions in colorectal cancer surgery; (**c**) conversion due to adhesions in rectal cancer surgery; (**d**) conversion due to adhesions in colorectal surgery for rectal prolapse/rectocele; (**e**) conversion due to adhesions in colorectal surgery for diverticular disease; (**f**) conversion due to adhesions in colorectal surgery performed by expert surgeons; (**g**) conversion due to adhesions in colorectal surgery performed by "early" surgeons.

3.5.2. Oesophagogastric Surgery

The results of the studies about oesophagogastric surgery are shown in Figure 4. Ten studies addressed oesophagogastric surgery [25,27,29,31,35,49,53,62,63,79], involving 3504 procedures, 2254 of which were laparoscopic and 1250 robotic. Of the included studies, five were about gastric cancer [27,49,62,63,79], four about morbid obesity [29,31,35,53] (two about Roux-en-Y gastric bypass [31,35], one about sleeve gastrectomy [29] and one about different surgical procedures for bariatric revisional surgery [53]) and one on Nissen fundoplication for reflux disease [25]. No statistically significant differences were found between the two groups in terms of conversion rate related to adhesions (OR 1.45, 95% CI 0.58–3.64, $p = 0.43$), with no heterogeneity among the included studies ($I^2 = 0\%$, $p = 0.47$).

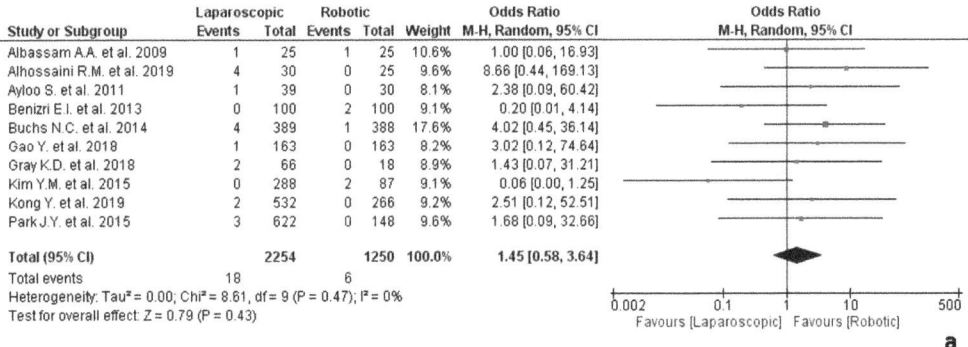

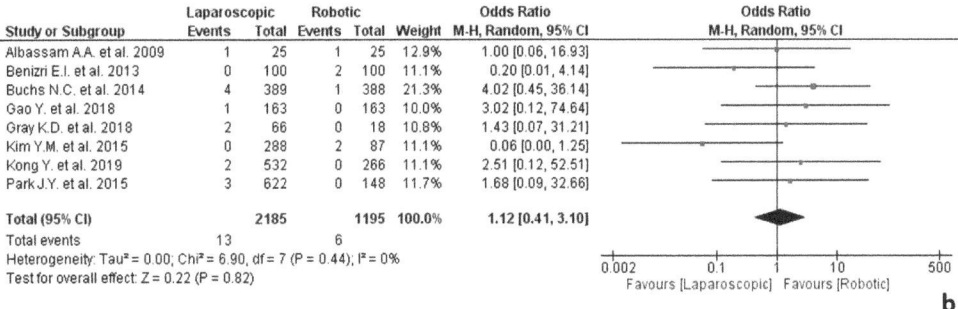

Figure 4. Results of the studies about oesophagogastric surgery: (**a**) conversion due to adhesions in oesophago-gastric surgery; (**b**) conversion due to adhesions in oesophagogastric surgery performed by expert surgeons.

Surgeons' expertise was reported by eight studies [25,31,35,49,53,62,63,79], that classified surgeons as experts. The other two studies did not report on these data [27,29]. The meta-analysis about surgeons' expertise showed that no statistically significant differences were found among the expert surgeon between robotic and laparoscopic conversion rate (OR 1.12, 95% CI 0.41–3.10, $p = 0.82$), with no heterogeneity among the studies ($I^2 = 0\%$, $p = 0.44$). The analysis about "novice" surgeons was not possible because none of the included studies reported these data.

3.5.3. Gynaecologic Surgery

The results of the studies about gynaecologic surgery are shown in Figure 5. Nineteen studies about gynaecologic surgery were included in the meta-analysis [34,38–40,44,47,50, 51,55,56,58,60,67,68,70,76,82,83,86]. Of the included studies, 18 reported data on hysterectomies performed for benign [50,60] or malignant conditions [34,39,40,44,47,51,55,56,58,67,

68,70,82,83,86] or the combination of malignancy and benign diseases [38] and one about salpingo-oophorectomy due to early ovarian cancer [76]. The included studies involved 3124 procedures, of which 1772 were laparoscopic and 1352 robotic, with no statistically significant difference between the two groups (OR 1.36, 95% CI 0.82–2.25, $p = 0.24$) in terms of conversion rate related to adhesions and no heterogeneity among the included studies ($I^2 = 0\%$, $p = 0.73$).

Fourteen studies classified the surgeons as "experts" [40,44,47,50,51,55,56,58,60,67,68,70,82,86], two as "novice" [34,83] and four did not report on these data [38,39,50,76]. No significant difference in terms of conversion rate related to adhesions was found between the two groups in the procedures performed by both expert or novice surgeons (OR 1.52, 95% CI 0.87–2.65, $p = 0.14$ and OR 1.18, 95% CI 0.12–11.43, $p = 0.89$), with no heterogeneity among the studies ($I^2 = 0\%$, $p = 0.77$ and $I^2 = 0\%$, $p = 0.37$).

3.5.4. Hepatobiliary Surgery

The results of the five hepatobiliary surgery studies are shown in Figure 6 [42,48,73,85,89]. Of the included studies, three [73,85,89] included 511 liver resections, 343 laparoscopic and 168 robotic, and all the studies classified surgeons as experts.

Cuendis-Velazquez A. et al. [41] and Gangemi et al. [48] reported hepaticojejunostomy performed for bile duct injury and cholecystectomy, respectively, so they were excluded from our analysis.

No differences were found in terms of conversion due to adhesions between the two groups (OR 1.41, 95% CI 0.15–13.30, $p = 0.76$), without a significant heterogeneity among the included studies ($I^2 = 41\%$, $p = 0.76$).

3.5.5. Pancreatic Surgery

The results of the studies about pancreatic surgery are shown in Figure 7. Six studies [13,26,36,66,69,75] reporting data about conversion due to adhesions in pancreatic surgery were included in the meta-analysis, involving 558 procedures, 333 laparoscopic and 225 robotic. Of the included studies, four [13,26,36,66] reported data on distal pancreatectomies for pancreatic tumours [13,36,66] or neuroendocrine tumours (pNETs) [26], one about pancreaticoduodenectomies for periampullary neoplasms [69] and one about distal pancreatectomies or pancreatic enucleations for benign and borderline tumours [75]. The analysis showed no statistically significant difference in terms of conversion rate related to adhesions between the two groups (OR 1.03, 95% CI 0.40–2.68, $p = 0.95$), with no heterogeneity among the studies ($I^2 = 0\%$, $p = 0.53$).

Surgeons were classified as "expert" in four studies [26,36,66,69] and as "novice" in one study [13], while one study [75] did not report on these data.

In the case of surgery performed by expert surgeons, the analysis showed no significant differences in terms of conversion due to adhesions between the two groups (OR 0.74, 95% CI 0.25–2.15, $p = 0.58$), with no heterogeneity among the studies ($I^2 = 0\%$, $p = 0.54$).

3.5.6. Urologic Surgery

The results of the studies about urologic surgery are shown in Figure 8. Five studies [28,32,54,88,93] included partial nephrectomies [28,32,54,88] for renal cancer or simple enucleation with single layer renorrhaphy for localized renal tumours [93] were included in the analysis, involving 1087 procedures, 557 laparoscopic and 530 robotic.

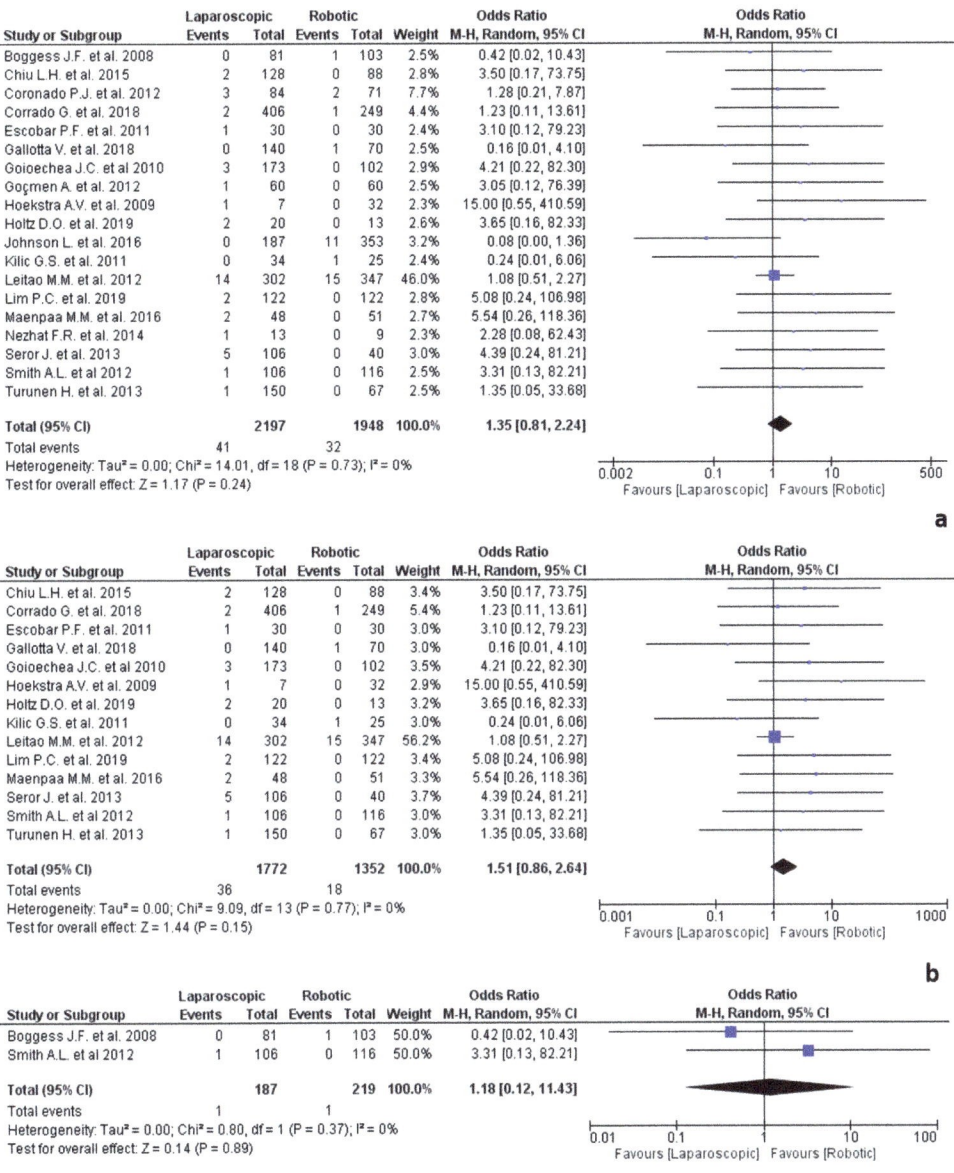

Figure 5. Results of the studies about gynaecologic surgery: (**a**) conversion due to adhesions in gynaecologic surgery; (**b**) conversion due to adhesions in gynaecologic surgery performed by expert surgeons; (**c**) conversion due to adhesions in gynaecologic surgery performed by "early" surgeons.

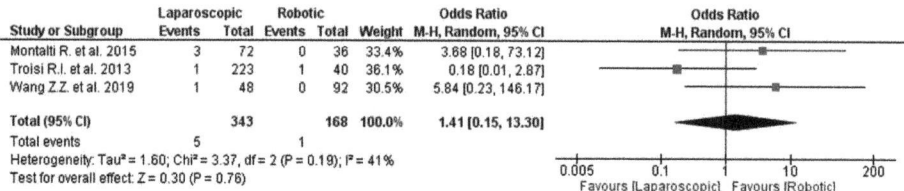

Figure 6. Conversion due to adhesions in hepatobiliary surgery.

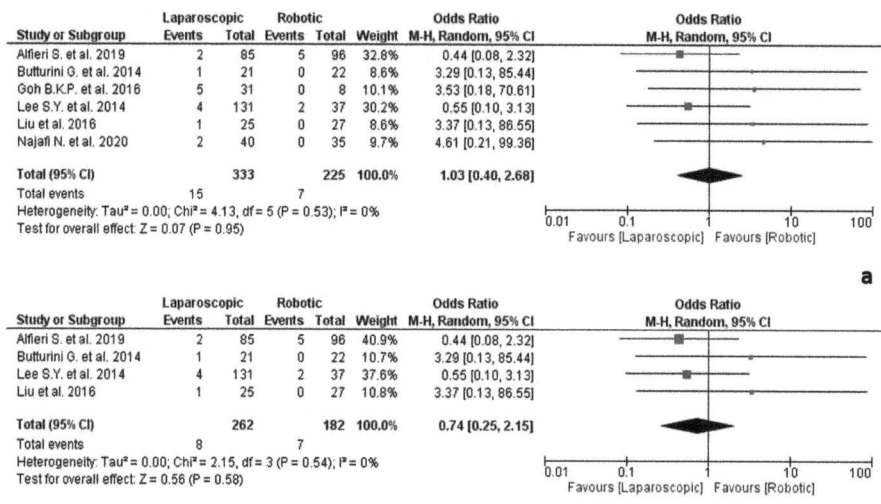

Figure 7. Results of the studies about pancreatic surgery: (**a**) conversion due to adhesions in pancreatic surgery; (**b**) conversion due to adhesions in pancreatic surgery performed by expert surgeons.

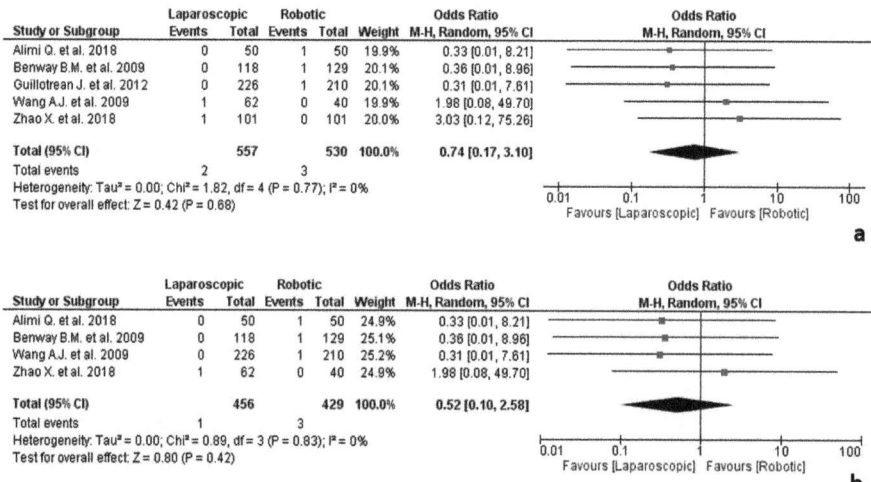

Figure 8. Results of the studies about urologic surgery: (**a**) conversion due to adhesions in urologic surgery; (**b**) conversion due to adhesions in urologic surgery performed by expert surgeons.

No statistical difference was found in the two groups in terms of conversion due to adhesions (OR 0.74, 95% CI 0.17–3.10, $p = 0.68$), with no heterogeneity among the studies ($I^2 = 0\%$, $p = 0.77$).

Four studies [28,32,88,93] classified surgeons as experts, while one study [54] did not report on these data.

The analysis of the studies about expert surgeons showed no significant differences between the two groups (OR 0.92, 95% CI 0.18–4.58, $p = 0.92$), with no heterogeneity among the studies ($I^2 = 0\%$, $p = 0.83$).

3.5.7. Endocrine Surgery

The results of the endocrine surgery studies are shown in Figure 9. Three studies [59,74,77] that addressed adrenalectomies for adrenal cancer were included in the analysis, involving 286 procedures, 155 laparoscopic and 131 robotic.

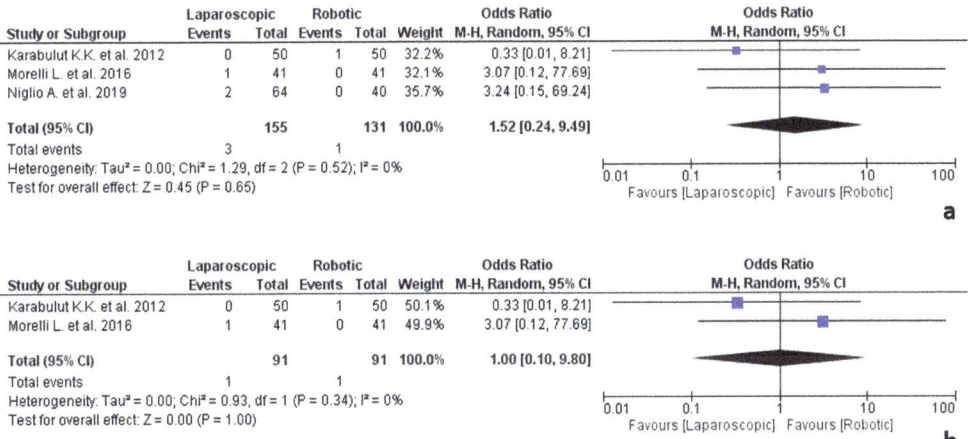

Figure 9. Results of the studies about endocrine surgery: (**a**) conversion due to adhesions in endocrine surgery; (**b**) conversion due to adhesions in endocrine surgery performed by expert surgeons.

No significant difference was found between the two groups in terms of conversion due to adhesions (OR 1.52, 95% CI 0.24–9.49, $p = 0.65$), with no heterogeneity among the studies ($I^2 = 0\%$, $p = 0.52$).

Surgeons' expertise was reported by two studies [59,74], classifying surgeons as experts. One study [77] did not report on these data.

Analysis of the studies about expert surgeons showed no significant differences between the two groups (OR 1.00, 95% CI 0.10–9.80, $p = 1.00$), with no heterogeneity among the studies ($I^2 = 0\%$, $p = 0.34$).

3.5.8. Other Surgical Fields

Khrucharoen et al. [64] described the median arcuate ligament (MAL) release for median arcuate ligament syndrome. Vasilescu et al. [87] reported splenectomy for hereditary spherocytosis. Warren et al. [90] described ventral hernia repair. These were individual studies for each respective surgical field, so it was not possible to perform a meta-analysis.

3.6. Publication Bias

Visual inspection of the funnel plot (Figure S1) showed symmetry, which was confirmed by Egger's linear regression test ($p = 0.12$), indicating no publication bias. In the subgroup analyses, a symmetrical distribution of the studies was observed in all surgical fields except from pancreatic surgery, in which the visual inspection of the funnel plot suggested an asymmetric distribution of studies around the mean and the Egger's test confirmed a significant publication bias ($p = 0.0029$).

4. Discussion

Since its introduction in the early 1990s, laparoscopic surgery has become the gold standard treatment of many benign and malignant conditions [100–103].

The advantages of a minimally invasive approach over an open approach are well proven [6,104], but laparoscopic surgery is technically challenging with a long learning curve.

Robotic surgery was introduced in the early 2000s to overcome these challenges of laparoscopic surgery, but to date, it is considered the gold standard treatment only for radical prostatectomy [6].

The efficacy and the feasibility of the robotic technique have been shown in various procedures across many surgical fields and demonstrate some benefits over the laparoscopic approach [3,4,105–110].

One of the reported benefits of robotic surgery is the lower rate of unplanned conversions to open surgery compared to laparoscopy [8–14,110]. This was, however, not supported by the results of an RCT on rectal cancer surgery and comparing conversions for all causes in robotic and laparoscopic procedures [15]. A cause–effect analysis is required to specifically target conversions related to adhesions and appraise the true impact of the robotic technique in comparison to laparoscopy in order to support the adoption of the robotic technique across all surgical fields.

By pooling together 14,329 patients, 6472 of whom were undergoing robotic surgery and 7857 laparoscopic surgery, we were able to observe that the robotic approach seems to be associated with a lower number of conversions due to abdominal adhesions compared to laparoscopic surgery, with an overall OR of 1.5.

However, to reduce the heterogeneity in the included studies, we performed subgroups analyses to assess if the statistical significance was confirmed in each surgical field.

Our subgroups analysis performed on colorectal patients confirmed the reduced conversion rate due to adhesions in the robotic surgery population, as obtained in the overall analysis, with an OR of 2.22 (95% CI 1.18–4.19, $p = 0.01$). Furthermore, the analysis on different colorectal procedures showed that this significance was present only in colorectal procedures performed in cancer patients (OR 2.62, 95% CI 1.20–5.72, $p = 0.02$), while the colorectal procedures for other diseases did not significantly impact the results (OR 1.72, 95% CI 0.27–11.16, $p = 0.57$ for rectal prolapse and OR 1.36, 95% CI 0.10–18.02, $p = 0.81$ for diverticular disease).

One potential explanation of these findings is that surgery for colorectal cancer often requires access to various quadrants of the abdomen: frequently both the supra- and the infra-mesocolic spaces. Thus, the presence of adhesions in those cases could significantly affect this type of surgical procedure, more than other speciality procedures that are confined to one compartment in the abdomen or the pelvis.

Evaluating the role of surgeons' experience was of paramount importance, being a potential confounding factor considering the study's primary endpoint (conversion to open). We performed this subgroup analysis to ensure that the results of the two techniques were comparable and not affected by different experience levels.

Our results showed that the robotic approach significantly reduced the conversion rate in the case of expert surgeons (OR 1.48, 95% CI 1.03–2.12, $p = 0.03$), while no significant difference was found in the case of procedures performed by "novice" surgeons (OR 1.53, 95% CI 0.44–5.28, $p = 0.50$). This finding was also observed in the overall conversion analysis and in the colorectal surgery subgroup.

In the analysis on the colorectal surgery subgroup performed by expert surgeons, a statistically significant difference favouring robotic surgery was observed (OR 2.34, 95% CI 1.07–5.11, $p = 0.03$), while no statistically significant difference was observed among colorectal (OR 1.35, 95% CI 0.25–7.40, $p = 0.73$) "novice" surgeons. One possible explanation of these results is that the benefits of the robotic approach in colorectal surgery are maximised and become evident only after completing the learning curve.

However, the criteria to define the expertise remains heterogeneous. In fact, only five studies reported the number of procedures [45,46,61,65,84] performed by the surgeons, and none of the studies provided an exact definition of the various steps of the surgical procedure. We attempted to apply rigorous criteria to evaluate the quality of the techniques, but none of the studies reported on surgeons' credentialing, standardisation of techniques and objective evaluation and monitoring of surgeons' skills. Nevertheless, the pooled data in this study highlight the importance of optimal training in robotic surgery in order to achieve the maximum benefits for the patients.

Our study has several strengths. To date, this is the first meta-analysis on the risk of conversion due to intraabdominal adhesions comparing robotic and laparoscopic surgery. In this setting, clinical decisions of adopting one technique over the other could be supported by our meta-analysis, which comprises a large number of studies and cases and therefore enhances the external validity and generalizability.

Based on these results, we could encourage the use of robotic surgery in patients with known or suspected abdominal adhesions and due to undergo a colorectal cancer resection.

However, several limitations should also be acknowledged. By only including studies published in English with full text, a language bias could not be excluded. Results from retrospective studies inevitably contained potential selection bias, confounding bias and missing data bias.

We could not fully adjust for confounding factors, including the causes and the extent and severity of the adhesions. Additionally, in the included studies, the definition of expertise is heterogeneous, with an increased risk of surgeons-dependent performance bias.

Further efforts are required to implement a quality assurance framework when reporting on advanced surgical skills [21].

No ad hoc studies were currently available specifically addressing the role of robotic versus laparoscopic surgery determining conversion related to adhesions.

Additionally, the definition of conversion to open was not adequately standardised; in fact, only nine studies provide this information. [13,35,41,43,45,46,50,78,84] and an optimal information prevalence of conversions for adhesions cannot be obtained.

5. Conclusions

Limitations notwithstanding, this state-of-the-art review provides a lens through which to scrutinise and appraise the currently available evidence on abdominal robotic and laparoscopic surgery with a focus on conversion rates due to intraabdominal adhesions.

Our study should not be interpreted as an arbitrary conclusion that any planned colorectal intervention with certain or presumed adhesions should be treated by a robotic approach. Instead, our findings should support surgeons in the process of selecting the optimal technique and highlight the potential advantages of the robotic approach when performing surgery with a high risk of necessitating complex adhesiolysis.

Supplementary Materials: The following supporting information can be downloaded at: https://www.mdpi.com/article/10.3390/jpm12020307/s1. Figure S1: Forest plot analysis of the included studies.

Author Contributions: M.M. (Marco Milone), conceptualisation of the study and supervision; M.M. (Michele Manigrasso), P.A., A.D. and S.V., data curation and investigation; M.M. (Michele Manigrasso) and M.C.G., formal analysis; M.M. (Michele Manigrasso), S.V., G.R., M.C.G., R.I.T. and G.D.D.P., drafting of the article; U.E., M.M. (Marco Milone), R.I.T., G.D.D.P. and N.K.F., review and editing of the article; M.M. (Marco Milone), M.M. (Michele Manigrasso), P.A., A.D., U.E., M.C.G., G.R., S.V., R.I.T., G.D.D.P. and N.K.F., final approval. All authors have read and agreed to the published version of the manuscript.

Funding: This research received no external funding.

Institutional Review Board Statement: The study was conducted according to the guidelines of the Declaration of Helsinki. Ethical review and approval were not required for a systematic review and meta-analysis.

Informed Consent Statement: Informed consent was obtained from all subjects involved in the study.

Data Availability Statement: The data presented in this study are available on request from the corresponding author.

Conflicts of Interest: The authors declare no conflict of interest.

References

1. Milone, M.; Manigrasso, M.; Vertaldi, S.; Velotti, N.; Aprea, G.; Maione, F.; Gennarelli, N.; De Simone, G.; De Conno, B.; Pesce, M.; et al. Robotic versus laparoscopic approach to treat symptomatic achalasia: Systematic review with meta-analysis. *Dis. Esophagus* **2019**, *32*, 1–8. [CrossRef] [PubMed]
2. Chen, K.; Pan, Y.; Zhang, B.; Maher, H.; Wang, X.F.; Cai, X.J. Robotic versus laparoscopic Gastrectomy for gastric cancer: A systematic review and updated meta-analysis. *BMC Surg.* **2017**, *17*, 93. [CrossRef] [PubMed]
3. Gavriilidis, P.; Wheeler, J.; Spinelli, A.; de'Angelis, N.; Simopoulos, C.; Di Saverio, S. Robotic vs laparoscopic total mesorectal excision for rectal cancers: Has a paradigm change occurred? A systematic review by updated meta-analysis. *Colorectal Dis.* **2020**, *22*, 1506–1517. [CrossRef] [PubMed]
4. Solaini, L.; Bazzocchi, F.; Cavaliere, D.; Avanzolini, A.; Cucchetti, A.; Ercolani, G. Robotic versus laparoscopic right colectomy: An updated systematic review and meta-analysis. *Surg. Endosc.* **2017**, *32*, 1104–1110. [CrossRef]
5. Milone, M.; Manigrasso, M.; Velotti, N.; Torino, S.; Vozza, A.; Sarnelli, G.; Aprea, G.; Maione, F.; Gennarelli, N.; Musella, M.; et al. Completeness of total mesorectum excision of laparoscopic versus robotic surgery: A review with a meta-analysis. *Int. J. Colorectal Dis.* **2019**, *34*, 983–991. [CrossRef]
6. Ng, A.T.; Tam, P.C. Current status of robot-assisted surgery. *Hong Kong Med. J.* **2014**, *20*, 241–250. [CrossRef]
7. Ceccarelli, G.; Andolfi, E.; Biancafarina, A.; Rocca, A.; Amato, M.; Milone, M.; Scricciolo, M.; Frezza, B.; Miranda, E.; De Prizio, M.; et al. Robot-assisted surgery in elderly and very elderly population: Our experience in oncologic and general surgery with literature review. *Aging Clin. Exp. Res.* **2017**, *29* (Suppl. 1), 55–63. [CrossRef]
8. Park, D.A.; Lee, D.H.; Kim, S.W.; Lee, S.H. Comparative safety and effectiveness of robot-assisted laparoscopic hysterectomy versus conventional laparoscopy and laparotomy for endometrial cancer: A systematic review and meta-analysis. *Eur. J. Surg. Oncol.* **2016**, *42*, 1303–1314. [CrossRef]
9. Huang, Y.J.; Kang, Y.N.; Huang, Y.M.; Wu, A.T.; Wang, W.; Wei, P.L. Effects of laparoscopic vs robotic-assisted mesorectal excision for rectal cancer: An update systematic review and meta-analysis of randomized controlled trials. *Asian J. Surg.* **2019**, *42*, 657–666. [CrossRef]
10. Nota, C.L.; Rinkes, I.H.B.; Molenaar, I.Q.; van Santvoort, H.C.; Fong, Y.; Hagendoorn, J. Robot-assisted laparoscopic liver resection: A systematic review and pooled analysis of minor and major hepatectomies. *HPB* **2016**, *18*, 113–120. [CrossRef]
11. Albright, B.B.; Witte, T.; Tofte, A.N.; Chou, J.; Black, J.D.; Desai, V.B.; Erekson, E.A. Robotic versus laparoscopic hysterectomy for benign disease: A systematic review and meta-analysis of randomized trials. *J. Minim. Invasive Gynecol.* **2016**, *23*, 18–27. [CrossRef] [PubMed]
12. Ind, T.; Laios, A.; Hacking, M.; Nobbenhuis, M. A comparison of operative outcomes between standard and robotic laparoscopic surgery for endometrial cancer: A systematic review and meta-analysis. *Int. J. Med Robot. Comput. Assist. Surg.* **2017**, *13*, e1851. [CrossRef] [PubMed]
13. Goh, B.K.; Chan, C.Y.; Soh, H.L.; Lee, S.Y.; Cheow, P.C.; Chow, P.K.; Ooi, L.L.; Chung, A.Y. A comparison between robotic-assisted laparoscopic distal pancreatectomy versus laparoscopic distal pancreatectomy. *Int. J. Med. Robot.* **2017**, *13*, e1733. [CrossRef] [PubMed]
14. Qu, L.; Zhiming, Z.; Xianglong, T.; Yuanxing, G.; Yong, X.; Rong, L.; Yee, L.W. Short- and mid-term outcomes of robotic versus laparoscopic distal pancreatosplenectomy for pancreatic ductal adenocarcinoma: A retrospective propensity score-matched study. *Int. J. Surg.* **2018**, *55*, 81–86. [CrossRef] [PubMed]
15. Jayne, D.; Pigazzi, A.; Marshall, H.; Croft, J.; Corrigan, N.; Copeland, J.; Quirke, P.; West, N.; Rautio, T.; Thomassen, N.; et al. Effect of robotic-assisted vs conventional laparoscopic surgery on risk of conversion to open laparotomy among patients undergoing resection for rectal cancer: The ROLARR randomized clinical trial. *JAMA* **2017**, *318*, 1569–1580. [CrossRef]
16. Bhama, A.R.; Wafa, A.M.; Ferraro, J.; Collins, S.; Mullard, A.J.; Vandewarker, J.F.; Krapohl, G.; Byrn, J.C.; Cleary, R.K. Comparison of risk factors for unplanned conversion from laparoscopic and robotic to open colorectal surgery using the Michigan surgical quality collaborative (MSQC) database. *J. Gastrointest. Surg.* **2016**, *20*, 1223–1230. [CrossRef]
17. Jones, N.; Fleming, N.D.; Nick, A.M.; Munsell, M.F.; Rallapalli, V.; Westin, S.N.; Meyer, L.A.; Schmeler, K.M.; Ramirez, P.T.; Soliman, P.T. Conversion from robotic surgery to laparotomy: A case-control study evaluating risk factors for conversion. *Gynecol. Oncol.* **2014**, *134*, 238–242. [CrossRef]
18. Unger, C.A.; Lachiewicz, M.P.; Ridgeway, B. Risk factors for robotic gynecologic procedures requiring conversion to other surgical procedures. *Int. J. Gynaecol. Obstet.* **2016**, *135*, 299–303. [CrossRef]

19. Page, M.J.; McKenzie, J.E.; Bossuyt, P.M.; Boutron, I.; Hoffmann, T.C.; Mulrow, C.D.; Shamseer, L.; Tetzlaff, J.M.; Akl, E.A.; Brennan, S.E.; et al. The PRISMA 2020 statement: An updated guideline for reporting systematic reviews. *BMJ* 2021, *372*, n71. [CrossRef]
20. Stroup, D.F.; Berlin, J.A.; Morton, S.C.; Olkin, I.; Williamson, G.D.; Rennie, D.; Moher, D.; Becker, B.J.; Sipe, T.A.; Thacker, S.B. Meta-analysis of observational studies in epidemiology: A proposal for reporting. Meta-analysis of observational studies in epidemiology (MOOSE) group. *JAMA* 2000, *283*, 2008–2012. [CrossRef]
21. Francis, N.K.; Curtis, N.J.; Crilly, L.; Noble, E.; Dyke, T.; Hipkiss, R.; Dalton, R.; Allison, A.; Salib, E.; Ockrim, J. Does the number of operating specialists influence the conversion rate and outcomes after laparoscopic colorectal cancer surgery? *Surg. Endosc.* 2018, *32*, 3652–3658. [CrossRef] [PubMed]
22. Foster, J.D.; Mackenzie, H.; Nelson, H.; Hanna, G.B.; Francis, N.K. Methods of quality assurance in multicenter trials in laparoscopic colorectal surgery: A systematic review. *Ann. Surg.* 2014, *260*, 220–229. [CrossRef] [PubMed]
23. Wells, G.A.; Shea, B.; O'Connell, D.; Peterson, J.; Welch, V.; Losos, M.; Tugwell, P.; Ottawa Hospital Research Institute. The Newcastle-Ottawa Scale (NOS) for Assessing the Quality of Nonrandomized Studies in Meta-Analyses. Available online: http://www.ohri.ca/programs/clinical_epidemiology/oxford.html (accessed on 1 December 2021).
24. Higgins, J.P.; Altman, D.G.; Gøtzsche, P.C.; Jüni, P.; Moher, D.; Oxman, A.D.; Savović, J.; Schulz, K.F.; Weeks, L.; Sterne, J.A.; et al. The Cochrane collaboration's tool for assessing risk of bias in randomised trials. *BMJ* 2011, *343*, d5928. [CrossRef] [PubMed]
25. Albassam, A.A.; Mallick, M.S.; Gado, A.; Shoukry, M. Nissen fundoplication, robotic-assisted versus laparoscopic procedure: A comparative study in children. *Eur. J. Pediatr. Surg.* 2009, *19*, 316–319. [CrossRef]
26. Alfieri, S.; Butturini, G.; Boggi, U.; Pietrabissa, A.; Morelli, L.; Vistoli, F.; Damoli, I.; Peri, A.; Fiorillo, C.; The Italian Robotic pNET Group; et al. Short-term and long-term outcomes after robot-assisted versus laparoscopic distal pancreatectomy for pancreatic neuroendocrine tumors (pNETs): A multicenter comparative study. *Langenbeck's Arch. Surg.* 2019, *404*, 459–468. [CrossRef]
27. Alhossaini, R.M.; Altamran, A.A.; Cho, M.; Roh, C.; Seo, W.J.; Choi, S.; Son, T.; Kim, H.-I.; Hyung, W.J. Lower rate of conversion using robotic-assisted surgery compared to laparoscopy in completion total gastrectomy for remnant gastric cancer. *Surg. Endosc.* 2020, *34*, 847–852. [CrossRef]
28. Alimi, Q.; Peyronnet, B.; Sebe, P.; Cote, J.-F.; Kammerer-Jacquet, S.-F.; Khene, Z.-E.; Pradere, B.; Mathieu, R.; Verhoest, G.; Guillonneau, B.; et al. Comparison of short-term functional, oncological, and perioperative outcomes between laparoscopic and robotic partial nephrectomy beyond the learning curve. *J. Laparoendosc. Adv. Surg. Tech.* 2018, *28*, 1047–1052. [CrossRef]
29. Ayloo, S.; Buchs, N.C.; Addeo, P.; Bianco, F.M.; Giulianotti, P.C. Robot-assisted sleeve gastrectomy for super-morbidly obese patients. *J. Laparoendosc. Adv. Surg. Tech.* 2011, *21*, 295–299. [CrossRef]
30. Baek, J.H.; Pastor, C.; Pigazzi, A. Robotic and laparoscopic total mesorectal excision for rectal cancer: A case-matched study. *Surg. Endosc.* 2011, *25*, 521–525. [CrossRef]
31. Benizri, E.I.; Renaud, M.; Reibel, N.; Germain, A.; Ziegler, O.; Zarnegar, R.; Ayav, A.; Bresler, L.; Brunaud, L. Perioperative outcomes after totally robotic gastric bypass: A prospective nonrandomized controlled study. *Am. J. Surg.* 2013, *206*, 145–151. [CrossRef]
32. Benway, B.M.; Bhayani, S.B.; Rogers, C.G.; Dulabon, L.M.; Patel, M.N.; Lipkin, M.; Wang, A.J.; Stifelman, M.D. Robot assisted partial nephrectomy versus laparoscopic partial nephrectomy for renal tumors: A multi-institutional analysis of perioperative outcomes. *J. Urol.* 2009, *182*, 866–872. [CrossRef] [PubMed]
33. Bilgin, I.A.; Bas, M.; Benlice, C.; Esen, E.; Ozben, V.; Aytac, E.; Baca, B.; Hamzaoglu, I.; Karahasanoglu, T. Totally laparoscopic and totally robotic surgery in patients with left-sided colonic diverticulitis. *Int. J. Med. Robot.* 2020, *16*, e2068. [CrossRef] [PubMed]
34. Boggess, J.F.; Gehrig, P.A.; Cantrell, L.; Shafer, A.; Ridgway, M.; Skinner, E.N.; Fowler, W.C. A comparative study of 3 surgical methods for hysterectomy with staging for endometrial cancer: Robotic assistance, laparoscopy, laparotomy. *Am. J. Obstet. Gynecol.* 2008, *199*, 360.e1–360.e9. [CrossRef] [PubMed]
35. Buchs, N.C.; Morel, P.; Azagury, D.; Jung, M.K.; Chassot, G.; Huber, O.; Hagen, M.E.; Pugin, F.L. Laparoscopic versus robotic Roux-en-Y gastric bypass: Lessons and long-term follow-up learned from a large prospective monocentric study. *Obes. Surg.* 2014, *24*, 2031–2039. [CrossRef] [PubMed]
36. Butturini, G.; Damoli, I.; Crepaz, L.; Malleo, G.; Marchegiani, G.; Daskalaki, D.; Esposito, A.; Cingarlini, S.; Salvia, R.; Bassi, C. A prospective non-randomised single-center study comparing laparoscopic and robotic distal pancreatectomy. *Surg. Endosc.* 2015, *29*, 3163–3170. [CrossRef] [PubMed]
37. Cassini, D.; Depalma, N.; Grieco, M.; Cirocchi, R.; Manoochehri, F.; Baldazzi, G. Robotic pelvic dissection as surgical treatment of complicated diverticulitis in elective settings: A comparative study with fully laparoscopic procedure. *Surg. Endosc.* 2019, *33*, 2583–2590. [CrossRef] [PubMed]
38. Chiu, L.H.; Chen, C.H.; Tu, P.C.; Chang, C.W.; Yen, Y.K.; Liu, W.M. Comparison of robotic surgery and laparoscopy to perform total hysterectomy with pelvic adhesions or large uterus. *J. Minim. Access Surg.* 2015, *11*, 87–93.
39. Coronado, P.J.; Herraiz, M.A.; Magrina, J.F.; Fasero, M.; Vidart, J.A. Comparison of perioperative outcomes and cost of robotic-assisted laparoscopy, laparoscopy and laparotomy for endometrial cancer. *Eur. J. Obstet. Gynecol. Reprod. Biol.* 2012, *165*, 289–294. [CrossRef]
40. Corrado, G.; Vizza, E.; Cela, V.; Mereu, L.; Bogliolo, S.; Legge, F.; Ciccarone, F.; Mancini, E.; Gallotta, V.; Baiocco, E.; et al. Laparoscopic versus robotic hysterectomy in obese and extremely obese patients with endometrial cancer: A multi-institutional analysis. *Eur. J. Surg. Oncol.* 2018, *44*, 1935–1941. [CrossRef]

41. Crippa, J.; Grass, F.; Achilli, P.; Mathis, K.L.; Kelley, S.R.; Merchea, A.; Colibaseanu, D.T.; Larson, D.W. Risk factors for conversion in laparoscopic and robotic rectal cancer surgery. *Br. J. Surg.* **2020**, *107*, 560–566. [CrossRef]
42. Cuendis-Velázquez, A.; Trejo-Ávila, M.; Bada-Yllán, O.; Cárdenas-Lailson, E.; Morales-Chávez, C.; Fernández-Álvarez, L.; Romero-Loera, S.; Rojano-Rodríguez, M.; Valenzuela-Salazar, C.; Moreno-Portillo, M. A new era of bile duct repair: Robotic-assisted versus laparoscopic hepaticojejunostomy. *J. Gastrointest. Surg.* **2019**, *23*, 451–459. [CrossRef] [PubMed]
43. Elliott, P.A.; McLemore, E.C.; Abbass, M.A.; Abbas, M.A. Robotic versus laparoscopic resection for sigmoid diverticulitis with fistula. *J. Robot. Surg.* **2015**, *9*, 137–142. [CrossRef] [PubMed]
44. Escobar, P.F.; Frumovitz, M.; Soliman, P.T.; Frasure, H.E.; Fader, A.N.; Schmeler, K.M.; Ramirez, P.T. Comparison of single-port laparoscopy, standard laparoscopy, and robotic surgery in patients with endometrial cancer. *Ann. Surg. Oncol.* **2012**, *19*, 1583–1588. [CrossRef] [PubMed]
45. Esen, E.; Aytac, E.; Ağcaoğlu, O.; Zenger, S.; Balik, E.; Baca, B.; Hamzaoğlu, I.; Karahasanoğlu, T.; Buğra, D. Totally robotic versus totally laparoscopic surgery for rectal cancer. *Surg. Laparosc. Endosc. Percutaneous Tech.* **2018**, *28*, 245–249. [CrossRef]
46. Feroci, F.; Vannucchi, A.; Bianchi, P.P.; Cantafio, S.; Garzi, A.; Formisano, G.; Scatizzi, M. Total mesorectal excision for mid and low rectal cancer: Laparoscopic vs robotic surgery. *World J. Gastroenterol.* **2016**, *22*, 3602–3610. [CrossRef]
47. Gallotta, V.; Conte, C.; Federico, A.; Vizzielli, G.; Alletti, S.G.; Tortorella, L.; Anchora, L.P.; Cosentino, F.; Chiantera, V.; Fagotti, A.; et al. Robotic versus laparoscopic radical hysterectomy in early cervical cancer: A case matched control study. *Eur. J. Surg. Oncol.* **2018**, *44*, 754–759. [CrossRef]
48. Gangemi, A.; Danilkowicz, R.; Elli, F.E.; Bianco, F.; Masrur, M.; Giulianotti, P.C. Could ICG-aided robotic cholecystectomy reduce the rate of open conversion reported with laparoscopic approach? A head to head comparison of the largest single institution studies. *J. Robot. Surg.* **2017**, *11*, 77–82. [CrossRef]
49. Gao, Y.; Xi, H.; Qiao, Z.; Li, J.; Zhang, K.; Xie, T.; Shen, W.; Cui, J.; Wei, B.; Chen, L. Comparison of robotic- and laparoscopic-assisted gastrectomy in advanced gastric cancer: Updated short- and long-term results. *Surg. Endosc.* **2019**, *33*, 528–534. [CrossRef]
50. Göçmen, A.; Şanlıkan, F.; Uçar, M.G. Robot-assisted hysterectomy vs total laparoscopic hysterectomy: A comparison of short-term surgical outcomes. *Int. J. Med. Robot.* **2012**, *8*, 453–457. [CrossRef]
51. Cardenas-Goicoechea, J.; Adams, S.; Bhat, S.B.; Randall, T.C. Surgical outcomes of robotic-assisted surgical staging for endometrial cancer are equivalent to traditional laparoscopic staging at a minimally invasive surgical center. *Gynecol. Oncol.* **2010**, *117*, 224–228. [CrossRef]
52. Gorgun, E.; Ozben, V.; Costedio, M.; Stocchi, L.; Kalady, M.; Remzi, F. Robotic versus conventional laparoscopic rectal cancer surgery in obese patients. *Colorectal Dis.* **2016**, *18*, 1063–1071. [CrossRef] [PubMed]
53. Gray, K.D.; Moore, M.D.; Elmously, A.; Bellorin, O.; Zarnegar, R.; Dakin, G.; Pomp, A.; Afaneh, C. Perioperative outcomes of laparoscopic and robotic revisional bariatric surgery in a complex patient population. *Obes. Surg.* **2018**, *28*, 1852–1859. [CrossRef] [PubMed]
54. Guillotreau, J.; Haber, G.-P.; Autorino, R.; Miocinovic, R.; Hillyer, S.; Hernandez, A.; Laydner, H.; Yakoubi, R.; Isac, W.; Long, J.-A.; et al. Robotic partial nephrectomy versus laparoscopic cryoablation for the small renal mass. *Eur. Urol.* **2012**, *61*, 899–904. [CrossRef] [PubMed]
55. Hoekstra, A.V.; Jairam-Thodla, A.; Rademaker, A.; Singh, D.K.; Buttin, B.M.; Lurain, J.R.; Schink, J.C.; Lowe, M.P. The impact of robotics on practice management of endometrial cancer: Transitioning from traditional surgery. *Int. J. Med. Robot.* **2009**, *5*, 392–397. [CrossRef]
56. Holtz, D.O.; Miroshnichenko, G.; Finnegan, M.O.; Chernick, M.; Dunton, C.J. Endometrial cancer surgery costs: Robot vs laparoscopy. *J. Minim. Invasive Gynecol.* **2010**, *17*, 500–503. [CrossRef]
57. Ielpo, B.; Duran, H.; Diaz, E.; Fabra, I.; Caruso, R.; Malavé, L.; Ferri, V.; Nuñez, J.; Ruiz-Ocaña, A.; Jorge, E.; et al. Robotic versus laparoscopic surgery for rectal cancer: A comparative study of clinical outcomes and costs. *Int. J. Colorectal Dis.* **2017**, *32*, 1423–1429. [CrossRef]
58. Johnson, L.; Bunn, W.D.; Nguyen, L.; Rice, J.; Raj, M.; Cunningham, M.J. Clinical comparison of robotic, laparoscopic, and open hysterectomy procedures for endometrial cancer patients. *J. Robot. Surg.* **2017**, *11*, 291–297. [CrossRef]
59. Karabulut, K.; Agcaoglu, O.; Aliyev, S.; Siperstein, A.; Berber, E. Comparison of intraoperative time use and perioperative outcomes for robotic versus laparoscopic adrenalectomy. *Surgery* **2012**, *151*, 537–542. [CrossRef]
60. Kilic, G.S.; Moore, G.; Elbatanony, A.; Radecki, C.; Phelps, J.Y.; Borahay, M.A. Comparison of perioperative outcomes of total laparoscopic and robotically assisted hysterectomy for benign pathology during introduction of a robotic program. *Obstet. Gynecol. Int.* **2011**, *2011*, 683703. [CrossRef]
61. Kim, J.C.; Lee, J.L.; Yoon, Y.S.; Kim, C.W.; Park, I.J.; Lim, S.B. Robotic left colectomy with complete mesocolectomy for splenic flexure and descending colon cancer, compared with a laparoscopic procedure. *Int. J. Med. Robot.* **2018**, *14*, e1918. [CrossRef]
62. Kim, Y.-W.; Reim, D.; Park, J.Y.; Eom, B.W.; Kook, M.-C.; Ryu, K.W.; Yoon, H.M. Role of robot-assisted distal gastrectomy compared to laparoscopy-assisted distal gastrectomy in suprapancreatic nodal dissection for gastric cancer. *Surg. Endosc.* **2016**, *30*, 1547–1552. [CrossRef]
63. Kong, Y.; Cao, S.; Liu, X.; Li, Z.; Wang, L.; Lu, C.; Shen, S.; Zhu, H.; Zhou, Y. Short-term clinical outcomes after laparoscopic and robotic gastrectomy for gastric cancer: A propensity score matching analysis. *J. Gastrointest. Surg.* **2020**, *24*, 531–539. [CrossRef] [PubMed]

64. Khrucharoen, U.; Juo, Y.Y.; Chen, Y.; Jimenez, J.C.; Dutson, E.P. Short- and intermediate-term clinical outcome comparison between laparoscopic and robotic-assisted median arcuate ligament release. *J. Robot. Surg.* **2020**, *14*, 123–129. [CrossRef] [PubMed]
65. Law, W.L.; Foo, D.C.C. Comparison of short-term and oncologic outcomes of robotic and laparoscopic resection for mid- and distal rectal cancer. *Surg. Endosc.* **2017**, *31*, 2798–2807. [CrossRef] [PubMed]
66. Lee, S.Y.; Allen, P.J.; Sadot, E.; D'Angelica, M.I.; DeMatteo, R.P.; Fong, Y.; Jarnagin, W.R.; Kingham, T.P. Distal pancreatectomy: A single institution's experience in open, laparoscopic, and robotic approaches. *J. Am. Coll. Surg.* **2015**, *220*, 18–27. [CrossRef]
67. Leitao, M.M., Jr.; Briscoe, G.; Santos, K.; Winder, A.; Jewell, E.L.; Hoskins, W.J.; Chi, D.S.; Abu-Rustum, N.R.; Sonoda, Y.; Brown, C.L.; et al. Introduction of a computer-based surgical platform in the surgical care of patients with newly diagnosed uterine cancer: Outcomes and impact on approach. *Gynecol. Oncol.* **2012**, *125*, 394–399. [CrossRef]
68. Lim, P.C.; Kang, E.; Park, D.H. A comparative detail analysis of the learning curve and surgical outcome for robotic hysterectomy with lymphadenectomy versus laparoscopic hysterectomy with lymphadenectomy in treatment of endometrial cancer: A case-matched controlled study of the first one hundred twenty two patients. *Gynecol. Oncol.* **2011**, *120*, 413–418.
69. Liu, R.; Zhang, T.; Zhao, Z.M.; Tan, X.L.; Zhao, G.D.; Zhang, X.; Xu, Y. The surgical outcomes of robot-assisted laparoscopic pancreaticoduodenectomy versus laparoscopic pancreaticoduodenectomy for periampullary neoplasms: A comparative study of a single center. *Surg. Endosc.* **2017**, *31*, 2380–2386. [CrossRef]
70. Mäenpää, M.M.; Nieminen, K.; Tomás, E.I.; Laurila, M.; Luukkaala, T.H.; Mäenpää, J.U. Robotic-assisted vs traditional laparoscopic surgery for endometrial cancer: A randomized controlled trial. *Am. J. Obstet. Gynecol.* **2016**, *215*, 588.e1–588.e7. [CrossRef]
71. Mantoo, S.; Podevin, J.; Regenet, N.; Rigaud, J.; Lehur, P.A.; Meurette, G. Is robotic-assisted ventral mesh rectopexy superior to laparoscopic ventral mesh rectopexy in the management of obstructed defaecation? *Colorectal Dis.* **2013**, *15*, e469–e475. [CrossRef]
72. Mehmood, R.K.; Parker, J.; Bhuvimanian, L.; Qasem, E.; Mohammed, A.A.; Zeeshan, M.; Grugel, K.; Carter, P.; Ahmed, S. Short-term outcome of laparoscopic versus robotic ventral mesh rectopexy for full-thickness rectal prolapse. Is robotic superior? *Int. J. Colorectal Dis.* **2014**, *29*, 1113–1118. [CrossRef] [PubMed]
73. Montalti, R.; Scuderi, V.; Patriti, A.; Vivarelli, M.; Troisi, R.I. Robotic versus laparoscopic resections of posterosuperior segments of the liver: A propensity score-matched comparison. *Surg. Endosc.* **2016**, *30*, 1004–1013. [CrossRef] [PubMed]
74. Morelli, L.; Tartaglia, D.; Bronzoni, J.; Palmeri, M.; Guadagni, S.; Gennai, A.; Bianchini, M.; Bastiani, L.; Moglia, A.; Fommei, E.; et al. Robotic assisted versus pure laparoscopic surgery of the adrenal glands: A case-control study comparing surgical techniques. *Langenbeck's Arch. Surg.* **2016**, *401*, 999–1006. [CrossRef] [PubMed]
75. Najafi, N.; Mintziras, I.; Wiese, D.; Albers, M.B.; Maurer, E.; Bartsch, D.K. A retrospective comparison of robotic versus laparoscopic distal resection and enucleation for potentially benign pancreatic neoplasms. *Surg. Today* **2020**, *50*, 872–880. [CrossRef] [PubMed]
76. Nezhat, F.R.; Finger, T.N.; Vetere, P.; Radjabi, A.R.; Vega, M.; Averbuch, L.; Khalil, S.; Altinbas, S.K.; Lax, D. Comparison of perioperative outcomes and complication rates between conventional versus robotic-assisted laparoscopy in the evaluation and management of early, advanced, and recurrent stage ovarian, fallopian tube, and primary peritoneal cancer. *Int. J. Gynecol. Cancer* **2014**, *24*, 600–607. [CrossRef]
77. Niglio, A.; Grasso, M.; Costigliola, L.; Zenone, P.; De Palma, M. Laparoscopic and robot-assisted transperitoneal lateral adrenalectomy: A large clinical series from a single center. *Updates Surg.* **2020**, *72*, 193–198. [CrossRef]
78. Ozben, V.; De Muijnck, C.; Karabork, M.; Ozoran, E.; Zenger, S.; Bilgin, I.A.; Aytac, E.; Baca, B.; Balik, E.; Hamzaoglu, I.; et al. The da Vinci Xi system for robotic total/subtotal colectomy vs. conventional laparoscopy: Short-term outcomes. *Tech. Coloproctol.* **2019**, *23*, 861–868. [CrossRef]
79. Park, J.Y.; Ryu, K.W.; Reim, D.; Eom, B.W.; Yoon, H.M.; Rho, J.Y.; Choi, I.J.; Kim, Y.-W. Robot-assisted gastrectomy for early gastric cancer: Is it beneficial in viscerally obese patients compared to laparoscopic gastrectomy? *World J. Surg.* **2015**, *39*, 1789–1797. [CrossRef]
80. Ramji, K.M.; Cleghorn, M.C.; Josse, J.M.; MacNeill, A.; O'brien, C.; Urbach, D.; Quereshy, F.A. Comparison of clinical and economic outcomes between robotic, laparoscopic, and open rectal cancer surgery: Early experience at a tertiary care center. *Surg. Endosc.* **2016**, *30*, 1337–1343. [CrossRef]
81. Rencuzogullari, A.; Gorgun, E.; Costedio, M.; Aytac, E.; Kessler, H.; Abbas, M.A.; Remzi, F.H. Case-matched comparison of robotic versus laparoscopic proctectomy for inflammatory bowel disease. *Surg. Laparosc. Endosc. Percutaneous Tech.* **2016**, *26*, e37–e40. [CrossRef]
82. Seror, J.; Bats, A.S.; Huchon, C.; Bensaïd, C.; Douay-Hauser, N.; Lécuru, F. Laparoscopy vs robotics in surgical management of endometrial cancer: Comparison of intraoperative and postoperative complications. *J. Minim. Invasive Gynecol.* **2014**, *21*, 120–125. [CrossRef] [PubMed]
83. Smith, A.L.; Krivak, T.C.; Scott, E.M.; Rauh-Hain, J.A.; Sukumvanich, P.; Olawaiye, A.B.; Richard, S.D. Dual-console robotic surgery compared to laparoscopic surgery with respect to surgical outcomes in a gynecologic oncology fellowship program. *Gynecol. Oncol.* **2012**, *126*, 432–436. [CrossRef] [PubMed]
84. Spinoglio, G.; Bianchi, P.P.; Marano, A.; Priora, F.; Lenti, L.M.; Ravazzoni, F.; Petz, W.; Borin, S.; Ribero, D.; Formisano, G.; et al. Robotic versus laparoscopic right colectomy with complete mesocolic excision for the treatment of colon cancer: Perioperative outcomes and 5-year survival in a consecutive series of 202 patients. *Ann. Surg. Oncol.* **2018**, *25*, 3580–3586. [CrossRef]
85. Troisi, R.I.; Patriti, A.; Montalti, R.; Casciola, L. Robot assistance in liver surgery: A real advantage over a fully laparoscopic approach? Results of a comparative bi-institutional analysis. *Int. J. Med. Robot.* **2013**, *9*, 160–166. [CrossRef] [PubMed]

86. Turunen, H.; Pakarinen, P.; Sjöberg, J.; Loukovaara, M. Laparoscopic vs robotic-assisted surgery for endometrial carcinoma in a centre with long laparoscopic experience. *J. Obstet. Gynaecol.* **2013**, *33*, 720–724. [CrossRef]
87. Vasilescu, C.; Stanciulea, O.; Tudor, S. Laparoscopic versus robotic subtotal splenectomy in hereditary spherocytosis. Potential advantages and limits of an expensive approach. *Surg. Endosc.* **2012**, *26*, 2802–2809. [CrossRef]
88. Wang, A.J.; Bhayani, S.B. Robotic partial nephrectomy versus laparoscopic partial nephrectomy for renal cell carcinoma: Single-surgeon analysis of >100 consecutive procedures. *Urology* **2009**, *73*, 306–310. [CrossRef]
89. Wang, Z.Z.; Tang, W.B.; Hu, M.G.; Zhao, Z.M.; Zhao, G.D.; Li, C.G.; Tan, X.L.; Zhang, X.; Lau, W.Y.; Liu, R. Robotic vs laparoscopic hemihepatectomy: A comparative study from a single center. *J. Surg. Oncol.* **2019**, *120*, 646–653. [CrossRef]
90. Warren, J.A.; Cobb, W.S.; Ewing, J.A.; Carbonell, A.M. Standard laparoscopic versus robotic retromuscular ventral hernia repair. *Surg. Endosc.* **2017**, *31*, 324–332. [CrossRef]
91. Wong, M.T.; Meurette, G.; Rigaud, J.; Regenet, N.; Lehur, P.A. Robotic versus laparoscopic rectopexy for complex rectocele: A prospective comparison of short-term outcomes. *Dis. Colon. Rectum.* **2011**, *54*, 342–346. [CrossRef]
92. Yamaguchi, T.; Kinugasa, Y.; Shiomi, A.; Tomioka, H.; Kagawa, H.; Yamakawa, Y. Robotic-assisted vs. conventional laparoscopic surgery for rectal cancer: Short-term outcomes at a single center. *Surg. Today* **2016**, *46*, 957–962. [CrossRef] [PubMed]
93. Zhao, X.; Lu, Q.; Campi, R.; Ji, C.; Guo, S.; Liu, G.; Zhang, S.; Li, X.; Gan, W.; Minervini, A.; et al. Endoscopic robot-assisted simple enucleation versus laparoscopic simple enucleation with single-layer renorrhaphy in localized renal tumors: A propensity score-matched analysis from a high-volume centre. *Urology* **2018**, *121*, 97–103. [CrossRef] [PubMed]
94. Friedrich, J.O.; Adhikari, N.K.; Beyene, J. Inclusion of zero total event trials in meta-analyses maintains analytic consistency and incorporates all available data. *BMC Med. Res. Methodol.* **2007**, *7*, 5. [CrossRef] [PubMed]
95. Furukawa, T.A.; Barbui, C.; Cipriani, A.; Brambilla, P.; Watanabe, N. Imputing missing standard deviations in meta-analyses can provide accurate results. *J. Clin. Epidemiol.* **2006**, *59*, 7–10. [CrossRef] [PubMed]
96. DerSimonian, R.; Laird, N. Meta-analysis in clinical trials. *Control Clin. Trials* **1986**, *7*, 177–188. [CrossRef]
97. Higgins, J.P.; Thompson, S.G.; Deeks, J.J.; Altman, D.G. Measuring inconsistency in meta-analyses. *BMJ* **2003**, *327*, 557–560. [CrossRef]
98. Thompson, S.G.; Sharp, S.J. Explaining heterogeneity in meta-analysis: A comparison of methods. *Stat. Med.* **1999**, *18*, 2693–2708. [CrossRef]
99. Egger, M.; Davey Smith, G.; Schneider, M.; Minder, C. Bias in meta-analysis detected by a simple, graphical test. *BMJ* **1997**, *315*, 629–634. [CrossRef]
100. Milone, M.; Manigrasso, M.; Burati, M.; Elmore, U.; Gennarelli, N.; Giglio, M.C.; Maione, F.; Musella, M.; Conte, V.L.; Milone, F.; et al. Intracorporeal versus extracorporeal anastomosis after laparoscopic gastrectomy for gastric cancer. A systematic review with meta-analysis. *J. Visc. Surg.* **2019**, *156*, 305–318. [CrossRef]
101. Milone, M.; Vignali, A.; Milone, F.; Pignata, G.; Elmore, U.; Musella, M.; De Placido, G.; Mollo, A.; Fernandez, L.M.S.; Coretti, G.; et al. Colorectal resection in deep pelvic endometriosis: Surgical technique and post-operative complications. *World J. Gastroenterol.* **2015**, *21*, 13345–13351. [CrossRef]
102. Milone, M.; Manigrasso, M.; Burati, M.; Velotti, N.; Milone, F.; De Palma, G.D. Surgical resection for rectal cancer. Is laparoscopic surgery as successful as open approach? A systematic review with meta-analysis. *PLoS ONE* **2018**, *13*, e0204887. [CrossRef]
103. Milone, M.; Elmore, U.; Vignali, A.; Gennarelli, N.; Manigrasso, M.; Burati, M.; Milone, F.; De Palma, G.D.; DelRio, P.; Rosati, R. Recovery after intracorporeal anastomosis in laparoscopic right hemicolectomy: A systematic review and meta-analysis. *Langenbeck's Arch. Surg.* **2018**, *403*, 1–10. [CrossRef] [PubMed]
104. Sato, K.; Inomata, M.; Kakisako, K.; Shiraishi, N.; Adachi, Y.; Kitano, S. Surgical technique influences bowel function after low anterior resection and sigmoid colectomy. *Hepatogastroenterology* **2003**, *50*, 1381–1384. [PubMed]
105. Papanikolaou, I.G. Robotic surgery for colorectal cancer: Systematic review of the literature. *Surg. Laparosc. Endosc. Percutaneous Tech.* **2014**, *24*, 478–483. [CrossRef] [PubMed]
106. Wong, D.J.; Wong, M.J.; Choi, G.H.; Wu, Y.M.; Lai, P.B.; Goh, B.K.P. Systematic review and meta-analysis of robotic versus open hepatectomy. *ANZ J. Surg.* **2019**, *89*, 165–170. [CrossRef]
107. Advincula, A.P.; Song, A. The role of robotic surgery in gynecology. *Curr. Opin. Obstet. Gynecol.* **2007**, *19*, 331–336. [CrossRef]
108. Boylu, U.; Oommen, M.; Raynor, M.; Lee, B.R.; Thomas, R. Robot-assisted laparoscopic radical prostatectomy in patients with previous abdominal surgery: A novel laparoscopic adhesiolysis technique. *J. Endourol.* **2010**, *24*, 229–232. [CrossRef]
109. Petros, F.G.; Patel, M.N.; Kheterpal, E.; Siddiqui, S.; Ross, J.; Bhandari, A.; Diaz, M.; Menon, M.; Rogers, C.G. Robotic partial nephrectomy in the setting of prior abdominal surgery. *BJU Int.* **2011**, *108*, 413–419. [CrossRef]
110. Gkegkes, I.D.; Mamais, I.A.; Iavazzo, C. Robotics in general surgery: A systematic cost assessment. *J. Minim. Access Surg.* **2017**, *13*, 243–255. [CrossRef]

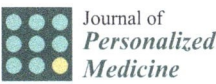

Journal of
Personalized
Medicine

Review

Update on Robotic Total Mesorectal Excision for Rectal Cancer

Simona Giuratrabocchetta [1,*], Giampaolo Formisano [1], Adelona Salaj [1], Enrico Opocher [2], Luca Ferraro [1], Francesco Toti [1] and Paolo Pietro Bianchi [1]

1. Division of General and Robotic Surgery, Dipartimento di Scienze della Salute, Università di Milano, ASST Santi Paolo e Carlo, 20142 Milano, Italy; giampaolo.formisano@asst-santipaolocarlo.it (G.F.); adelona.salaj@asst-santipaolocarlo.it (A.S.); luca.ferraro@asst-santipaolocarlo.it (L.F.); francesco.toti@asst-santipaolocarlo.it (F.T.); PaoloPietro.Bianchi@unimi.it (P.P.B.)
2. Division of General and HPB Surgery, Dipartimento di Scienze della Salute, Università di Milano, ASST Santi Paolo e Carlo, 20142 Milano, Italy; enrico.opocher@unimi.it
* Correspondence: simona.giuratrabocchetta@asst-santipaolocarlo.it or simonagiura@live.it

Abstract: The minimally invasive treatment of rectal cancer with Total Mesorectal Excision is a complex and challenging procedure due to technical and anatomical issues which could impair postoperative, oncological and functional outcomes, especially in a defined subgroup of patients. The results from recent randomized controlled trials comparing laparoscopic versus open surgery are still conflicting and trans-anal bottom-up approaches have recently been developed. Robotic surgery represents the latest consistent innovation in the field of minimally invasive surgery that may potentially overcome the technical limitations of conventional laparoscopy thanks to an enhanced dexterity, especially in deep narrow operative fields such as the pelvis. Results from population-based multicenter studies have shown the potential advantages of robotic surgery when compared to its laparoscopic counterpart in terms of reduced conversions, complication rates and length of stay. Costs, often advocated as one of the main drawbacks of robotic surgery, should be thoroughly evaluated including both the direct and indirect costs, with the latter having the potential of counterbalancing the excess of expenditure directly related to the purchase and maintenance of robotic equipment. Further prospectively maintained or randomized data are still required to better delineate the advantages of the robotic platform, especially in the subset of most complex and technically challenging patients from both an anatomical and oncological standpoint.

Keywords: robotic surgery; rectal cancer; total mesorectal excision; robotic low anterior resection

Citation: Giuratrabocchetta, S.; Formisano, G.; Salaj, A.; Opocher, E.; Ferraro, L.; Toti, F.; Bianchi, P.P. Update on Robotic Total Mesorectal Excision for Rectal Cancer. *J. Pers. Med.* **2021**, *11*, 900. https://doi.org/10.3390/jpm11090900

Academic Editor: Marco Milone

Received: 10 July 2021
Accepted: 6 September 2021
Published: 8 September 2021

Publisher's Note: MDPI stays neutral with regard to jurisdictional claims in published maps and institutional affiliations.

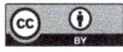

Copyright: © 2021 by the authors. Licensee MDPI, Basel, Switzerland. This article is an open access article distributed under the terms and conditions of the Creative Commons Attribution (CC BY) license (https://creativecommons.org/licenses/by/4.0/).

1. Introduction

Surgery for rectal cancer remains challenging due to its critical anatomical, oncological and technical issues. Total Mesorectal Excision (TME), first described by Heald in 1982 [1], is the gold standard for the treatment of rectal cancer; a precise dissection along an avascular embryologically based plane is performed in order to achieve good oncological and functional results. However, a debate still exists on the best surgical approach for TME, especially in challenging patients (i.e., low-lying tumors, high BMI, prior chemoradiotherapy and unfavorable pelvimetry) and the trans-anal approach has been described over the last years to overcome the limitations of conventional laparoscopy [2–5].

Laparoscopic surgery for colon cancer can achieve comparable oncological outcomes and superior short-term postoperative outcomes when compared to open surgery [6–8]. As far as rectal cancer is concerning, some randomized controlled trials have validated laparoscopic surgery to be as safe and effective oncologically as the open approach, with better postoperative outcomes [9–14], while others have failed to prove its non-inferiority from an oncological standpoint [15,16], even at a 2-year follow up [17]. These data show that laparoscopic TME still remains technically challenging, due to the technical limitations of conventional laparoscopy. Moreover, the complexity of TME is mainly increased in patients with a narrow pelvis, male and/or obese patients and patients with bulky tumors and all these factors could potentially negatively affect operative time, specimen quality, complication rate and, ultimately, survival.

Robotic surgery may potentially overcome these drawbacks thanks to its 3D high-definition vision, the use of a stable camera and the wrist-like movement of the instruments allowing seven degrees of freedom and tremor filtration. The wristed tip of the robotic instrument allows for correct triangulation, traction and countertraction even deep in the pelvis for optimal tissue handling. The first report about robotic TME was in 2006 by Pigazzi et al. [18]. Since then, several papers comparing robotic rectal surgery (RRS)/TME with laparoscopic rectal surgery (LRS) and open rectal surgery (ORS) have been published. Although the largest and only available Randomized Controlled Trial (RCT) published to date [19] failed to demonstrate superiority in the conversion rate for robotic compared to laparoscopic rectal surgery, robotic surgery may have a positive impact in most challenging cases [19] and several population-based studies have shown benefits in terms of conversions, complications, functional outcomes and length of hospital stay [20–29]. This paper aims to describe the surgical technique of robotic TME and review the recent literature on robotic rectal surgery, focusing on short-term, oncological, functional outcomes and costs.

2. Surgical Technique

The procedure is a full-robotic TME, performed with the Davinci Xi Surgical Platform (Intuitive Surgical Inc., Sunnyvale, CA, USA). Compared to previous robotic platforms, this system allows for an easier setup and multiquadrant access, faster docking and simple OR setup (boom-mounted rotating arms).

2.1. Patient Positioning and Docking

The patient is placed supine in a modified lithotomy position with arms alongside the body and abducted legs positioned in adjustable stirrups. The patient is carefully secured with a dedicated patient soft foam pad (Pink Pad, Xodus Medical Inc., New Kensington, PA, USA) to prevent sliding in steep Trendelemburg. The first assistant stands on the patient's right side and the cart is placed at the patient's left side, docked from the left lower quadrant over the left hip (Figure 1). The patient is then placed in a 20–25° Trendelemburg position with a 20–25° right tilt (Figure 2).

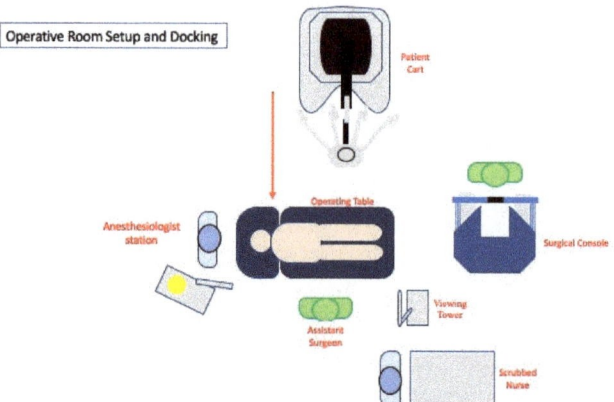

Figure 1. Operative room setup.

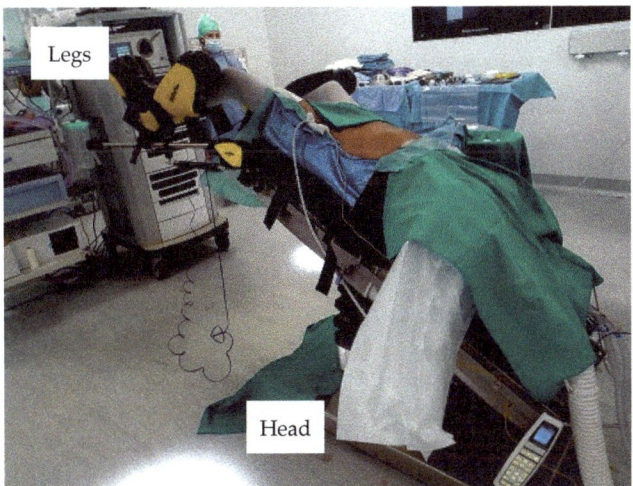

Figure 2. Patient positioning.

A Verres needle is inserted in the left hypochondrium (Palmer's point) for the induction of 12 mmHg pneumoperitoneum. A 12 mm optical port is inserted in the right flank. Four 8 mm robotic trocars are then inserted along a straight line that is parallel to and about 4 cm cranial to the costofemoral line; a distance of 6–8 cm between each port is maintained. An additional 8 mm robotic port is placed in the left flank and will be used for the TME and vascular control. A 5 mm laparoscopic port may be introduced in the right hypochondrium to optimize the assistant's tractions, if required (Figure 3).

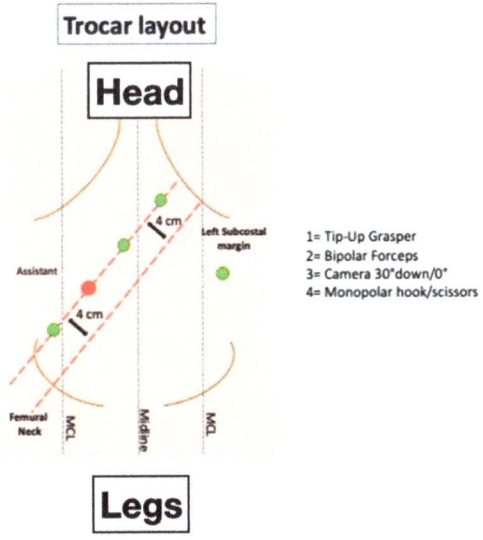

Figure 3. Trocar layout for a fully robotic TME.

The cart is deployed for docking from the patient's left side. In order to define the correct cart position, a green laser is emitted from the overhead boom to the optical port and the guided docking procedure is completed.

2.2. Step-By-Step Technique

A tip-up fenestrated grasper, Bipolar forceps and a permanent cautery hook (or Monopolar curved scissors) are mounted in R1, R2 and R4, respectively.

Full-robotic TME is essentially based on three steps:

- Vascular control;
- TME;
- Splenic flexure mobilization.

2.3. Vascular Control

The sigmoid colon is lifted up with the robotic grasper in R1 (8 mm robotic trocar in the left flank). The peritoneum is then incised at the level of the sacral promontory to access the avascular presacral mesorectal plane, where the hypogastric nerves are identified and preserved and a medial to lateral dissection is performed to identify the left ureter and gonadal vessels. The superior rectal artery is identified as a landmark and the dissection continues in a bottom-to-up fashion. The origin of inferior mesenteric artery (IMA) is thus identified with the surrounding lymphatic tissue, dissected at its origin and divided with Hem-o-lok® clips.

The medial to lateral dissection is performed underneath the inferior mesenteric vein (IMV) and the Toldt–Gerota plane is identified as a landmark.

The IMV is dissected, isolated and transected using Hem-o-lok® clips (Teleflex, Wayne, PA, USA). The dissection continues downward in a medial-to-lateral fashion, with the R1-grasper lifting the descending-sigmoid mesocolon and the assistant surgeon providing countertraction on the Gerota's fascia. Coloparietal detachment is then completed along the white line of Toldt.

2.4. TME

TME is carried out according to the Heald's embryologically based principles along the avascular plane in order to preserve the hypogastric nerve and the sacral venous plexus. Frequent repositioning of the grasper in R1 is fundamental to maintain the right countertraction for dissection.

The dissection starts posteriorly along the plane between the endopelvic visceral fascia and endopelvic parietal fascia. R1 is used to provide upward traction on the mesorectum, with the wrist joint in a L-shape to allow for a larger area of retraction; the assistant maintains a cranial traction on the sigmoid colon and R2 and R4 are the operative arms, with a bipolar grasper and a monopolar hook. The right lateral and the anterior plane are then dissected up to the seminal vesicles in a counterclockwise fashion; R1 is now used to lift the peritoneum of the Douglas pouch and vagina and the seminal vesicles and prostate are freed and protected. The left lateral pelvic fascia is then dissected up to its lower portion until the pelvic nerve plexus is identified and the "bare rectum area" is visualized. The mesorectal dissection is performed in a cylindric fashion until past the level of the lesion and the access to the levator ani plane is gained (Figure 4). During this phase in the lower mesorectum, a 0° camera may be helpful to achieve a better visualization. Rectal transection is performed with a robotic stapler after the evaluation of the vascular perfusion of the rectal stump through the integrated fluorescence imaging system. Stapled end-to-end low/ultralow colorectal anastomosis or manual coloanal anastomosis are performed according to the tumor distance from the anal verge. A transabdominal robotic top-down targeted transection of the levator ani plane may be performed if an abdominoperineal/extralevator abdominoperineal excision is required.

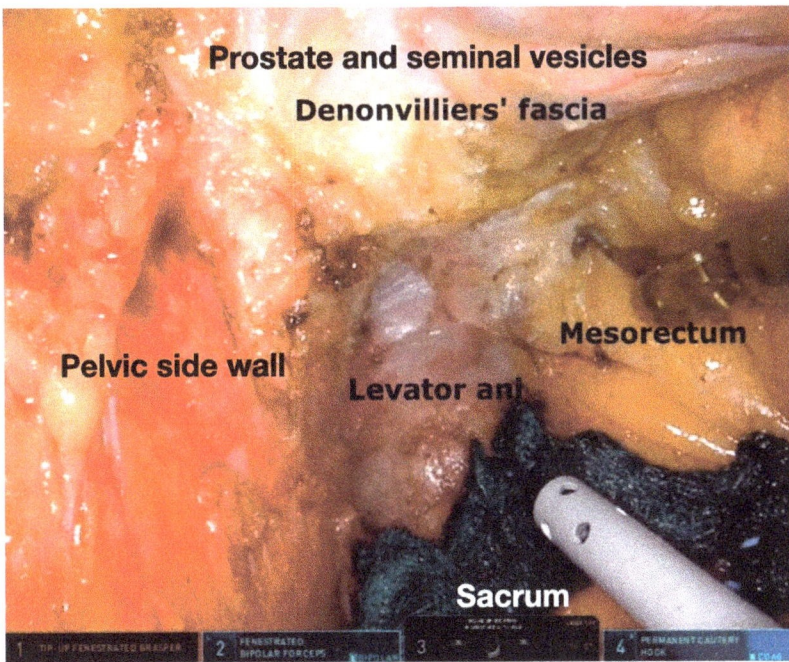

Figure 4. Final view after Total Mesorectal Excision.

2.5. Splenic Flexure Mobilization

Splenic flexure mobilization is performed in the vast majority of the patients to provide for tension-free colorectal anastomosis, with a few exceptions in the case of a very long and redundant sigmoid colon. During this step of the procedure, the robotic grasper in R1 is moved to the epigastric trocar.

Splenic flexure takedown is performed with a one-inch one-inch bottom-up approach.

The Toldt–Gerota plane previously developed and the IMV are identified. The transverse colon is lifted up with a R1-grasper and the lesser sac is opened through the incision of the transverse mesocolic root at the level of the anterior pancreatic border, gaining access to the lesser sac (one-inch one-inch bottom-up approach) [30,31] (Figure 5). The assistant keeps holding the transverse colon and the R1 grabs the posterior side of the stomach to achieve optimal exposure. A medial-to-lateral approach is carried out along the pancreatic body. The splenic flexure is then retracted medially by the assistant and the mobilization is completed from the inferior splenic pole to the previous plane along to the white line of Toldt. Coloparietal and coloepiploic detachment are performed and splenic flexure takedown is thus completed.

Different approaches have been described for splenic flexure takedown, depending on the surgeons' preference, with different trocar layouts and table tilting (i.e., reverse Trendelemburg). Some authors are used to performing this step laparoscopically; thus, the robot is docked for the core of the procedure, namely TME [32].

Regardless of the surgical approach (robotic or laparoscopic), four ways to mobilize the splenic flexure have been described [33]. The medial approach (medial-to-lateral) involves an extensive dissection of the medial plane separating the descending mesocolon from the Toldt fascia; the sovramesocolic approach (top-to-bottom) starts with a gastrocolic ligament transection to enter the lesser sac; the lateral approach begins with coloparietal detachment along the white line of Toldt; finally, the "one inch-one inch" approach allows access to the lesser sac in a bottom-to-up fashion through the transection of the transverse mesocolic root along the pancreatic fusion fascia.

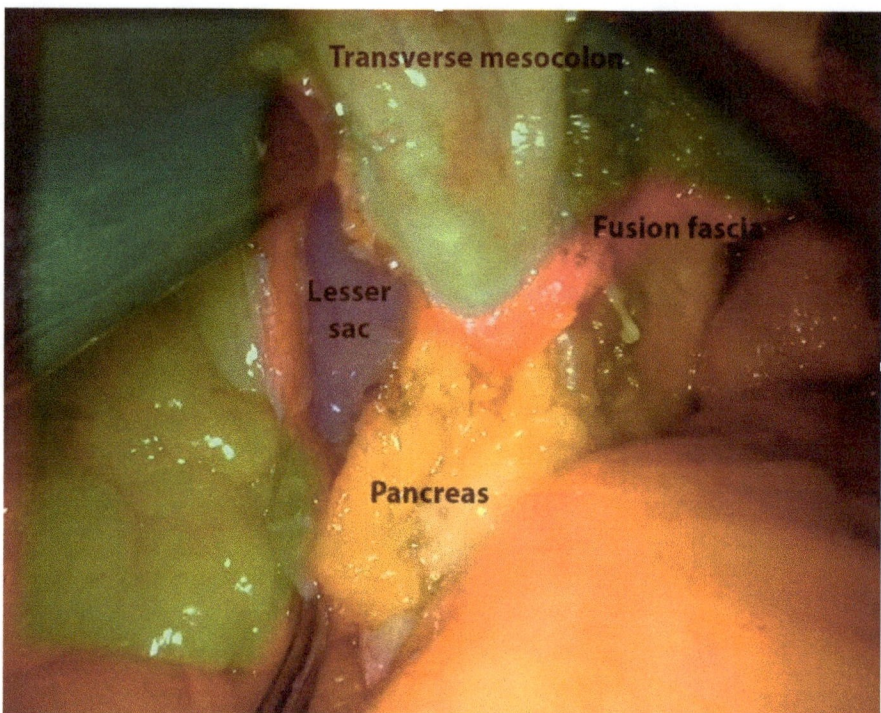

Figure 5. Splenic flexure takedown—**bottom** to **up** approach.

In our experience, a full-robotic low anterior resection is performed. Splenic flexure takedown can be challenging and the robotic approach could represent a valuable tool in facilitating this step of the procedure when compared to conventional laparoscopy. Moreover, the new robotic platform (DaVinci Xi system) is capable of extensive multiquadrant access and significantly reduces external arm collisions and docking time and allows the procedure to be performed without any change in table tilting/docking (steep Trendelenburg position with right tilt for splenic flexure takedown, vascular control and TME).

The bottom-up approach, with stable exposure and traction exerted by the third arm on the transverse mesocolon, allows for easy access into the lesser sac and dissection along embryological planes (pancreatic fusion fascia) over the body and tail of the pancreas, thus preserving the integrity of the proper mesocolic fascia and its blood supply as well.

3. Discussion and Literature Review

The potential advantages of RRS compared to conventional LRS have been widely discussed in many studies with different levels of evidence. Due to the limited space and maneuverability of instruments and the influence of tremor fulcrum effects as well, performing laparoscopic surgery in a narrow pelvis could be challenging. Technical improvements in robotic instruments and technology may provide advantages in vision, ergonomics, dexterity and wristed articulation, leading to a better surgical performance and consequently potential better short-term, oncological, functional outcomes as well.

3.1. Intraoperative and Short-Term Postoperative Outcomes

Data from the meta-analysis and RCTs reported a longer operative time for the robotic approach compared to laparoscopy and open surgery [19–27,34–43]. This was mainly attributed to time-consuming double-docking procedures and the changing of the robotic instruments. Over the last few years, the increased use of the DaVinci Xi platform with its technology improvements seems to be associated with a significant reduction in operative time [28,44], which is almost comparable to laparoscopy. This could be mainly due both to the improvements in the technology itself (endoscope inserted in any arm, multiquadrant access, longer instruments), leading to a significantly decreased docking time and instrument switch and the improvement in the surgeon's learning curve that flattens with time and experience.

As far as the conversion rate is concerned, the ROLARR trial [19] failed to demonstrate superiority in the conversion rate for RRS compared to LRS. However, meta-analysis [35,45], many population-based studies and a national database [20–26] including thousands of patients showed a significantly lower conversion rate in the robotic group compared to laparoscopy, especially in rectal surgery and in the high-risk patients subgroup (male, neoadjuvant radiochemotherapy, T3N1 patients) [20,21,46], probably reflecting what actually happens in daily practice. Those data have been confirmed by a recent large retrospective cohort study and a logistic regression analysis involving 600 patients [47,48] showing that the type of surgery (laparoscopic vs. robotic approach) and obese patients are independent risk factors for conversion.

Although no significant statistical difference has been seen in the complication rate among robotic, laparoscopic and open groups in some studies [28,35,36,45,49,50], other papers have reported data trending in favor of robotic surgery. The ROLARR trial reported a similar complication rate in both the robotic and laparoscopic group, 14% vs. 16.5%, respectively, related in particular to anastomotic leakage, 9.9% and 12.2%, respectively [19]. In a recent meta-analysis, Simillis et al. [27] reported lower wound infections due to shorter skin incisions and less contamination. The same results have been reported in large population-based studies, including about 11,000 patients with a lower overall septic complication rate (1.6% in robot vs. 3.1% in lap, p value = 0.02) and a lower wound dehiscence rate (0.1% in robot vs. 0.7% in lap, p value = 0.05) in the robotic group [21,23,24]. As complications increase, postoperative morbidity and mortality proportionally increase as well, mostly in low-volume hospitals and if surgery is performed by a less trained surgeon [46].

The aforementioned population-based studies [23–26] also reported a significant reduction in the length of stay in favor of the robotic group (3.8–4.8 vs. 4.7–6.3 days, $p < 0.001$, robotic vs. laparoscopic group, respectively), that is probably strictly related to the reduction in the conversion and complication rates [31]. The same figures have been reported as far as a shorter time to first flatus is concerned [27].

3.2. Functional Outcomes

Functional outcomes are among the most important issues related to pelvic surgery since they could ultimately impact and affect patients' postoperative quality of life. This topic has been widely investigated by comparing the functional outcomes in the RRS and LRS groups, based on the assumption that a better 3D visualization of anatomical structures and more precise movements may enable the surgeon to preserve the autonomic nerves and function. Although most reports are from case-series, with different measurements, follow-ups and small sample sizes, two recent meta-analyses [51,52] reported better functional results after robotic surgery for rectal cancer when compared to conventional laparoscopy. Regarding urinary function in men at 6 months after surgery, the IPSS (International Prostatic Symptoms Score) was significantly improved in the RRS group compared to the LRS group and these data were confirmed at a 12-month follow-up. IIEF (International Index of Erectile Function) scores were significantly in favor of the RRS group at 6- and 12-months post-operation. Mixed urinary and sexual function outcomes were also reported for women in many case series, with no significant differences in meta-analysis results. The available evidence of the potential functional benefits of robotic surgery over traditional laparoscopy after rectal cancer resection should be confirmed by high-quality randomized or prospective multicenter studies adequately powered for functional outcomes and patient-reported outcomes and quality of life.

3.3. Oncological Outcomes

Circumferential resection margin (CRM), distal resection margin (DRM) and the mesorectal grading system according to the Quirke criteria [53] are universally considered as valuable surrogates for long-term local recurrence rates and oncological outcomes as shown by several studies [10,54–59].

The ROLARR Trial reported a CRM positivity of 5.1% and 6.3% in the robotic and laparoscopic group, respectively, with no statistically significant difference between the two groups. DRM involvement and the pathological assessment of the quality of the plane of surgery were also comparable [19]. Another RCT from Korea [43] reported the same figures, with no statistically significant difference between robotic and laparoscopic surgery as far as pathological outcomes are concerned.

A recent metanalysis [58] has shown that robotic surgery is the better way to achieve a complete TME. Nevertheless, the lack of quality and heterogeneity among the included studies must be underlined. Based on the quality of the available evidence and according to pathological outcomes as surrogates for long-term oncological results, it cannot be concluded that robotic surgery is actually superior to its laparoscopic counterpart.

The survival data from the ROLARR trial are still unavailable and reports of long-term oncologic outcomes for robotic rectal surgery remain limited due to the relatively recent uptake of robotic surgery. Park et al. [59] found no differences in the 5-year OS, DSF and LR rates. Similar results were reported by Cho et al. in a case matched series of 278 patients [60], with a 5-year OS of 92.2% and a DFS of 81.8% in the robotic group. More recently, Kim et al. [61] showed that robotic surgery was a significant positive prognostic factor for OS and cancer-specific survival in a multivariate analysis. Recently, Park et al., in their retrospective single-center propensity score-matched analysis focusing only on mid-low rectal cancers, reported that robotic surgery had similar overall 5-year survival figures when compared to laparoscopic surgery. However, they found robotic surgery to be beneficial in a subgroup of patients who received preoperative chemoradiation and had ypT3–4 tumors after neoadjuvant treatment. The 5-year distant and local recurrence rates were 44.8% and 5.0% in the laparoscopic group and 9.8% and 9.8% in the robotic group, respectively and reached statistical significance. These data suggest that robotic surgery may be beneficial in most complex cases with high-risk features of recurrence [62].

The ongoing European RESET trial [63] (prospective, observational, case-matched, four-cohort patients) has been designed to analyze TME outcomes with open, laparoscopic, robotic and trans-anal approaches in a complex subset of patients from both an anatomical and oncological standpoint (distance from the anal verge, intertuberous distance, obesity and T stage). The preliminary results are still awaited.

3.4. Costs

One of the most critical issues for robotic surgery remains the cost, with institutions and payers being concerned about acquisition, maintenance, equipment and implementation. Actually, most of the available studies in different surgical specialties and subspecialties show higher costs related to robotic surgery when compared to its laparoscopic counterpart [32,64,65]. Unfortunately, to date, most of the studies have focused only on the direct costs related to the purchase and maintenance of the robot, along with the related instrumentation per procedure. Although short-term outcomes such as conversions, length of stay and complications seem to be favorable in the robotic surgery groups compared to conventional laparoscopy, these data are rarely taken into account and analyzed as a "total" and inclusive episode cost with a reduced financial burden related to hospitalization, medications and follow-up visits that may reduce the overall costs and counterbalance the excess of expenditure related to robotic equipment. The indirect costs related to the higher conversion rate compared to open surgery, with a prolonged length of stay, postoperative complication management and a delayed return to daily activities are rarely investigated, although they have a significant negative impact on the overall financial burden for each Institution. Cleary et al. [66] in an observational study from a linked data registry including clinical data from the Michigan Surgical Quality Collaborative (2012–2015) specifically showed that the conversion to open surgery significantly increases the payments associated with minimally invasive colorectal surgery. Since conversion rates are lower in robotic versus laparoscopic surgery, the excess expenditures attributable to robotics are attenuated by the consideration of the cost of conversions itself [66,67]. Moreover, as data show that the conversion rate is significantly lower in large volume hospitals, it seems that this variable may impact on indirect costs as well [46]. Therefore, large case series per institution, multidisciplinary team utilization and, ideally, the presence of industry competition are key factors that could reduce the financial burden and make robotic surgery a cost-effective technique.

4. Conclusions

Rectal surgery remains challenging, especially in male patients, obese patients and patients with a narrow pelvis and bulking tumors. Robotic technology applied to pelvic surgery may potentially offer clinical and oncological benefits, due to the more precise visualization and dissection along the embryological planes. To date, population-based studies with large sample sizes and metanalyses comparing robotic and laparoscopic surgery have reported better statistically significant results in terms of conversion rates, complications, length of stay and functional outcomes. The excess of expenditures related to robotic surgery may be balanced and mitigated by better short-term results that should be included in future cost analysis studies. Results of prospective multicenter studies focusing on technically challenging patients with high-risk features for recurrence are awaited.

Funding: This research received no external funding.

Institutional Review Board Statement: Not applicable.

Informed Consent Statement: Not applicable.

Data Availability Statement: Not applicable.

Conflicts of Interest: The authors declare no conflict of interest.

References

1. Heald, R.J.; Husband, E.M.; Ryall, R.D.H. The mesorectum in rectal cancer surgery—The clue to pelvic recurrence? *J. Br. Surg.* **2005**, *69*, 613–616. [CrossRef]
2. Lacy, A.M.; Tasende, M.M.; Delgado, S.; Fernandez-Hevia, M.; Jimenez, M.; De Lacy, B.; Castells, A.; Bravo, R.; Wexner, S.D.; Heald, R.J. Transanal Total Mesorectal Excision for Rectal Cancer: Outcomes after 140 Patients. *J. Am. Coll. Surg.* **2015**, *221*, 415–423. [CrossRef]
3. González-Abós, C.; De Lacy, F.B.; Guzmán, Y.; Nogueira, S.T.; Otero-Piñeiro, A.; Almenara, R.; Lacy, A.M. Transanal total mesorectal excision for stage II or III rectal cancer: Pattern of local recurrence in a tertiary referral center. *Surg. Endosc.* **2021**, 1–9. [CrossRef]
4. Deijen, C.L.; Velthuis, S.; Tsai, A.; Mavroveli, S.; Klerk, E.S.M.D.L.-D.; Sietses, C.; Tuynman, J.B.; Lacy, A.M.; Hanna, G.B.; Bonjer, H.J. COLOR III: A multicentre randomised clinical trial comparing transanal TME versus laparoscopic TME for mid and low rectal cancer. *Surg. Endosc.* **2016**, *30*, 3210–3215. [CrossRef]
5. Roodbeen, S.X.; Penna, M.; MacKenzie, H.; Kusters, M.; Slater, A.; Jones, O.M.; Lindsey, I.; Guy, R.J.; Cunningham, C.; Hompes, R. Transanal total mesorectal excision (TaTME) versus laparoscopic TME for MRI-defined low rectal cancer: A propensity score-matched analysis of oncological outcomes. *Surg. Endosc.* **2019**, *33*, 2459–2467. [CrossRef] [PubMed]
6. Guillou, P.J.; Quirke, P.; Thorpe, H.; Walker, J.; Jayne, D.G.; Smith, A.M.; Heath, R.M.; Brown, J.M. Short-term endpoints of conventional versus laparoscopic-assisted surgery in patients with colorectal cancer (MRC CLASICC trial): Multicentre, randomised controlled trial. *Lancet* **2005**, *365*, 1718–1726. [CrossRef]
7. Hazebroek, E.J.; The Color Study. COLOR: A randomized clinical trial comparing laparoscopic and open resection for colon cancer. *Surg. Endosc.* **2002**, *16*, 949–953. [CrossRef]
8. Clinical Outcomes of Surgical Therapy Study Group; Nelson, H.; Sargent, D.; Wieand, H.S.; Fleshman, J.; Anvari, M.; Stryker, S.J.; Beart, R.W.; Hellinger, M.; Flanagan, R.; et al. A Comparison of Laparoscopically Assisted and Open Colectomy for Colon Cancer. *N. Engl. J. Med.* **2004**, *350*, 2050–2059. [CrossRef] [PubMed]
9. Kearney, D.E.; Coffey, J.C. A Randomized Trial of Laparoscopic versus Open Surgery for Rectal Cancer. *N. Engl. J. Med.* **2015**, *373*, 194. [CrossRef]

10. Van der Pas, M.H.; Haglind, E.; Cuesta, M.A.; Fürst, A.; Lacy, A.M.; Hop, W.C.; Bonjer, H.J.; COlorectal cancer Laparoscopic or Open Resection II (COLOR II) Study Group. Laparoscopic versus open surgery for rectal cancer (COLOR II): Short-term outcomes of a randomised, phase 3 trial. *Lancet Oncol.* **2013**, *14*, 210–218. [CrossRef]
11. Jayne, D.G.; Guillou, P.J.; Thorpe, H.; Quirke, P.; Copeland, J.; Smith, A.M.; Heath, R.M.; Brown, J.M. Randomized Trial of Laparoscopic-Assisted Resection of Colorectal Carcinoma: 3-Year Results of the UK MRC CLASICC Trial Group. *J. Clin. Oncol.* **2007**, *25*, 3061–3068. [CrossRef] [PubMed]
12. Jayne, D.G.; Thorpe, H.C.; Copeland, J.; Quirke, P.; Brown, J.M.; Guillou, P.J. Five-year follow-up of the Medical Research Council CLASICC trial of laparoscopically assisted versus open surgery for colorectal cancer. *J. Br. Surg.* **2010**, *97*, 1638–1645. [CrossRef] [PubMed]
13. Jeong, S.-Y.; Park, J.W.; Nam, B.H.; Kim, S.; Kang, S.-B.; Lim, S.-B.; Choi, H.S.; Kim, D.-W.; Chang, H.J.; Kim, D.Y.; et al. Open versus laparoscopic surgery for mid-rectal or low-rectal cancer after neoadjuvant chemoradiotherapy (COREAN trial): Survival outcomes of an open-label, non-inferiority, randomised controlled trial. *Lancet Oncol.* **2014**, *15*, 767–774. [CrossRef]
14. Kang, S.-B.; Park, J.W.; Jeong, S.-Y.; Nam, B.H.; Choi, H.S.; Kim, D.-W.; Lim, S.-B.; Lee, T.-G.; Kim, D.Y.; Kim, J.-S.; et al. Open versus laparoscopic surgery for mid or low rectal cancer after neoadjuvant chemoradiotherapy (COREAN trial): Short-term outcomes of an open-label randomised controlled trial. *Lancet Oncol.* **2010**, *11*, 637–645. [CrossRef]
15. Stevenson, A.R.L.; Solomon, M.; Lumley, J.W.; Hewett, P.; Clouston, A.; Gebski, V.; Davies, L.; Wilson, C.; Hague, W.; Simes, J. Effect of Laparoscopic-Assisted Resection vs Open Resection on Pathological Outcomes in Rectal Cancer: The ALaCaRT Randomized Clinical Trial. *JAMA* **2015**, *314*, 1356–1363. [CrossRef]
16. Fleshman, J.W.; Branda, M.E.; Sargent, D.J.; Boller, A.M.; George, V.; Abbas, M.A.; Peters, W.R.; Maun, D.; Chang, G.; Herline, A.J.; et al. Effect of Laparoscopic-Assisted Resection vs Open Resection of Stage II or III Rectal Cancer on Pathologic Outcomes: The ACOSOG Z6051 Randomized Clinical Trial. *JAMA* **2015**, *314*, 1346–1355. [CrossRef]
17. Fleshman, J.; Branda, M.E.; Sargent, D.J.; Boller, A.M.; George, V.V.; Abbas, M.A.; Peters, W.R.; Maun, D.C.; Chang, G.J.; Herline, A.; et al. Disease-free Survival and Local Recurrence for Laparoscopic Resection Compared with Open Resection of Stage II to III Rectal Cancer: Follow-up Results of the ACOSOG Z6051 Randomized Controlled Trial. *Ann. Surg.* **2019**, *269*, 589–595. [CrossRef]
18. Pigazzi, A.; Ellenhorn, J.D.I.; Ballantyne, G.H.; Paz, I.B. Robotic-assisted laparoscopic low anterior resection with total mesorectal excision for rectal cancer. *Surg. Endosc.* **2006**, *20*, 1521–1525. [CrossRef]
19. Jayne, D.; Pigazzi, A.; Marshall, H.; Croft, J.; Corrigan, N.; Copeland, J.; Quirke, P.; West, N.; Rautio, T.; Thomassen, N.; et al. Effect of Robotic-Assisted vs Conventional Laparoscopic Surgery on Risk of Conversion to Open Laparotomy Among Patients Undergoing Resection for Rectal Cancer: The ROLARR Randomized Clinical Trial. *JAMA* **2017**, *318*, 1569–1580. [CrossRef] [PubMed]
20. Sun, Z.; Kim, J.; Adam, M.A.; Nussbaum, D.P.; Speicher, P.J.; Mantyh, C.R.; Migaly, J. Minimally Invasive Versus Open Low Anterior Resection: Equivalent Survival in a National Analysis of 14,033 Patients With Rectal Cancer. *Ann. Surg.* **2016**, *263*, 1152–1158. [CrossRef] [PubMed]
21. Bhama, A.R.; Obias, V.; Welch, K.B.; Vandewarker, J.F.; Cleary, R.K. A comparison of laparoscopic and robotic colorectal surgery outcomes using the American College of Surgeons National Surgical Quality Improvement Program (ACS NSQIP) database. *Surg. Endosc.* **2015**, *30*, 1576–1584. [CrossRef]
22. Tam, M.S.; Kaoutzanis, C.; Mullard, A.J.; Regenbogen, S.E.; Franz, M.G.; Hendren, S.; Krapohl, G.; Vandewarker, J.F.; Lampman, R.M.; Cleary, R.K. A population-based study comparing laparoscopic and robotic outcomes in colorectal surgery. *Surg. Endosc.* **2016**, *30*, 455–463. [CrossRef]
23. Al-Mazrou, A.M.; Chiuzan, C.; Kiran, R.P. The robotic approach significantly reduces length of stay after colectomy: A propensity score-matched analysis. *Int. J. Color. Dis.* **2017**, *32*, 1415–1421. [CrossRef] [PubMed]
24. Altieri, M.S.; Yang, J.; Telem, D.A.; Zhu, J.; Halbert, C.; Talamini, M.; Pryor, A.D. Robotic approaches may offer benefit in colorectal procedures, more controversial in other areas: A review of 168,248 cases. *Surg. Endosc.* **2015**, *30*, 925–933. [CrossRef]
25. Benlice, C.; Aytac, E.; Costedio, M.; Kessler, H.; Abbas, M.A.; Remzi, F.H.; Gorgun, E. Robotic, laparoscopic, and open colectomy: A case-matched comparison from the ACS-NSQIP. *Int. J. Med. Robot. Comput. Assist. Surg.* **2017**, *13*, e1783. [CrossRef]
26. Al-Temimi, M.H.; Chandrasekaran, B.; Agapian, J.; Peters, W.R.; Wells, K.O. Robotic versus laparoscopic elective colectomy for left side diverticulitis: A propensity score–matched analysis of the NSQIP database. *Int. J. Color. Dis.* **2019**, *34*, 1385–1392. [CrossRef] [PubMed]
27. Simillis, C.; Lal, N.; Thoukididou, S.N.; Kontovounisios, C.; Smith, J.J.; Hompes, R.; Adamina, M.; Tekkis, P.P. Open Versus Laparoscopic Versus Robotic Versus Transanal Mesorectal Excision for Rectal Cancer: A Systematic Review and Network Meta-analysis. *Ann. Surg.* **2019**, *270*, 59–68. [CrossRef]
28. Polat, F.; Willems, L.H.; Dogan, K.; Rosman, C. The oncological and surgical safety of robot-assisted surgery in colorectal cancer: Outcomes of a longitudinal prospective cohort study. *Surg. Endosc.* **2019**, *33*, 3644–3655. [CrossRef]
29. Phan, K.; Kahlaee, H.R.; Kim, S.H.; Toh, J.W.T. Laparoscopic vs. robotic rectal cancer surgery and the effect on conversion rates: A meta-analysis of randomized controlled trials and propensity-score-matched studies. *Tech. Coloproctol.* **2019**, *23*, 221–230. [CrossRef]
30. Formisano, G.; Marano, A.; Bianchi, P.P.; Spinoglio, G. Challenges with robotic low anterior resection. *Minerva Chir.* **2015**, *70*, 341–354. [PubMed]

31. Esposito, S.; Formisano, G.; Giuliani, G.; Misitano, P.; Krizzuk, D.; Salvischiani, L.; Bianchi, P.P. Update on robotic surgery for rectal cancer treatment. *Ann. Laparosc. Endosc. Surg.* **2017**, *2*, 132. [CrossRef]
32. Park, S.Y.; Lee, S.M.; Park, J.S.; Kim, H.J.; Choi, G.S. Robot Surgery Shows Similar Long-term Oncologic Outcomes as Laparoscopic Surgery for Mid/Lower Rectal Cancer but Is Beneficial to ypT3/4 After Preoperative Chemoradiation. *Dis. Colon. Rectum.* **2021**, *64*, 812–821. [CrossRef] [PubMed]
33. Petz, W.; Ribero, D.; Bertani, E.; Polizzi, M.L.; Spinoglio, G. Notes of robotic surgical technique: Four ways to mobilize splenic flex-ure. *Minerva Chir.* **2016**, *71*, 345–348. [PubMed]
34. Xiong, B.; Ma, L.; Huang, W.; Zhao, Q.; Cheng, Y.; Liu, J. Robotic Versus Laparoscopic Total Mesorectal Excision for Rectal Cancer: A Meta-analysis of Eight Studies. *J. Gastrointest. Surg.* **2015**, *19*, 516–526. [CrossRef] [PubMed]
35. Xiong, B.; Ma, L.; Zhang, C.; Cheng, Y. Robotic versus laparoscopic total mesorectal excision for rectal cancer: A meta-analysis. *J. Surg. Res.* **2014**, *188*, 404–414. [CrossRef] [PubMed]
36. Trastulli, S.; Farinella, E.; Cirocchi, R.; Cavaliere, D.; Avenia, N.; Sciannameo, F.; Gullà, N.; Noya, G.; Boselli, C. Robotic resection compared with laparoscopic rectal resection for cancer: Systematic review and meta-analysis of short-term outcome. *Color. Dis.* **2012**, *14*, e134–e156. [CrossRef]
37. Sun, Y.; Xu, H.; Li, Z.; Han, J.; Song, W.; Wang, J.; Xu, Z. Robotic versus laparoscopic low anterior resection for rectal cancer: A meta-analysis. *World J. Surg. Oncol.* **2016**, *14*, 1–8. [CrossRef]
38. Holmer, C.; Kreis, M.E. Systematic review of robotic low anterior resection for rectal cancer. *Surg. Endosc.* **2018**, *32*, 569–581. [CrossRef]
39. Lee, S.H.; Kim, D.H.; Lim, S.W. Robotic versus laparoscopic intersphincteric resection for low rectal cancer: A systematic review and meta-analysis. *Int. J. Color. Dis.* **2018**, *33*, 1741–1753. [CrossRef]
40. Ohtani, H.; Maeda, K.; Nomura, S.; Shinto, O.; Mizuyama, Y.; Nakagawa, H.; Nagahara, H.; Shibutani, M.; Fukuoka, T.; Amano, R.; et al. Meta-analysis of Robot-assisted Versus Laparoscopic Surgery for Rectal Cancer. *In Vivo* **2018**, *32*, 611–623. [CrossRef]
41. Prete, F.; Pezzolla, A.; Prete, F.; Testini, M.; Marzaioli, R.; Patriti, A.; Jimenez-Rodriguez, R.M.; Gurrado, A.; Strippoli, G.F.M. Robotic Versus Laparoscopic Minimally Invasive Surgery for Rectal Cancer: A Systematic Review and Meta-analysis of Randomized Controlled Trials. *Ann. Surg.* **2018**, *267*, 1034–1046. [CrossRef]
42. Cui, Y.; Li, C.; Xu, Z.; Wang, Y.; Sun, Y.; Xu, H.; Li, Z.; Sun, Y. Robot-assisted versus conventional laparoscopic operation in anus-preserving rectal cancer: A meta-analysis. *Ther. Clin. Risk Manag.* **2017**, *13*, 1247–1257. [CrossRef]
43. Kim, M.J.; Park, S.C.; Park, J.W.; Chang, H.J.; Kim, D.Y.; Nam, B.-H.; Sohn, D.K.; Oh, J.H. Robot-assisted Versus Laparoscopic Surgery for Rectal Cancer: Phase II Open Label Prospective Randomized Controlled Trial. *Ann. Surg.* **2018**, *267*, 243–251. [CrossRef]
44. Morelli, L.; Guadagni, S.; Di Franco, G.; Palmeri, M.; Caprili, G.; D'Isidoro, C.; Cobuccio, L.; Marciano, E.; Di Candio, G.; Mosca, F. Use of the new da Vinci Xi® during robotic rectal resection for cancer: A pilot matched-case comparison with the da Vinci Si®. *Int. J. Med. Robot. Comput. Assist. Surg.* **2016**, *13*, e1728. [CrossRef]
45. Araujo, S.E.A.; Seid, V.E.; Klajner, S. Robotic surgery for rectal cancer: Current immediate clinical and oncological outcomes. *World J. Gastroenterol.* **2014**, *20*, 14359–14370. [CrossRef]
46. Ackerman, S.J.; Daniel, S.; Baik, R.; Liu, E.; Mehendale, S.; Tackett, S.; Hellan, M. Comparison of complication and conversion rates between robotic-assisted and laparoscopic rectal resection for rectal cancer: Which patients and providers could benefit most from robotic-assisted surgery? *J. Med. Econ.* **2017**, *21*, 254–261. [CrossRef] [PubMed]
47. Crippa, J.; Grass, F.; Dozois, E.J.; Mathis, K.L.; Merchea, A.; Colibaseanu, D.T.; Kelley, S.R.; Larson, D.W. Robotic Surgery for Rectal Cancer Provides Advantageous Outcomes Over Laparoscopic Approach: Results From a Large Retrospective Cohort. *Ann. Surg.* **2020**. [CrossRef] [PubMed]
48. Crippa, J.; Grass, F.; Achilli, P.; Mathis, K.L.; Kelley, S.R.; Merchea, A.; Colibaseanu, D.T.; Larson, D.W. Risk factors for conversion in laparoscopic and robotic rectal cancer surgery. *J. Br. Surg.* **2020**, *107*, 560–566. [CrossRef] [PubMed]
49. Katsuno, H.; Hanai, T.; Masumori, K.; Koide, Y.; Ashida, K.; Matsuoka, H.; Tajima, Y.; Endo, T.; Mizuno, M.; Cheong, Y.; et al. Robotic Surgery for Rectal Cancer: Operative Technique and Review of the Literature. *J. Anus Rectum Colon* **2020**, *4*, 14–24. [CrossRef]
50. Bianchi, P.P.; Ceriani, C.; Locatelli, A.; Spinoglio, G.; Zampino, M.G.; Sonzogni, A.M.; Crosta, C.; Andreoni, L.B. Robotic versus laparoscopic total mesorectal excision for rectal cancer: A comparative analysis of oncological safety and short-term outcomes. *Surg. Endosc.* **2010**, *24*, 2888–2894. [CrossRef] [PubMed]
51. Fleming, C.A.; Cullinane, C.; Lynch, N.; Killeen, S.; Coffey, J.C.; Peirce, C.B. Urogenital function following robotic and laparoscopic rectal cancer surgery: Meta-analysis. *J. Br. Surg.* **2021**, *108*, 128–137. [CrossRef]
52. Kowalewski, K.F.; Seifert, L.; Ali, S.; Schmidt, M.W.; Seide, S.; Haney, C.; Tapking, C.; Shamiyeh, A.; Kulu, Y.; Hackert, T.; et al. Functional outcomes after laparoscopic versus robotic-assisted rectal resection: A systematic review and meta-analysis. *Surg. Endosc.* **2021**, *35*, 81–95. [CrossRef]
53. Quirke, P.; Steele, R.J.; Monson, J.; Grieve, R.; Khanna, S.; Couture, J.; O'Callaghan, C.; Myint, A.S.; Bessell, E.; Thompson, L.C.; et al. Effect of the plane of surgery achieved on local recurrence in patients with operable rectal cancer: A prospective study using data from the MRC CR07 and NCIC-CTG CO16 randomised clinical trial. *Lancet* **2009**, *373*, 821–828. [CrossRef]
54. Baik, S.H.; Kwon, H.Y.; Kim, J.S.; Hur, H.; Sohn, S.K.; Cho, C.H.; Kim, H. Robotic Versus Laparoscopic Low Anterior Resection of Rectal Cancer: Short-Term Outcome of a Prospective Comparative Study. *Ann. Surg. Oncol.* **2009**, *16*, 1480–1487. [CrossRef]

55. Kim, J.Y.; Kim, N.-K.; Lee, K.Y.; Hur, H.; Min, B.S.; Kim, J.H. A Comparative Study of Voiding and Sexual Function after Total Mesorectal Excision with Autonomic Nerve Preservation for Rectal Cancer: Laparoscopic Versus Robotic Surgery. *Ann. Surg. Oncol.* **2012**, *19*, 2485–2493. [CrossRef]
56. Nagtegaal, I.; van Krieken, J. The role of pathologists in the quality control of diagnosis and treatment of rectal cancer—An overview. *Eur. J. Cancer* **2002**, *38*, 964–972. [CrossRef]
57. Nagtegaal, I.D.; Quirke, P. What Is the Role for the Circumferential Margin in the Modern Treatment of Rectal Cancer? *J. Clin. Oncol.* **2008**, *26*, 303–312. [CrossRef] [PubMed]
58. Milone, M.; Manigrasso, M.; Velotti, N.; Torino, S.; Vozza, A.; Sarnelli, G.; Aprea, G.; Maione, F.; Gennarelli, N.; Musella, M.; et al. Completeness of total mesorectum excision of laparoscopic versus robotic surgery: A review with a meta-analysis. *Int. J. Color. Dis.* **2019**, *34*, 983–991. [CrossRef] [PubMed]
59. Park, E.J.; Cho, M.S.; Baek, S.J.; Hur, H.; Min, B.S.; Baik, S.H.; Lee, K.Y.; Kim, N.-K. Long-term Oncologic Outcomes of Robotic Low Anterior Resection for Rectal Cancer: A comparative study with laparoscopic surgery. *Ann. Surg.* **2015**, *261*, 129–137. [CrossRef]
60. Cho, M.S.; Baek, S.J.; Hur, H.; Min, B.S.; Baik, S.H.; Lee, K.Y.; Kim, N.-K. Short and Long-Term Outcomes of Robotic versus Laparoscopic Total Mesorectal Excision for Rectal Cancer: A case-matched retrospective study. *Medicine* **2015**, *94*, e522. [CrossRef] [PubMed]
61. Kim, J.; Baek, S.-J.; Kang, D.-W.; Roh, Y.-E.; Lee, J.W.; Kwak, H.-D.; Kwak, J.M.; Kim, S.-H. Robotic Resection is a Good Prognostic Factor in Rectal Cancer Compared with Laparoscopic Resection: Long-term Survival Analysis Using Propensity Score Matching. *Dis. Colon Rectum* **2017**, *60*, 266–273. [CrossRef]
62. Fung, A.K.; Aly, E.H. Robotic colonic surgery: Is it advisable to commence a new learning curve? *Dis. Colon Rectum* **2013**, *56*, 786–796. [CrossRef] [PubMed]
63. Rouanet, P.; Gourgou, S.; Gögenur, I.; Jayne, D.; Ulrich, A.; Rautio, T.; Spinoglio, G.; Bouazza, N.; Moussion, A.; Ruiz, M.G. Rectal Surgery Evaluation Trial: Protocol for a parallel cohort trial of outcomes using surgical techniques for total mesorectal excision with low anterior resection in high-risk rectal cancer patients. *Color. Dis.* **2019**, *21*, 516–522. [CrossRef] [PubMed]
64. Higgins, R.M.; Frelich, M.J.; Bosler, M.E.; Gould, J.C. Cost analysis of robotic versus laparoscopic general surgery procedures. *Surg. Endosc.* **2016**, *31*, 185–192. [CrossRef] [PubMed]
65. Khorgami, Z.; Li, W.T.; Jackson, T.N.; Howard, C.A.; Sclabas, G.M. The cost of robotics: An analysis of the added costs of robotic-assisted versus laparoscopic surgery using the National Inpatient Sample. *Surg. Endosc.* **2018**, *33*, 2217–2221. [CrossRef] [PubMed]
66. Cleary, R.K.; Mullard, A.J.; Ferraro, J.; Regenbogen, S.E. The cost of conversion in robotic and laparoscopic colorectal surgery. *Surg. Endosc.* **2018**, *32*, 1515–1524. [CrossRef] [PubMed]
67. Regenbogen, S.E.; Veenstra, C.M.; Hawley, S.T.; Banerjee, M.; Ward, K.C.; Kato, I.; Morris, A.M. The personal financial burden of complications after colorectal cancer surgery. *Cancer* **2014**, *120*, 3074–3081. [CrossRef]

Update on Robotic Rectal Prolapse Treatment

Giampaolo Formisano [1], Luca Ferraro [1,*], Adelona Salaj [1], Simona Giuratrabocchetta [1], Andrea Pisani Ceretti [2], Enrico Opocher [2] and Paolo Pietro Bianchi [1]

[1] Division of General and Robotic Surgery, Dipartimento di Scienze della Salute, Università di Milano, 20142 Milano, Italy; giampaoloformisano@hotmail.com (G.F.); adelona.87@gmail.com (A.S.); simona.giuratrabocchetta@gmail.com (S.G.); PaoloPietro.Bianchi@unimi.it (P.P.B.)
[2] Division of General and HPB Surgery, Dipartimento di Scienze della Salute, Università di Milano, 20142 Milano, Italy; andreapisaniceretti@yahoo.it (A.P.C.); enrico.opocher@unimi.it (E.O.)
* Correspondence: Lucaferraro.md@gmail.com; Tel.: +39-3921548621

Abstract: Rectal prolapse is a condition that can cause significant social impairment and negatively affects quality of life. Surgery is the mainstay of treatment, with the aim of restoring the anatomy and correcting the associated functional disorders. During recent decades, laparoscopic abdominal procedures have emerged as effective tools for the treatment of rectal prolapse, with the advantages of faster recovery, lower morbidity, and shorter length of stay. Robotic surgery represents the latest evolution in the field of minimally invasive surgery, with the benefits of enhanced dexterity in deep narrow fields such as the pelvis, and may potentially overcome the technical limitations of conventional laparoscopy. Robotic surgery for the treatment of rectal prolapse is feasible and safe. It could reduce complication rates and length of hospital stay, as well as shorten the learning curve, when compared to conventional laparoscopy. Further prospectively maintained or randomized data are still required on long-term functional outcomes and recurrence rates.

Keywords: robotic surgery; robotic ventral rectopexy; rectal prolapse; pelvic organ prolapse treatment

1. Introduction

Pelvic organs prolapse, including rectal prolapse (RP), is a condition that mainly affects women in middle and advanced age and can involve both the anterior and posterior compartments. A multidisciplinary approach is traditionally required, involving urologists, gynecologists, and colorectal surgeons [1]. Depending on the anatomy and the type of prolapse, symptoms may vary from urinary or fecal incontinence to obstructed defecation, pelvic pain, and sexual dysfunction. This condition may significantly worsen the quality of life (QoL) and represent an important social and economic burden in the setting of an aging population.

Surgery is the mainstay of treating this complex disease, and several abdominal and perineal approaches have been described to date. However, since multiple options are available, treatment may be surgeon-dependent and is influenced by many factors. Therefore, a tailored, multidisciplinary approach is recommended, with abdominal procedures usually performed in younger, healthier patients and perineal procedures offered to higher-risk individuals.

External rectal prolapse or symptomatic internal rectal prolapse with rectocele or enterocele are commonly treated with ventral rectopexy in fit patients.

The abdominal approach aims to reduce rectal mobility by fixation with or without excision of the redundant colon. Rectopexy is associated with lower recurrence risk than simple rectal mobilization, with a similar rate of overall complications [2]. Fixation of the prolapsed rectum to the sacral promontory is the key to restore the physiological anatomy of the pelvic floor. This goal can be achieved by simple suturing, as first described by D. Cutait in 1959 [3], or using a mesh fixed anteriorly, posteriorly, laterally, or all over the rectum. Many techniques have been described, such as the Ripstein rectopexy, based on the anterior fixation of a mesh below the sacral promontory, or the Wells procedure, with the detachment of the lateral ligaments of the rectum.

Both these approaches are associated with a significant complication rates and are currently abandoned [4,5].

There is no evidence as to whether associated sigmoidectomy results in better functional outcomes compared to a simple rectopexy. Resection rectopexy is thought to improve complaints of constipation, reducing the possible kinking of the redundant colon. However, it is a matter of fact that the creation of an anastomosis may increase the risk of severe complications [6–8]. Ventral rectopexy is typically performed laparoscopically and involves the anterior placement of a mesh to the sacral promontory, as described by D'Hoore [9]. It is favored over posterior mesh rectopexy since it reduces autonomic nerve injuries by avoiding postero-lateral dissection of the rectum. This approach thus reduces impairment of rectal motility that could potentially and ultimately lead to ongoing functional disfunction and impaired quality of life [10,11].

Since the introduction of the minimally invasive treatment for rectal prolapse in the early 90 s [12], the uptake of laparoscopy has been progressively growing to treat this condition. The benefits of the minimally invasive approach are well known in terms of faster recovery and normal return to daily activities, lower morbidity, decreased postoperative pain, shorter length of stay, and lower blood loss and the laparoscopic approach as the preferred technique has been recommended by several authors [13–16]. Laparoscopy has shown similar outcomes compared to the open technique for the surgical treatment of rectal prolapse [14,17]. A meta-analysis by Sajid et al. in 2010 reported no statistically significant difference between 688 patients treated with an open or laparoscopic approach in terms of recurrence, functional outcomes, and complication rate. Moreover, they reported a shorter length of hospital stay in the laparoscopic group [18]. However, the laparoscopic approach can be challenging, especially in the deep and narrow pelvis or in the setting of morbid obesity.

Since its introduction, the uptake of robotic surgery in several fields of general surgery has constantly grown. Robotic assistance is rapidly increasing in pelvic floor surgery because of its advantages in complex maneuvers such as dissection and intracorporeal suturing in the deep narrow pelvis. The technical features of the available robotic platforms may potentially overcome the limitations of conventional laparoscopy, thanks to enhanced dexterity, a stable optical platform, and exposure (third arm) that allows for a "precision" surgery to be performed. Adequate traction and counter traction allow for optimal surgical field exposure following embryological planes with minimal tissue trauma and blood loss [19]. Moreover, it has the potential of shortening the learning curve even regarding rectal mesh rectopexy, as demonstrated in other surgical procedures [20,21]. This study aims to describe the surgical technique of robotic ventral rectopexy and to review the available literature on intraoperative, short-term postoperative, and long-term functional outcomes.

2. Surgical Technique

The patient is placed in the lithotomy position. The arms are folded at the sides, taking care to provide adequate padding along the pressure points. An anti-slipping soft foam dedicated pad should be placed directly under the patient to conduct the operation safely. This device facilitates the steep Trendelenburg position often required to ensure adequate pelvic exposure.

A Verres needle is inserted at Palmer's point in the left hypochondrium to create the pneumoperitoneum. Access to the peritoneal cavity is achieved by a first assistant 12-mm optical trocar placed in the right flank under direct vision. The costo-femoral line is the landmark used to place three 8 mm robotic trocars along a parallel straight line, approximately 4 cm lateral to the previous one. Finally, an additional 8 mm robotic trocar is positioned in the left flank. Figure 1 shows the trocar layout. Limited laparoscopic lysis is performed when adhesions are encountered to permit the safe positioning of the robotic trocars; the adhesiolysis is then completed under robotic assistance.

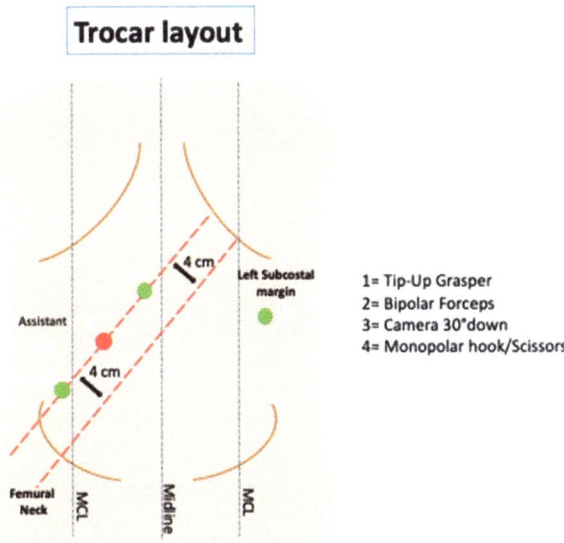

Figure 1. Trocar layout.

The patient is then positioned in a steep Trendelenburg and right tilt (20–25°), allowing the small bowel to be displaced under gravity, thus obtaining a good surgical field exposure. Next, the Da Vinci Xi® surgical system (Intuitive Surgical, Sunnyvale, CA, USA) is docked from the patient's left side. A full-robotic procedure is performed, with the assistant surgeon and scrub nurse standing on the patient's right side (Figure 2).

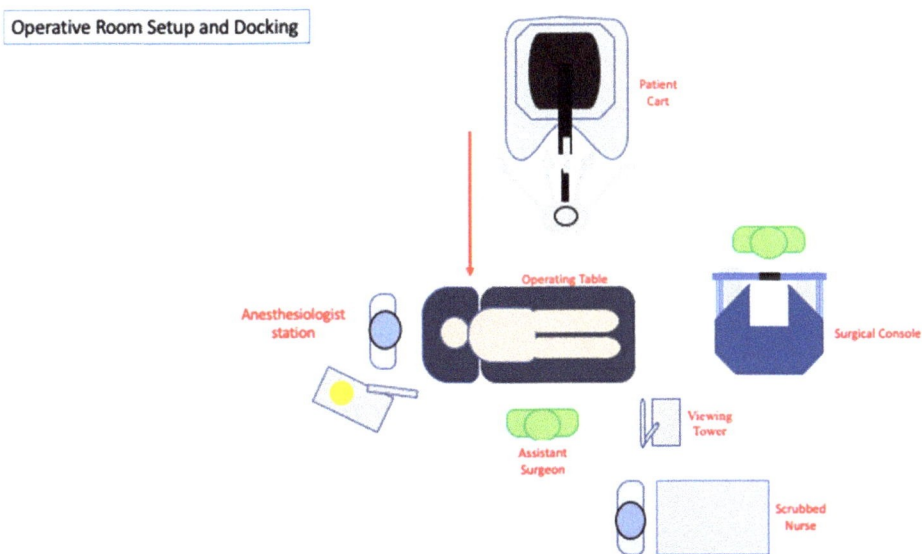

Figure 2. Operative room setup.

Tip-up grasper, bipolar forceps, and monopolar cautery hook/scissors (according to operating surgeon's preference) are mounted on robotic arm 1 (R1), arm 2 (R2), and arm 4 (R4), respectively. Robotic arm 3 (R3) is used for the 30° down scope.

The sigmoid colon is grasped and elevated anteriorly and cranially by the tip-up grasper in R1.

The peritoneum is entered by sharp dissection starting at the base of the rectosigmoid mesentery, identifying the avascular areolar plane along the sacral promontory. The right hypogastric nerve plexus and the ureter are then identified and preserved. The rectovaginal septum represents the limit to conduct the peritoneal incision.

At the level of the pouch of Douglas, the peritoneal incision is continued from right to left over the ventral aspect of the rectum.

A Breisky uterine and vaginal manipulator can identify and lift the posterior vaginal wall, thus facilitating the dissection along the anterior rectal wall. At this stage, the third arm is used as a retractor deep in the pelvis (lifting the posterior vaginal wall, once identified), and the assistant's atraumatic grasper lifts the rectum. The rectovaginal septum is entered, and anterior dissection is carried out all the way down to the levator ani plane, as inferiorly as possible, and laterally to the cardinal ligaments and pelvic sidewalls. The rectum is fully mobilized anteriorly, while the posterior and lateral attachments are left intact to preserve the autonomic nerves and optimize functional outcomes in the postoperative period.

A 14–18 cm long, 3–4 cm wide, light-weight macroporous polypropylene mesh is inserted into the abdominal cavity through the 12 mm assistant port. Biologic and titanium-coated polypropylene mesh can also be used. The mesh is positioned along the anterior wall of the rectum caudally and at the level of the sacral promontory cranially (Figures 3 and 4). Four interrupted stitches are used to secure the mesh along the anterior distal extraperitoneal surface of the rectum, using a 2-0 non-absorbable monofilament. The mesh is then fixated at the level of the sacral promontory with a 2-0 non-absorbable monofilament interrupted suture, taking care to preserve both the presacral venous plexus and the hypogastric nerves. The peritoneum is then closed with a reabsorbable barbed running suture (Figure 5). No drain is routinely left in place. Trocars are removed under direct vision, and the fascial defect of the 12-mm assistant port is closed with absorbable sutures.

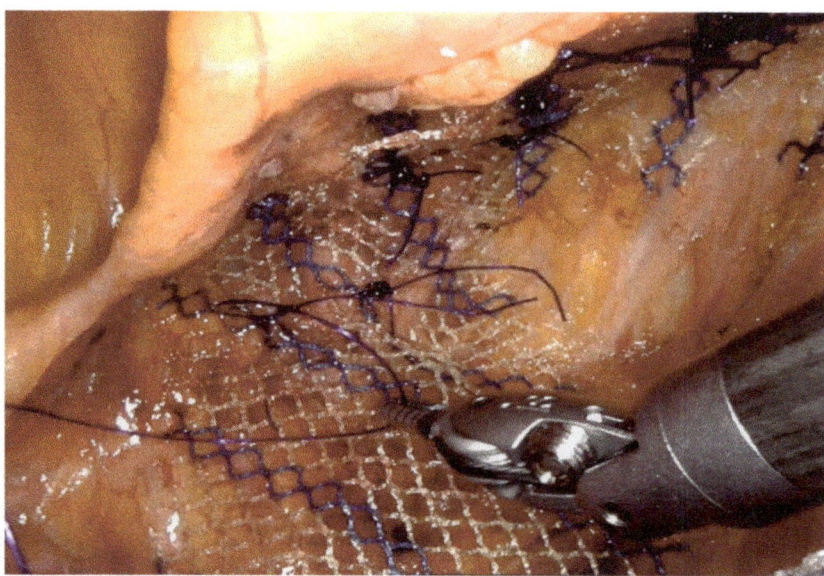

Figure 3. The mesh (macroporous polipropilene) is secured distally at the level of the anterior rectal wall with permanent sutures.

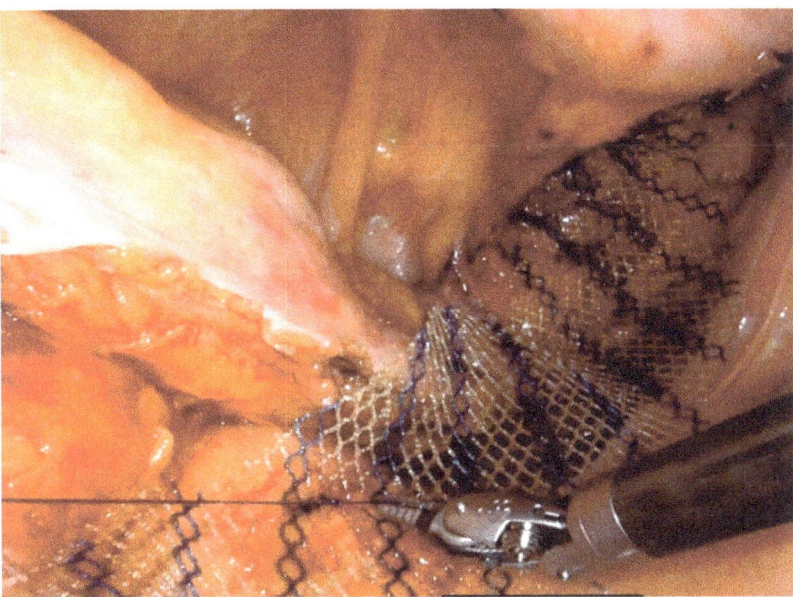

Figure 4. The mesh (macroporous polipropilene) is secured cranially at the level of the sacral promontory with permanent sutures.

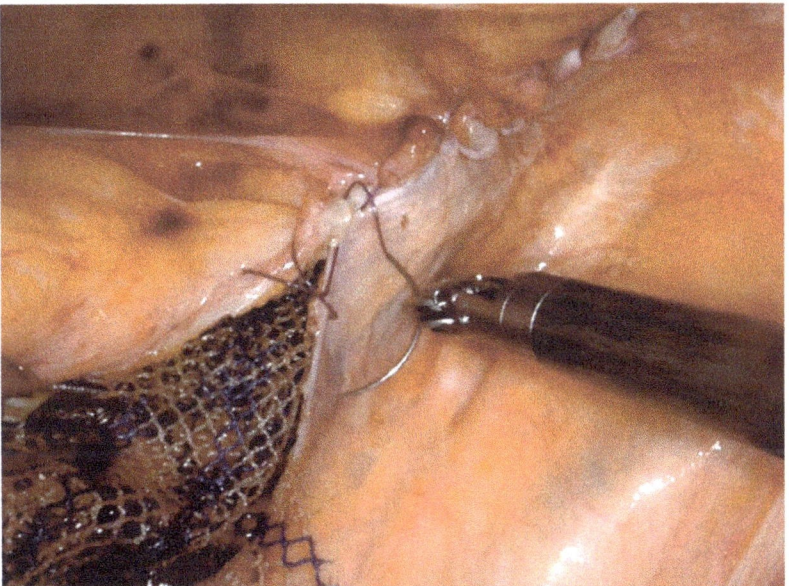

Figure 5. The peritoneum is closed with absorbable barbed running suture.

3. Discussion and Literature Review

Currently, minimally invasive surgery has widespread indications in colorectal surgery, with the robotic-assisted platform gaining extensive consensus due to its technical advantage in narrow and limited spaces [22].

Among all the various surgical options available for rectal prolapse treatment, ventral mesh rectopexy is the only technique that does not require a full rectal mobilization, with a limited anterior rectal preparation. This procedure has become the standard of care for patients with full-thickness rectal prolapse and deep enterocele [22–24]. However, it requires a good dissection of the anterior rectal surface from the prostate or the vagina and the fixation of a mesh within the narrow confines of the pelvis.

An important objective of rectal prolapse surgical treatment is to resolve or improve the functional symptoms (e.g., fecal incontinence, constipation, pain) by correcting the underlying anatomical defect. This goal should be obtained with an acceptable recurrence rate and at a reasonable cost.

The laparoscopic ventral rectopexy (LVR) is the treatment of choice for rectal prolapse nowadays [24]. LVR's use reflects widespread laparoscopy diffusion, although surgical robots have gained broad availability and have more indications in the modern surgical scenario.

To date, few studies have reported the outcomes of robotic ventral rectopexy (RVR), with most consisting of a small sample size. However, data in the literature reports that the robotic approach to rectal prolapse is feasible and safe, with outcomes almost on a par with the laparoscopic and open techniques [19,25,26].

In this section, we report on the currently available data on RVR, analyze the short-term, functional outcomes and recurrence of this approach, and look at data comparing the robotic approach with the laparoscopic approach.

3.1. Intraoperative and Short-Term Post-Operative Outcomes

Most authors report on the feasibility and safety of RVR, mainly due to the capability of the robot to conduct a fine dissection in deep and narrow space [27–29].

Features such as three-dimensional vision, restorable eye-hand-targeting, absence of depth misperception, tremor elimination, better definition of surgical planes, and robotic instrumentation wristing may facilitate the surgeon performing a correct anatomical dissection and mesh fixation in the pelvis [19].

Ventral mesh rectopexy is ideally suited for robotic surgery. The robotic platform ameliorates the visualization of the pelvis, facilitating the dissection and the suturing capability in narrow and confined spaces, allowing an optimal mesh placement to the rectovaginal septum. Indeed, the fixation of the mesh to the pelvic structures is technically more accessible, thus fastening the learning curve, with approximately twenty cases described to gain proficiency with the robotic technique compared to almost one hundred cases of the laparoscopic approach [30,31].

A recent systematic review by Albayati et al. [22] of five prospective cohort studies and one randomized controlled trial reports a significant increase in operating time for RVR compared to the laparoscopic approach. This finding is similar to that of a previous meta-analysis conducted by Ramage et al. [28]. A longer operative time is one of the main criticisms and on-vogue topics by the detractors of robotic surgery. However, it must be taken into account that these series usually show the outcomes of experienced laparoscopic surgeons compared to those of surgeons at the beginning of their robotic experience [25,30,32,33]. Indeed, recent series have described that the mean operative time for robotic rectopexy decreases with increased caseloads and experience [34,35]. These data have been confirmed by a recent metanalysis showing a non-significant trend towards longer operative times of robotic vs. laparoscopic ventral mesh rectopexy [36].

The previous systematic reviews report no statistically significant reduction of conversion rate associated with RVR [22,28]. This may be the consequence either of the exiguity of the pooled data or may be explained by the different operating surgeons' experience. Previous reviews and metanalysis of rectal prolapse treatment also describe an unclear benefit of reducing the conversion rate [36–38]. However, data in the literature show promising results in lowering the conversion rate of the robotic approach compared to open surgery in colorectal surgery [39–41].

Data in the literature show that RVR is safe and effective. Munz et al. [42], in the early 2000s, described no major complications in six patients treated robotically for rectal prolapse.

Germain et al. [35], in 2014, reported a morbidity rate of 1.7% after seventy-seven RVR. They did not reach statistical significance in the complication rate between elderly and young patients [35]. Recently, van Iersel et al. [43], in a large meta-analysis of twenty-seven studies, outlines post-operative morbidity ranging from 4.5% to 11% for the RVR reports, compared to the 0% to 23.5 that occurred in the LVR series. Bao et al. have recently documented a significant decrease in post-operative complications by 0.45 (95% confidence interval (CI), 0.24–0.83, $p = 0.009$) in the RVR group compared to the LVR group, with eight studies included in their metanalysis [38].

Robotic surgery is often criticized regarding the lack of tactile feedback during the manipulation of the anatomical structures, resulting in uncontrolled tractions leading to possible organ injuries during the procedure. In our long-lasting colorectal robotic experience, the misperception of force feedback during the dissection of the rectum from the sacral promontory and beyond is overcome thanks to increased visual feedback, which helps to recognize the anatomical landmarks better, facilitating the dissection and the respect of the hypogastric nerves, presacral venous plexus, and ureters. Moreover, the fixed third arm used for retraction permits a stable exposition of the surgical field, allowing a fine dissection throughout the operation. These features optimize the dissection along the embryological planes, as occur during total mesorectal excision.

Robotic surgery is associated with higher hospital costs compared to the laparoscopic technique. Several studies have shown how robotic surgery is related to higher costs than laparoscopy in rectal prolapse surgical treatment [44,45].

However, a recent study shows how RVR's expenditure is almost comparable to that of the laparoscopic approach after adjusting the costs for improved health-related quality of life [46]. Moreover, in their recent series, Albayati et al. [22] show a shorter length of hospital stay after RVR, which is a common finding after robotic surgery, thus increasing the cost-effectiveness and decreasing the overall expenditure of robotic surgery procedures [47]. The shorter length of stay could offset higher equipment expenditure and theatre costs related to robotic surgery, with faster recovery probably related to reduced pain, bleeding, and complications due to a more precise pelvic dissection [36].

3.2. Functional Outcomes

Ventral mesh rectopexy is associated with lower constipation and fecal incontinence than other trans-abdominal or perineal procedures [48,49].

This technique was initially ideated to reduce post-operative constipation related to the posterolateral detachment of the rectum, thus minimizing autonomic nerve injuries [9].

A limited anterior rectal dissection is associated with a minimal risk of damaging the parasympathetic fibers of the hypogastric plexus, with a reduced rate of post-operative functional impairments, as demonstrated in several studies [50].

De Hoog et al. [51] report a median Cleveland clinic constipation score (CCCS) gain of 3.2 points after RVR. This series reports no statistical difference in the functional outcomes (CCCS, Wexner Incontinence Score, Impact on daily life-score IDL) between the open, laparoscopic, and robotic approaches. Similar results are reported by other studies [19,42,44].

A recent clinical trial by Mehmood et al. [26] shows how the post-operative Wexner incontinence score is significantly lower in the RVR group compared to the laparoscopic group. Furthermore, they report that the Short Form Health Survey 36 (SF-36) questionnaires reach higher scoring with the robotic approach compared to laparoscopy [26]. Additionally, Mantoo et al. [33] report a significant improvement for obstructed defecation after RVR. These data, however, were not confirmed by a recent metanalysis that showed lower mean Wexner and fecal incontinence scores in the RVR group but without reaching statistical significance [38].

In fact, the small size of pooled data and the short duration of follow-up reported in those studies make it difficult to derive any conclusion from the available literature.

Moreover, patients' heterogeneity, different standards of outcome detection, and the lack of a systematic approach adopted for most studies need to be considered when analyzing these results.

3.3. Recurrences

Ventral mesh rectopexy shows similar recurrence rates and less functional post-operative complications than other abdominal approaches for rectal prolapse [48,49,52]. According to current data, the recurrence rate following RVR ranges between 0% up to 20% compared to 0% to 26.7% with the laparoscopic approach, never reaching statistical significance [22,43]. The use of a mesh to lift the middle compartment of the pelvis has been subject to discussion in recent years [53]. However, recent studies report a low rate of mesh-related complications, with mesh erosion percentage raging up to 4% of complications following ventral mesh rectopexy [54,55]. There are many different types of mesh available to use, generally divided into synthetic and biological. Synthetics are usually lightweight or heavyweight polypropylene mesh, with polyester and expanded polytetrafluoroethylene not being recommended due to a high rate of post-operative recurrence [24,31].

Biological meshes have been developed to reduce the risk of mesh erosion and infection thanks to the time-related deterioration with the regeneration of host tissue. Conversely, the degradation of the material may be associated with a higher percentage of recurrence. However, current data do not show a significant difference in both mesh-related complications and recurrence rate between the synthetic and biological grafts, suggesting the use of the latter in high-risk patients (diabetics, smokers, with previous pelvic radiation, with inflammatory bowel disease, with intraoperative finding of rectum or vaginal leak) [43,55,56].

Again, no consistent and robust long-term data are available to draw firm conclusions.

4. Conclusions

Robotic surgery is a safe and feasible approach for the treatment of rectal prolapse that may potentially lower complication rates and length of hospital stay, as well as shorten the learning curve thanks to its technological features. Consistent long-term prospective or randomized data are needed on recurrence and functional improvement of robotic surgical treatment of rectal prolapse compared to laparoscopic rectopexy.

Author Contributions: Conceptualization, G.F., L.F., E.O. and P.P.B.; methodology, L.F., E.O. and P.P.B.; draft preparation, L.F., S.G., A.S., A.P.C., E.O. and P.P.B.; validation, G.F., L.F., E.O. and P.P.B. All authors have read and agreed to the published version of the manuscript.

Funding: The authors received no funding or financial support for the research.

Institutional Review Board Statement: Not applicable.

Informed Consent Statement: Not applicable.

Data Availability Statement: Not applicable.

Conflicts of Interest: Giampaolo Formisano, Luca Ferraro, Adelona Salaj, Simona Giuratrabbocchetta, Enrico Opocher, and Andrea Pisani have no conflicts of interest or financial ties to disclose. Paolo Pietro Bianchi is a proctor for Intuitive Surgical Inc.

References

1. Wijffels, N.A.; Collinson, R.; Cunningham, C.; Lindsey, I. What is the natural history of internal rectal prolapse? *Color. Dis.* **2009**, *12*, 822–830. [CrossRef] [PubMed]
2. Karas, J.R.; Uranues, S.; Altomare, D.F.; Sokmen, S.; Krivokapic, Z.; Hoch, J.; Bartha, I.; Bergamaschi, R. No Rectopexy Versus Rectopexy Following Rectal Mobilization for Full-Thickness Rectal Prolapse: A Randomized Controlled Trial. *Dis. Colon Rectum* **2011**, *54*, 29–34. [CrossRef] [PubMed]
3. Cutait, D. Sacro-promontory fixation of the rectum for complete rectal prolapse. *Proc. R Soc. Med.* **1959**, *52*, 105.
4. Hrabe, J.; Gurland, B. Optimizing Treatment for Rectal Prolapse. *Clin. Colon Rectal Surg.* **2016**, *29*, 271–276. [CrossRef] [PubMed]

5. Novell, J.R.; Osborne, M.J.; Winslet, M.C.; Lewis, A.A. Prospective randomized trial of Ivalon sponge versus sutured rectopexy for full-thickness rectal prolapse. *Br. J. Surg.* **1994**, *81*, 904–906. [CrossRef] [PubMed]
6. Senapati, A.; Gray, R.; Middleton, L.J.; Harding, J.; Hills, R.; Armitage, N.C.M.; Buckley, L.; Northover, J.M.A. The PROSPER Collaborative Group PROSPER: A randomised comparison of surgical treatments for rectal prolapse. *Color. Dis.* **2013**, *15*, 858–868. [CrossRef]
7. Luukkonen, P.; Mikkonen, U. Abdominal rectopexy with sigmoidectomy vs. rectopexy alone for rectal prolapse: A prospective, randomized study. *Int. J. Color. Dis.* **1992**, *7*, 219–222. [CrossRef]
8. McKee, R.; Lauder, J.; Poon, F. A prospective randomized study of abdominal rectopexy with and without sig-moidectomy in rectal prolapse. *Surg. Gynecol. Obs.* **1992**, *174*, 148.
9. D'Hoore, A.; Cadoni, R.; Penninckx, F. Long-term outcome of laparoscopic ventral rectopexy for total rectal prolapse. *BJS* **2004**, *91*, 1500–1505. [CrossRef]
10. Varma, J.S. Autonomic influences on colorectal motility and pelvic surgery. *World J. Surg.* **1992**, *16*, 811–819. [CrossRef]
11. El Muhtaseb, M.S.; Bartolo, D.C.; Zayiae, D.; Salem, T. Colonic transit before and after resection rectopexy for full-thickness rectal prolapse. *Tech. Coloproctol.* **2014**, *18*, 273–276. [CrossRef]
12. Kim, D.-S.; Tsang, C.B.S.; Wong, D.W.; Lowry, A.C.; Goldberg, S.M.; Madoff, R.D. Complete rectal prolapse. *Dis. Colon Rectum* **1999**, *42*, 460–466. [CrossRef]
13. Kairaluoma, M.V.; Viljakka, M.T.; Kellokumpu, I.H. Open vs. Laparoscopic Surgery for Rectal Prolapse. *Dis. Colon Rectum* **2003**, *46*, 353–360. [CrossRef]
14. Kariv, Y.; Delaney, C.P.; Casillas, S.; Hammel, J.; Nocero, J.; Bast, J.; Brady, K.; Fazio, V.W.; Senagore, A.J. Long-term outcome after laparoscopic and open surgery for rectal prolapse. *Surg. Endosc.* **2005**, *20*, 35–42. [CrossRef] [PubMed]
15. Purkayastha, S.; Tekkis, P.; Athanasiou, T.; Aziz, O.; Paraskevas, P.; Ziprin, P.; Darzi, A. A Comparison of Open vs. Laparoscopic Abdominal Rectopexy for Full-Thickness Rectal Prolapse: A Meta-Analysis. *Dis. Colon Rectum* **2005**, *48*, 1930–1940. [CrossRef] [PubMed]
16. Kessler, H.; Hohenberger, W. Laparoscopic Resection Rectopexy for Rectal Prolapse. *Dis. Colon Rectum* **2005**, *48*, 1800–1801. [CrossRef]
17. Solomon, M.J.; Young, C.J.; Eyers, A.; Roberts, R.A. Randomized clinical trial of laparoscopic versus open abdominal rectopexy for rectal prolapse. *BJS* **2002**, *89*, 35–39. [CrossRef] [PubMed]
18. Sajid, M.S. Open versus laparoscopic repair of fullthickness rectal prolapse: A re-meta-analysis. *Colorectal Dis.* **2010**, *12*, 515–525. [CrossRef]
19. Ayav, A.; Bresler, L.; Hubert, J.; Brunaud, L.; Boissel, P. Robotic-assisted pelvic organ prolapse surgery. *Surg. Endosc.* **2005**, *19*, 1200–1203. [CrossRef]
20. Trastulli, S.; Cirocchi, R.; Desiderio, J.; Coratti, A.; Guarino, S.; Renzi, C.; Corsi, A.; Boselli, C.; Santoro, A.; Minelli, L.; et al. Robotic versus Laparoscopic Approach in Colonic Resections for Cancer and Benign Diseases: Systematic Review and Meta-Analysis. *PLoS ONE* **2015**, *10*, e0134062. [CrossRef] [PubMed]
21. Formisano, G.; Esposito, S.; Coratti, F.; Giuliani, G.; Salaj, A.; Bianchi, P.P. Structured training program in colorectal surgery: The robotic surgeon as a new paradigm. *Minerva Chir.* **2019**, *74*, 170–175. [CrossRef]
22. Albayati, S.; Chen, P.; Morgan, M.J.; Toh, J.W.T. Robotic vs. laparoscopic ventral mesh rectopexy for external rectal prolapse and rectal intussusception: A systematic review. *Tech. Coloproctol.* **2019**, *23*, 529–535. [CrossRef] [PubMed]
23. Faucheron, J.-L.; Trilling, B.; Girard, E.; Sage, P.-Y.; Barbois, S.; Reche, F. Anterior rectopexy for full-thickness rectal prolapse: Technical and functional results. *World J. Gastroenterol.* **2015**, *21*, 5049–5055. [CrossRef]
24. Van Der Schans, E.M.; Paulides, T.J.C.; Wijffels, N.A.; Consten, E.C.J. Management of patients with rectal prolapse: The 2017 Dutch guidelines. *Tech. Coloproctol.* **2018**, *22*, 589–596. [CrossRef] [PubMed]
25. Ruurda, J.P.; Visser, P.L.; Broeders, I.A. Analysis of procedure time in robot-assisted surgery: Comparative study in laparo-scopic cholecystectomy. *Comput. Aided. Surg.* **2003**, *8*, 24–29. [CrossRef] [PubMed]
26. Mehmood, R.K.; Parker, J.; Bhuvimanie, L.; Qasem, E.; Mohammed, A.A.; Zeeshan, M.; Grugel, K.; Carter, P.; Ahmed, S. Short-term outcome of laparoscopic versus robotic ventral mesh rectopexy for full-thickness rectal prolapse. Is robotic superior? *Int. J. Color. Dis.* **2014**, *29*, 1113–1118. [CrossRef]
27. Gurland, B. Ventral Mesh Rectopexy. *Dis. Colon Rectum* **2014**, *57*, 1446–1447. [CrossRef]
28. Ramage, L.; Georgiou, P.; Tekkis, P.; Tan, E. Is robotic ventral mesh rectopexy better than laparoscopy in the treatment of rectal prolapse and obstructed defecation? A meta-analysis. *Tech. Coloproctol.* **2015**, *19*, 381–389. [CrossRef]
29. Faucheron, J.-L.; Trilling, B.; Barbois, S.; Sage, P.-Y.; Waroquet, P.-A.; Reche, F. Day case robotic ventral rectopexy compared with day case laparoscopic ventral rectopexy: A prospective study. *Tech. Coloproctol.* **2016**, *20*, 695–700. [CrossRef] [PubMed]
30. Mäkelä-Kaikkonen, J.; Rautio, T.; Pääkkö, E.; Biancari, F.; Ohtonen, P.; Mäkelä, J. Robot-assisted versus laparoscopic ventral rectopexy for external, internal rectal prolapse and enterocele: A randomised controlled trial. *Color. Dis.* **2016**, *18*, 1010–1015. [CrossRef]
31. MacKenzie, H.; Dixon, A.R. Proficiency gain curve and predictors of outcome for laparoscopic ventral mesh rectopexy. *Surgery* **2014**, *156*, 158–167. [CrossRef]

32. Mäkelä-Kaikkonen, J.; Rautio, T.; Klintrup, K.; Takala, H.; Vierimaa, M.; Ohtonen, P.; Mäkelä, J. Robotic-assisted and laparoscopic ventral rectopexy in the treatment of rectal prolapse: A matched-pairs study of operative details and complications. *Tech. Coloproctol.* **2013**, *18*, 151–155. [CrossRef] [PubMed]
33. Mantoo, S.; Podevin, J.; Regenet, N.; Rigaud, J.; Lehur, P.-A.; Meurette, G. Is robotic-assisted ventral mesh rectopexy superior to laparoscopic ventral mesh rectopexy in the management of obstructed defaecation? *Color. Dis.* **2013**, *15*, e469–e475. [CrossRef] [PubMed]
34. Moghadamyeghaneh, Z.; Hanna, M.H.; Hwang, G.; Carmichael, J.C.; Mills, S.D.; Pigazzi, A.; Stamos, M.J. Surgical management of rectal prolapse: The role of robotic surgery. *World J. Surg. Proced.* **2015**, *5*, 99–105. [CrossRef]
35. Germain, A.; Perrenot, C.; Scherrer, M.-L.; Ayav, C.; Brunaud, L.; Ayav, A.; Bresler, L. Long-term outcome of robotic-assisted laparoscopic rectopexy for full-thickness rectal prolapse in elderly patients. *Color. Dis.* **2014**, *16*, 198–202. [CrossRef]
36. Flynn, J.; Larach, J.T.; Kong, J.C.H.; Warrier, S.K.; Heriot, A. Robotic versus laparoscopic ventral mesh rectopexy: A systematic review and meta-analysis. *Int. J. Color. Dis.* **2021**, 1–11. [CrossRef]
37. Rondelli, F.; Bugiantella, W.; Villa, F.; Sanguinetti, A.; Boni, M.; Mariani, E.; Avenia, N. Robot-assisted or conventional laparoscoic rectopexy for rectal prolapse? Systematic review and meta-analysis. *Int. J. Surg.* **2014**, *12*, S153–S159. [CrossRef]
38. Bao, X.; Wang, H.; Song, W.; Chen, Y.; Luo, Y. Meta-analysis on current status, efficacy, and safety of laparoscopic and robotic ventral mesh rectopexy for rectal prolapse treatment: Can robotic surgery become the gold standard? *Int. J. Color. Dis.* **2021**, 1–10. [CrossRef]
39. Prete, F.; Pezzolla, A.; Prete, F.; Testini, M.; Marzaioli, R.; Patriti, A.; Jimenez-Rodriguez, R.M.; Gurrado, A.; Strippoli, G.F.M. Robotic Versus Laparoscopic Minimally Invasive Surgery for Rectal Cancer. *Ann. Surg.* **2018**, *267*, 1034–1046. [CrossRef]
40. Bhama, A.R.; Obias, V.; Welch, K.B.; Vandewarker, J.F.; Cleary, R.K. A comparison of laparoscopic and robotic colorectal surgery outcomes using the American College of Surgeons National Surgical Quality Improvement Program (ACS NSQIP) database. *Surg. Endosc.* **2015**, *30*, 1576–1584. [CrossRef]
41. Formisano, G.; Giuliani, G.; Salaj, A.; Salvischiani, L.; Ferraro, L.; De Luca, M.; Bianchi, P.P. Robotic elective colectomy for diverticular disease: Short-term outcomes of 80 patients. *Int. J. Med Robot. Comput. Assist. Surg.* **2021**, *17*. [CrossRef]
42. Munz, Y.; Moorthy, K.; Kudchadkar, R.; Hernandez, J.; Martin, S.; Darzi, A.; Rockall, T. Robotic assisted rectopexy. *Am. J. Surg.* **2004**, *187*, 88–92. [CrossRef] [PubMed]
43. Van Iersel, J.J.; Paulides, T.J.C.; Verheijen, P.M.; Lumley, J.W.; Broeders, I.; Consten, E.C.J. Current status of laparoscopic and robotic ventral mesh rectopexy for external and internal rectal prolapse. *World J. Gastroenterol.* **2016**, *22*, 4977–4987. [CrossRef]
44. Heemskerk, J.; De Hoog, D.E.; Van Gemert, W.G.; Baeten, C.G.; Greve, J.W.; Bouvy, N.D. Robot-assisted vs. conventional laparo-scopic rectopexy for rectal prolapse: A comparative study on costs and time. *Dis. Colon Rectum.* **2007**, *50*, 1825–1830. [CrossRef] [PubMed]
45. Perrenot, C.; Germain, A.; Scherrer, M.-L.; Ayav, A.; Brunaud, L.; Bresler, L. Long-term Outcomes of Robot-assisted Laparoscopic Rectopexy for Rectal Prolapse. *Dis. Colon Rectum.* **2013**, *56*, 909–914. [CrossRef]
46. Mäkelä-Kaikkonen, J.; Rautio, T.; Ohinmaa, A.; Koivurova, S.; Ohtonen, P.; Sintonen, H.; Mäkelä, J. Cost-analysis and quality of life after laparoscopic and robotic ventral mesh rectopexy for posterior compartment prolapse: A randomized trial. *Tech. Coloproctol.* **2019**, *23*, 461–470. [CrossRef]
47. Salman, M.; Bell, T.; Martin, J.; Bhuva, K.; Grim, R.; Ahuja, V. Use, cost, complications, and mortality of robotic versus non-robotic general surgery procedures based on a nationwide database. *Am. Surg.* **2013**, *79*, 553–560. [CrossRef]
48. Madiba, T.E.; Baig, M.K.; Wexner, S.D. Surgical Management of Rectal Prolapse. *Arch. Surg.* **2005**, *140*, 63–73. [CrossRef]
49. Cadeddu, F.; Sileri, P.; Grande, M.; De Luca, E.; Franceschilli, L.; Milito, G. Focus on abdominal rectopexy for full-thickness rectal prolapse: Meta-analysis of literature. *Tech. Coloproctol.* **2011**, *16*, 37–53. [CrossRef]
50. Speakman, C.T.M.; Madden, M.V.; Nicholls, R.J.; Kamm, M.A. Lateral ligament division during rectopexy causes constipation but prevents recurrence: Results of a prospective randomized study. *BJS* **2005**, *78*, 1431–1433. [CrossRef] [PubMed]
51. De Hoog, D.E.; Heemskerk, J.; Nieman, F.H.; Van Gemert, W.G.; Baeten, C.G.; Bouvy, N.D. Recurrence and functional results after open versus conventional laparoscopic versus robot-assisted laparoscopic rectopexy for rectal prolapse: A case-control study. *Int. J. Colorectal Dis.* **2009**, *24*, 1201–1206. [CrossRef] [PubMed]
52. Gosselink, M.P.; Adusumilli, S.; Gorissen, K.J.; Fourie, S.; Tuynman, J.B.; Jones, O.M.; Cunningham, C.; Lindsey, I. Laparoscopic ventralrectopexy for fecal incontinence associated with high-grade internal rectal prolapse. *Dis. Colon Rectum.* **2013**, *56*, 1409–1414. [CrossRef] [PubMed]
53. Food and Drug Administration. FDA Safety Communication: Urogynecologic Surgical Mesh: Update on the Safety and Effectiveness of Transvaginal Placement for Pelvic Organ Prolapse. *Rev. Lit. Arts Am.* **2011**. Available online: URL:http://www.fda.gov/downloads/medicaldevices/safety/alertsandnotices/ucm262760.pdf (accessed on 6 April 2016).
54. Smart, N.; Pathak, S.; Boorman, P.; Daniels, I.R. Synthetic or biological mesh use in laparoscopic ventral mesh rectopexy—A systematic review. *Color. Dis.* **2013**, *15*, 650–654. [CrossRef]
55. Evans, C.; Stevenson, A.R.L.; Sileri, P.; Mercer-Jones, M.A.; Dixon, A.R.; Cunningham, C.; Jones, O.M.; Lindsey, I. A Multicenter Collaboration to Assess the Safety of Laparoscopic Ventral Rectopexy. *Dis. Colon Rectum* **2015**, *58*, 799–807. [CrossRef] [PubMed]
56. Mercer-Jones, M.A.; D'Hoore, A.; Dixon, A.R.; Lehur, P.; Lindsey, I.; Mellgren, A.; Stevenson, A.R.L. Consensus on ventral rectopexy: Report of a panel of experts. *Color. Dis.* **2014**, *16*, 82–88. [CrossRef] [PubMed]

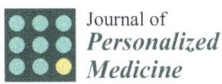

Journal of Personalized Medicine

Review

Review on Perioperative and Oncological Outcomes of Robotic Gastrectomy for Cancer

Giuseppe Giuliani *, Francesco Guerra, Lorenzo De Franco, Lucia Salvischiani, Roberto Benigni and Andrea Coratti

USL Toscana Sud Est, Misericordia Hospital, 58100 Grosseto, Italy; francesco.guerra@uslsudest.toscana.it (F.G.); lorenzogiacinto.defranco@uslsudest.toscana.it (L.D.F.); lucia.salvischiani@uslsudest.toscana.it (L.S.); roberto.benigni@uslsudest.toscana.it (R.B.); andrea.coratti@uslsudest.toscana.it (A.C.)
* Correspondence: giuseppe.giuliani@uslsudest.toscana.it

Abstract: Background. Minimally invasive gastrectomy is currently considered a valid option to treat gastric cancer and is gaining increasing acceptance. Recent reports have suggested that the application of robots may confer some advantages over conventional laparoscopy, but the role of robotic surgery in clinical practice is still uncertain. We aimed to critically review the relevant evidence comparing robotic to standard laparoscopic surgery in performing radical gastrectomy. Methods. The Pubmed/Medline electronic databases were searched through February 2021. Paper conference and the English language was the only restriction applied to our search strategy. Results. According to the existing data, robotic gastrectomy seems to provide some benefits in terms of blood loss, rate of conversion, procedure-specific postoperative morbidity, and length of hospital stay. Robotic gastrectomy is also associated with a longer duration of surgery and a higher economic burden as compared to its laparoscopic counterpart. No significant differences have been disclosed in terms of long-term survivals, while the number of lymph nodes retrieved with robotic gastrectomy is generally higher than that of laparoscopy. Conclusions. The current literature suggests that robotic radical gastrectomy appears as competent as the conventional laparoscopic procedure and may provide some clinical advantages. However, due to the relative paucity of high-level evidence, it is not possible to draw definitive conclusions.

Keywords: minimally invasive gastrectomy; robotic gastrectomy; laparoscopic gastrectomy; gastric cancer

1. Introduction

The employment of laparoscopic techniques in gastric surgery has diffused and evolved rapidly over the last two decades [1–3]. Minimally Invasive Gastrectomy (MIG) is now almost universally accepted as a valid option for the treatment of gastric cancer (GC) as it optimizes postoperative recovery without compromising the adequacy of resection and long-term oncological outcomes [1–6]. Recent NCCN guidelines (version 2.2021) for GC treatment indicate that MIG (including both conventional laparoscopic and robotic techniques) may be considered, for early and locally advanced cases, provided specific expertise in minimally invasive foregut procedures and lymphadenectomy are available [1–3,5–9].

The technical difficulties of laparoscopic surgery that are encountered in performing MIG have led some surgical teams to the use of robotic surgery [10,11]. Indeed, robotics has been originally introduced in clinical practice to overcome some of the intrinsic limitations of conventional laparoscopic and to broaden the range of application of minimally invasive surgery, and also in the field of the surgery of the stomach, several experiences have indicated excellent outcomes [3,5–9]. A recent study by Stewart et al. have investigated the adoption of robotic surgery in surgical oncology by analyzing the available data from the National Inpatient Sample (NIS) American database [12]. The authors showed that over 5 years (2010–2014), there was a 5-fold increase in the application of robotic surgery.

Of note, the application of robotic gastrectomy (RG) increased from 2% in 2010 to 6% in 2014. However, robotic surgery of the stomach is still in its early stages and its actual role in clinical practice is still to be defined [13,14]. Current evidence essentially indicates non-inferiority of RG to standard Laparoscopic Gastrectomy (LG), but general conclusions on whether RG provides clear advantages over LG are still difficult to draw, as available data is mainly derived from low-level analyses returning highly variable results [15–18]. Accordingly, this paper aims to analyze the existing evidence on RG for cancer with special emphasis on comparing the employ of robotic technology to conventional LG.

2. Methods

Institutional review board approval and written consent were not needed for this paper. The last version of PRISMA Statement (Ref) checklist for reporting systematic reviews and meta-analysis, was used as guide to aggregate the available scientific papers comparing RG and LG [19].

Two authors (GG, FG) performed an independent literature search up to APRIL 2021. The PubMed/MEDLINE electronic databases were queried with the following search strings: "robot-assisted surgery" and "laparoscopic" and "gastric cancer" or "gastric neoplasm" and "gastrectomy" or "gastric resection". All article typologies were considered eligible except for conference proceedings, case reports, and small series with less than ten patients. Reviews, meta-analyses, and original articles were included in our analysis based on the following features: novelty, caseload, topic, impact, and availability of raw data. Our search criteria were also restricted to the English language. Independently, the two authors screened titles and abstracts of the retrieved records. Full-text versions of the papers deemed suitable for inclusion were appraised, and relative references were screened to identify additional, eligible articles. Differences in opinion were discussed with the input of a third author (DFL).

Suitable studies were thus evaluated and pooled in the review if the following criteria were met:

- inclusion of adult patients undergoing robotic or laparoscopic total or distal gastrectomy for gastric cancer;
- robotic and standard laparoscopic approach comparator intervention;
- data on perioperative, post-operative, and oncological outcomes.

Continuous data are presented as mean ± standard deviation, whereas categorical data are expressed as absolute numbers and percentages.

3. Results

Our initial electronic search yielded 740 titles. Titles and abstracts were evaluated, and duplicate records were excluded. Full texts with relative bibliographies were thus appraised, and a total of 21 studies were eventually deemed suitable for inclusion and data extraction [4–6,8,13,15,17,18,20–32]. The selection process is given in Figure 1, while Table 1 describes the general characteristics of the included studies. There were 2 randomized controlled trial, 2 prospective study, 4 meta-analysis, 13 retrospective analyses.

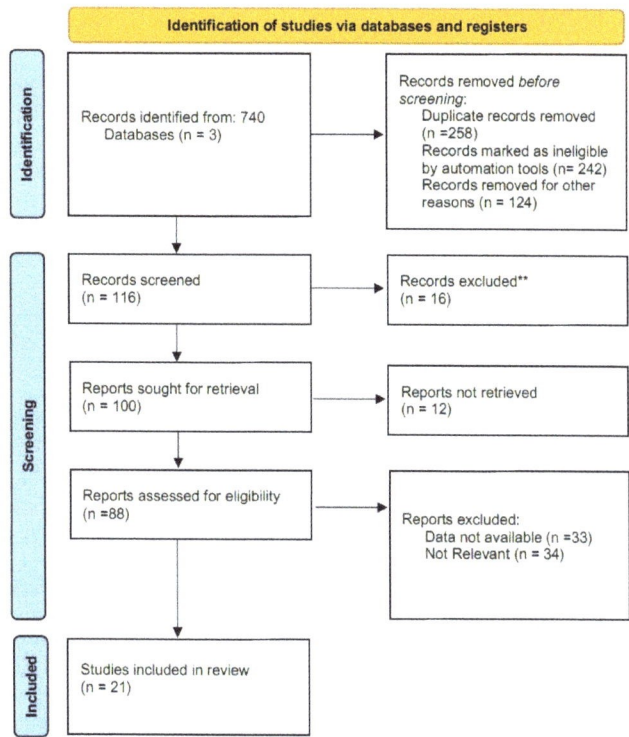

Figure 1. Search Strategy: Page MJ, McKenzie JE, Bossuyt PM, Boutron I, Hoffmann TC, Mulrow CD, et al. The PRISMA. 2020 statement: an updated guideline for reporting systematic reviews. *BMJ* **2021**, *372*, n71, doi:10.1136/bmj.n71.

Table 1. General characteristics of the included studies.

Author	Year	Study	Origin	Approach	n. Patients	Type of Resection
Kim HI et al.	2016	Prospective	Korea	LG/RG	434	TG/DG/PPG/PG
Chen K et al.	2017	Mata–Analysis	China	LG/RG	5953	TG/DG/PG
Pan HF et al.	2017	RCT	China	LG/RG	163	TG/DG/PG
Hendriksen BS et al.	2018	Retrospective	USA	LG/RG/OG	17.449	TG/ DG
Liu H et al.	2019	Retrospective	China	LG/RG	20	DG
Wang WJ et al.	2018	Retrospective	China	LG/RG	527	TG/DG
Uyama I et al.	2018	Prospective	Japan	RG	326	TG/DG/PG
Gao, Y Q et al.	2019	Retrospective	China	LG/RG	502	TG/DG/PG
Bobo Z et al.	2019	Mata–Analysis	China	LG/RG	4576	TG/DG
Hikage M et al.	2020	Retrospective	Japan	LG/RG	1208	TG / DG/PPG/PG
Guerrini GP et al.	2020	Mata–Analysis	Italy	LG/RG	17.712	TG/DG/PPG/PG
Yang P. et al.	2020	Mata–Analysis	China	LG/RG	4142	TG/DG
Li ZY et al.	2020	Retrospective	China	LG/RG	1476	DG
Alhossaini RM et al.	2020	Retrospective	Korea	LG/RG	55	CG
Bolger JC et al.	2021	Retrospective	Ireland	LG	258	TG/DG
Shin HJ et al.	2021	Retrospective	Korea	LG / RG	2084	TG/ DG
Nakauchi M et al.	2021	Retrospective	USA	LG/RG/OG	845	TG/DG/PG
Lu J et al.	2021	RCT	China	LG/RG	300	DG
Tian Y et al.	2021	Retrospective	China	LG/RG	1686	TG/DG
Kinoshita T et al.	2021	Retrospective	Japan	LG/RG	1172	TG/DG/PPG/PG
Choi S et al.	2021	Retrospective	Korea	LG/RG/OG	185	TG/DG

TG: Total Gastrectomy; RCT: Randomized Controlled Trial; DG: Distal Gastrectomy; PG: Proximal Gastrectomy; PPG: pylorus-preserving gastrectomy; CG: Completion Gastrectomy.

3.1. Perioperative Details

Regardless of the type of procedure, one of the main limitations of robotic surgery is operative time [12,18,19]. Several studies, including several meta-analyses, indicate that the duration of surgery for RG is invariably higher than for LG, for both total and distal gastrectomy [4,5,12,16,18–20]. However, such difference seems to be attenuated by the progress of specific experience with the technique. A recent study by Nakauchi et al., from the Memorial Sloan Kettering Cancer Center, reporting their experience with radical gastrectomy over 10 years. The authors started performing RG after an extensive experience with conventional LG. Interestingly, and in contrast with the majority of previous reports, the analysis of intraoperative outcomes showed that RG had a shorter operative time compared to LG [21].

Published studies comparing RG to LG almost regularly indicate that patients receiving MIG with the robot have reduced perioperative Estimated Blood Loss (EBL). High-level randomized studies mirror this evidence, which is in turn, consistent with recent meta-analyses appraising the issue [12,17,22].

Unplanned conversion into an open procedure has been conventionally utilized to evaluate the proficiency of minimally invasive surgery. A lower conversion rate has been reported as a theoretical advantage of robotic surgery over conventional laparoscopic surgery [33,34]. Emerging data from a recent meta-analysis, including 40 retrospective studies and 17.712 patients, demonstrated no statistical difference in conversion rate between RG and LG. [13]

However, a retrospective study comparing robotic and laparoscopic approaches for radical gastrectomy including 311 MIG, over ten-year experience from the Memorial Sloan Kettering Cancer Center, showed that RG had fewer conversion rate compared to LG (25.8% vs. 39.7%; $p = 0.010$) [21].

Compared to the laparoscopic approach, three-dimensional view, wrist movements and the stable traction of the robotic instruments provide a delicate and fine dissection that might explain the reduction of EBL as well as the trend of a lower conversion rate of RG.

3.2. Postoperative Outcomes

Currently, the only available RCTs comparing LG and RG are those published by Pan et al. [23] and Lu et al. [24]. Some 163 patients who underwent MIG with curative intent for AGC were included in the trial published in 2017 by Pan et al. RG was associated with significantly reduced blood losses and a higher number of yielded lymph nodes [23]. As for postoperative outcomes, patients in the RG group experienced significantly less postoperative pain and had an earlier functional recovery, including abbreviated length of hospital stay as compared to the LG group. On the other hand, the rate of postoperative complications favored RG over LG, but this difference did not disclose any statistical significance.

In the more recent trial by Lu et al., the authors compared the outcomes of patients receiving distal gastrectomy by surgeons with large expertise in MIG (>300 LG and 50 RG before trial initiation) [24]. In this trial, a total of 141 and 142 well-balanced patients were assigned to the RG group and the LG group, respectively. While no significant difference in the length of postoperative hospital stay was registered, interestingly, the overall incidence of postoperative morbidity was significantly lower for RG as compared to LG, mostly in terms of medical complications. Multivariate analysis demonstrated that RG was an independent protective factor for postoperative complications. The RG and LG groups did not differ significantly on the number of examined lymph nodes. However, the number of extra-perigastric stations (7–9, 11p and 12 a) was significantly higher following RG than LG, and the percentages of procedures resulting in lymph node noncompliance (defined as the absence of lymph nodes from more than one lymph node required station) was significantly lower for RG than LG (24.8% vs. 40.1%), mainly owing to different results for the extraperigastric regions.

A growing number of further, nonrandomized recent reports have suggested potential advantages of RG over LG in terms of postoperative complications [7,24–27]. Interestingly, such benefits seem to be enhanced in the setting of more technically demanding procedures, such as total and proximal MIG, completion of total gastrectomy for remnant gastric cancer, and MIG in patients who are obese or who present with advanced disease [5,13,26,28–30].

Kinoshita et al. very recently, published the results of an interesting retrospective, single-institutional, case-controlled study including nearly 1200 patients receiving MIG with either a robotic or conventional laparoscopic approach [26]. All included patients had primary, stage I-III gastric malignancy. All types of MIG were considered in the analysis, including a relatively high percentage of total gastrectomy (15–26%) and proximal gastrectomy (11–15%). Overall, although the two groups were well-matched in terms of general baseline characteristics, in the RG group there were more patients with advanced disease (clinical stage III) and there was a higher proportion of patients receiving total or proximal gastrectomy as compared to the LG group. Despite this, patients in the RG group had a significantly lower incidence of postoperative Clavien-Dindo grade II and III complications than those in the LG group [35]. A multivariate analysis of factors affecting postoperative morbidity, a robotic approach was significantly associated with reduced incidence of complications.

Alhossaini and colleagues retrospectively reviewed the outcomes of 55 patients who received minimally invasive completion gastrectomy for malignancy arising in the gastric remnant [28]. The authors compared 30 patients who had surgery with conventional laparoscopy with those whose procedure was accomplished with the robot. Overall, no significant differences were noted between the two groups of patients, neither in terms of perioperative data nor in terms of postoperative morbidity. Of note, though this data did not reach statistical significance ($p = 0.058$), there was a 13% rate of cases of unplanned conversion into an open procedure in the LG, while all RGs were completed in a minimally invasive technique.

A recent article by Wang et al. assessed the severity and rate of incidence of postoperative complications according to the Clavien—Dindo classification system following RG and LG for AGC [29]. The authors conducted a retrospective analysis of >500 MIGs which were matched between RG and LG with the propensity score matching method. RG was associated with a larger amount of examined lymph nodes as compared to LG (mean 40.8 vs. 37.1), while no differences were found in terms of perioperative blood loss and, of note, duration of surgery. Interestingly, they found that the incidence of overall and severe (defined as grade IIIa or greater events) morbidity following RG was significantly reduced as compared to LG (24.5% vs. 18.8%, and 8.9% vs. 17.5%, respectively, $p = 0.002$). This also translated into a shorter postoperative hospitalization for RG as compared to LG. In addition, at univariate analysis, together with age, BMI, advanced disease, duration of surgery, and total gastrectomy, LG was significantly associated with a higher risk of overall and severe morbidity.

3.3. Oncological Outcomes

Concerning long-term oncological outcomes, only limited data is still available [5,6,13,15,17,27]. One of the most robust data currently available is that by Shin et al., who recently published the results of a propensity score-weighted analysis of more than 2000 patients with GC receiving MIG (either LG or RG) with curative intent [5]. After patients matching, no differences were noted on the total number of harvested lymph nodes, while that of supra-pancreatic lymph nodes were higher in the RG. Interestingly, in terms of oncological findings, there was no statistically significant difference between LG and RG neither on OSs nor in DFSs at both unweighted and weighted analyses.

Analog findings have been indicated by Li et al., who reported on the long-term oncological outcomes of RG vs. LG in the treatment of patients with locally advanced GC [27]. Their study included nearly 1200 patients whose outcomes were compared between RG and LG using one-to-one propensity score matching. The 3-year DFS rates favoured RG (76%) over LG (70%) without statistical significance ($p = 0.07$). As for 3-year OS, there was a nonsignificant benefit following RG (77%) as compared to LG (73%).

Some of reviews have also investigated potential differences between RG and conventional LG, without identifying any significant advantage of one technique over the other [13,14,17]. The latest meta-analysis comparing the oncological outcomes of RG vs. LG has been published by Yang et al. and colleagues and combines the data reported in 11 articles including a total of nearly 4100 patients [17]. Overall, there was a nonsignificant OR of 0.98 and 0.53 favoring RG over LG in terms of 3-year and 5-year OS, respectively. Similarly, data on recurrences indicated that the two groups of treatment did not differ significantly (OR = 0.88).

It is well-known that the number of harvested lymph nodes and surgical margins are currently considered as most appropriate indicators of oncologically adequate resections [13]. Most comparisons between RG and LG, indicate that the median amount of lymph nodes harvested is higher during RG than LG [18,21,24,25,30]. The currently two available randomized trials upon the argument, as already mentioned, support an advantage of RG over LG on lymphadenectomy [23,24]. Other observational reports and several recent meta-analyses echo such findings [8,13,14,25,30], also in obese patients. Choi et al. recently published a study that compared short and long terms outcomes of open, laparoscopic, and robotic radical gastrectomy with D2 lymphadenectomy in obese patients. Among 185 patients with a median BMI of 26.5 kg/m^2, there were 69 open, 62 laparoscopic, and 54 robotic procedures. RG resulted in a greater mean number of retrieved lymph nodes, and a higher rate of lymph nodes harvest compliance compared to LG and OG.

With the purpose to evaluate the impact of MIS on survival in the United States, Hendriksen et al. analyzed the data of >17,000 patients who underwent gastrectomy for adenocarcinoma between 2010 and 2015 [6]. Overall, after propensity score matching, MIG resulted in a significantly improved 5-year survival compared to open surgery. Interestingly, while no difference was disclosed for long-term survival between patients receiving LG vs. RG, the percentage of patients receiving adequate lymph nodes sampling was significantly higher for RG (60%) as compared to LG (51%).

However, the most recent publication by Guerrini et al. represents the largest meta-analysis currently available and combines the results of 40 retrospective studies including nearly 18,000 patients receiving either laparoscopic or robotic MIG [13]. Concerning oncological outcomes, RG demonstrated a significantly increased mean number of yielded lymph nodes as compared to LG.

3.4. Costs

In general, the economic burden of robot-assisted surgery is substantially higher than that of conventional laparoscopic surgery and previous reports consistently indicate that costs associated with RG are higher as compared to standard laparoscopic MIG [13–15,18,32]. In the above-mentioned RCT by Lu et al. a specific analysis of costs was reported. The increased cost was found in RG as compared to LG in terms of total and indirect costs [24]. Interestingly, the direct cost of RG was significantly lower than that of LG, with specific economic advantages on surgical procedures, hospitalization, laboratory and radiology tests, and perioperative transfusions.

Actually, robotic surgery is evolving rapidly, and probably a reliable evaluation of its actual economic impact on clinical practice should include some indirect aspects, most of which are not fully predictable at present [36,37]. The effect due to possible differences between RG and LG on postoperative morbidity, length of hospitalization, and incidence of unplanned conversion should be considered over time [34,36,37]. In addition, given the exponential evolution of robotic surgery, it is likely that different robotic systems will enter the market in the near future resulting in more competition and lower purchase and maintenance costs of robotic platforms [34,36–38].

4. Discussion

The studies included in our updates on robotic gastrectomy for cancer demonstrate superior surgical outcomes of RG as compared to LG, especially in terms of perioperative blood losses, rates of conversion, procedure-related postoperative morbidity, and length of hospital stay. On the other hand, the duration of surgery and costs associated with the application of robotic surgery are consistently higher than those of LG [23–25,28,30]. Finally, RG is generally associated with a greater lymph node yield, while long-term outcomes seem to be substantially comparable [5,13,14,17].

Operative time is considered one of the limitations of the robotic approach: several studies demonstrated a longer operative time for RG than for LG [4,5,13,17,20]. However, such difference seems to be attenuated by the progress of specific experience with the technique. Recently Nakauchi et al. reported their experience with radical gastrectomy over 10 years from the Memorial Sloan Kettering Cancer Center. The authors compared OG with MIG and RG with LG. Interestingly, and in contrast with the majority of previous reports, the analysis of intraoperative outcomes showed that RG had a shorter operative time compared to LG (212 vs. 240 min $p < 0.001$) [21]. They concluded that this finding may reflect their institutional experience because the authors started performing RG after an extensive experience with conventional LG (more than 100 LG).

A lower conversion rate has been reported as a theoretical advantage of robotic surgery over conventional laparoscopic surgery [33,34].

Conversion negatively impacts postoperative outcomes, may postpone the initiation of adjuvant treatments, and ultimately translate into poorer long-term survivals [33,34,39].

We recently conducted a meta-analysis of available randomized evidence comparing robotic and conventional laparoscopic surgery to identify possible differences in the rate of unplanned conversion to open surgery [34]. From twelve trials, 1867 patients undergoing surgery with curative intent for abdominal malignancy were included in the analysis. The study included 443 patients treated for gastric cancer, both distal and total gastrectomy. Overall, the rate of conversion was 4.8%, 3.1%, and 6.5% being the relative incidence for robotic and laparoscopic surgery, respectively. At meta-analysis, this difference was significant, with an OR of 0.56 favoring robotic over laparoscopic surgery ($p = 0.03$).

Robotic gastrectomy compared to the laparoscopic conventional approach is associated with a lower incidence of postoperative complications. In the RCT published by Pan et al. in 2017, this difference did not reach statistical significance [23]. Nevertheless, in the more recent trial by Lu et al., in which a total of 141 and 142 well-balanced patients were assigned to the RG group and the LG group, respectively the overall incidence of postoperative morbidity was significantly lower for RG as compared to LG, mostly in terms of medical complications. Furthermore, at multivariate analysis the authors demonstrated that RG was an independent protective factor for postoperative complications [24].

However, these findings seem to be enhanced in the setting of more technically demanding procedures, such as total and proximal gastrectomy, completion total gastrectomy for remnant gastric cancer, as well as in patients who are obese or who present with advanced disease [5,13,26–28].

Pancreatic morbidity deserves a specific consideration when specific post-operative complications after MIG are analyzed. Pancreatic injury due to intraoperative manipulation during dissection and specifically lymphadenectomy may lead to acute pancreatitis, associated or not with pancreatic fistula formation [40–42]. The real incidence of such events is probably underestimated in clinical practice and likely difficult to ascertain. Still, pancreas-related morbidity following gastrectomy should be taken into consideration in the assessment of radical MIG, owing to the potential to significantly aggravate the postoperative course of patients [40–42]. The available evidence on the incidence of pancreas-related complications following radical MIG was investigated in a specific meta-analysis conducted by our group and published in 2018 [41]. RG was compared with LG on the relative incidence of postoperative acute pancreatitis and postoperative pancreatic fistula (POPF). A slight advantage of RG over LG was disclosed, albeit with marginal statistical significance. By analyzing more than 2000 patients from 8 comparative studies, the incidence of pancreatic events following MIG was 2.2%, ranging from 0.8% to 16.2%. Despite patients in the LG tended to have higher BMI and more advanced disease, 1.7%, and 2.5% were the relative rates of pancreas-related morbidity for RG and LG, respectively. In particular, the incidence of POPF favored RG over LG (2.7% vs. 3.8%) with an OR of 0.8, albeit without statistical significance ($p = 0.69$).

Although, long-term outcomes seem to be substantially comparable after RG and LG [17,27], interestingly, Choi et al. comparing long-term oncological outcomes (with a median follow-up of 56 months) of open, laparoscopic, and robotic radical gastrectomy with D2 lymphadenectomy in obese patients, demonstrated that RG compared to OG and LG was a protective factor for recurrence-free survival at multivariable analysis [30].

This finding may reflect the greater mean number of retrieved lymph nodes that seems to be associated with the robotic approach [6,8,13,14,23–25,30]. Three-dimensional video system, wrist movements, the stable traction of the robotic instruments as well as ICG fluorescent lymphography may explain the superior lymphadenectomy performance associated with RG [43].

In conclusion, in the last years, there has been probably too much enthusiasm around the introduction of the robot in surgical practice. Actually, despite possible specific merits over conventional LG, the relative lack of high-level evidence still precludes the possibility to reach definitive conclusions [8,13,14,24]. Randomized studies are difficult to run, as most referral centers dedicated to MIG have consolidated experience either in LG or in RG, and different levels of specific expertise are likely to affect monocentric comparisons [29,34]. Actually, both laparoscopic and robotic MIG can be recommended for selected patients at centers with specific technical expertise, as they are associated with fewer morbidity while resulting in long-term outcomes which are equivalent to those of open surgery [3,4,16,21]. Available data from RCT is scarce and most retrospective reports are still biased by some confounding factors. As a consequence, the question of whether RG presents significant advantages over conventional LG for GC remains an avenue for further research.

Author Contributions: Conceptualization, G.G. and F.G.; methodology, L.D.F.; software, R.B.; validation, L.S., and A.C.; formal analysis, G.G.; investigation, F.G.; resources, L.D.F.; data curation, R.B.; writing–original draft preparation, G.G.; writing—review and editing, F.G.; visualization, L.S.; supervision, A.C. All authors have read and agreed to the published version of the manuscript.

Funding: This research received no external funding.

Institutional Review Board Statement: Not applicable.

Informed Consent Statement: Not applicable.

Conflicts of Interest: The authors declare that they have no conflict of interest in the present manuscript. No grant or other sources of funding have been received for the drawing up of this manuscript, which is not submitted or under consideration elsewhere.

References

1. Kim, H.H.; Han, S.U.; Kim, M.C.; Kim, W.; Lee, H.J.; Ryu, S.W.; Cho, G.S.; Kim, C.Y.; Yang, H.-K.; Park, D.J.; et al. Effect of laparoscopic distal gastrectomy vs open distal gastrectomy on long-term surviv-al among patients with stage I gastric cancer: The KLASS-01 randomized clinical trial. *JAMA Oncol.* **2019**, *5*, 506–513. [CrossRef]
2. Liu, F.; Huang, C.; Xu, Z.; Su, X.; Zhao, G.; Ye, J.; Du, X.; Huang, H.; Hu, J.; Li, G.; et al. Chinese Laparoscopic Gastrointestinal Surgery Study (CLASS) Group. Morbidity and Mortality of Laparoscopic vs Open Total Gastrectomy for Clinical Stage I Gastric Cancer: The CLASS02 Multicenter Randomized Clinical Trial. *JAMA Oncol.* **2020**, *6*, 1590–1597. [CrossRef]
3. Bracale, U.; Merola, G.; Pignata, G.; Andreuccetti, J.; Dolce, P.; Boni, L.; Cassinotti, E.; Olmi, S.; Uccelli, M.; Gualtierotti, M.; et al. Laparoscopic gastrectomy for stage II and III advanced gastric cancer: Long-term follow-up data from a Western multicenter retrospective study. *Surg. Endosc.* **2021**, 1–12. [CrossRef]
4. Bolger, J.C.; Al Azzawi, M.; Whooley, J.; Bolger, E.M.; Trench, L.; Allen, J.; Kelly, M.E.; Brosnan, C.; Arumugasamy, M.; Robb, W.B. Surgery by a minimally invasive approach is associated with improved textbook outcomes in oesophageal and gastric cancer. *Eur. J. Surg. Oncol.* **2021**, *17*. [CrossRef]

5. Shin, H.-J.; Son, S.-Y.; Wang, B.; Roh, C.K.; Hur, H.; Han, S.-U. Long-term Comparison of Robotic and Laparoscopic Gastrectomy for Gastric Cancer. *Ann. Surg.* **2021**, *274*, 128–137. [CrossRef] [PubMed]
6. Hendriksen, B.S.; Brooks, A.J.; Hollenbeak, C.S.; Taylor, M.D.; Reed, M.F.; Soybel, D.I. The Impact of Minimally Invasive Gastrectomy on Survival in the USA. *J. Gastrointest. Surg.* **2019**, *24*, 1000–1009. [CrossRef] [PubMed]
7. NCCN Clinical Practice Guidelines in Oncology (Version 2.2021) for Gastric Cancer. Available online: http://www.nccn.org/professionals/physician_gls/PDF/occult.pdf (accessed on 3 April 2021).
8. Hikage, M.; Fujiya, K.; Kamiya, S.; Tanizawa, Y.; Bando, E.; Notsu, A.; Mori, K.; Terashima, M. Robotic Gastrectomy Compared with Laparoscopic Gastrectomy for Clinical Stage I/II Gastric Cancer Patients: A Propensity Score-Matched Analysis. *World J. Surg.* **2021**, 1–12. [CrossRef]
9. Park, Y.K.; Yoon, H.M.; Kim, Y.-W.; Park, J.Y.; Ryu, K.W.; Lee, Y.-J.; Jeong, O.; Yoon, K.Y.; Lee, J.H.; Lee, S.E.; et al. Laparoscopy-assisted versus Open D2 Distal Gastrectomy for Advanced Gastric Cancer. *Ann. Surg.* **2018**, *267*, 638–645. [CrossRef] [PubMed]
10. Giulianotti, P.C.; Coratti, A.; Angelini, M.; Sbrana, F.; Cecconi, S.; Balestracci, T.; Caravaglios, G. Robotics in general surgery: Per-sonal experience in a large community hospital. *Arch. Surg.* **2003**, *138*, 777–784. [CrossRef] [PubMed]
11. Hashizume, M.; Sugimachi, K. Robot-assisted gastric surgery. *Surg. Clin. N. Am.* **2003**, *83*, 1429–1444. [CrossRef]
12. Stewart, C.L.; Ituarte, P.H.G.; Melstrom, K.A.; Warner, S.G.; Melstrom, L.G.; Lai, L.L.; Fong, Y.; Woo, Y. Robotic surgery trends in general surgical oncology from the National Inpatient Sample. *Surg. Endosc.* **2018**, *33*, 2591–2601. [CrossRef]
13. Guerrini, G.P.; Esposito, G.; Magistri, P.; Serra, V.; Guidetti, C.; Olivieri, T.; Catellani, B.; Assirati, G.; Ballarin, R.; Di Sandro, S.; et al. Robotic versus laparoscopic gastrectomy for gastric cancer: The largest meta-analysis. *Int. J. Surg.* **2020**, *82*, 210–228. [CrossRef]
14. Kim, Y.M.; Hyung, W.J. Current status of robotic gastrectomy for gastric cancer: Comparison with laparoscopic gastrectomy. *Updat. Surg.* **2021**, *73*, 853–863. [CrossRef]
15. Gao, Y.; Xi, H.; Qiao, Z.; Li, J.; Zhang, K.; Xie, T.; Shen, W.; Cui, J.; Wei, B.; Chen, L. Comparison of robotic- and laparoscopic-assisted gastrectomy in advanced gastric cancer: Up-dated short- and long-term results. *Surg. Endosc.* **2019**, *33*, 528–534. [CrossRef] [PubMed]
16. Amore Bonapasta, S.; Guerra, F.; Linari, C.; Annecchiarico, M.; Boffi, B.; Calistri, M.; Coratti, A. Robot-assisted gastrectomy for cancer. *Chirurg* **2017**, *88* (Suppl. 1), 12–18. [CrossRef] [PubMed]
17. Yang, P.; Wu, H.-Y.; Lin, X.-F.; Li, W. Pooled analysis of the oncological outcomes in robotic gastrectomy versus laparoscopic gastrectomy for gastric cancer. *J. Minimal Access Surg.* **2021**, *17*, 287. [CrossRef] [PubMed]
18. Bobo, Z.; Xin, W.; Jiang, L.; Quan, W.; Liang, B.; Xiangbing, D.; Ziqiang, W. Robotic gastrectomy versus laparoscopic gastrectomy for gastric cancer: Meta-analysis and trial sequential analysis of prospective observational studies. *Surg. Endosc.* **2019**, *33*, 1033–1048. [CrossRef] [PubMed]
19. Page, M.J.; McKenzie, J.E.; Bossuyt, P.M.; Boutron, I.; Hoffmann, T.C.; Mulrow, C.D.; Shamseer, L.; Tetzlaff, J.M.; Akl, E.A.; Brennan, S.E.; et al. The PRISMA 2020 statement: An updated guideline for reporting systematic reviews. *BMJ* **2021**, *372*, n71. [CrossRef]
20. Liu, H.; Kinoshita, T.; Tonouchi, A.; Kaito, A.; Tokunaga, M. What are the reasons for a longer operation time in robotic gastrectomy than in laparoscopic gastrectomy for stomach cancer? *Surg. Endosc.* **2019**, *33*, 192–198. [CrossRef] [PubMed]
21. Nakauchi, M.; Vos, E.; Janjigian, Y.Y.; Ku, G.Y.; Schattner, M.A.; Nishimura, M.; Gonen, M.; Coit, D.G.; Strong, V.E. Comparison of Long- and Short-term Outcomes in 845 Open and Minimally Invasive Gastrectomies for Gastric Cancer in the United States. *Ann. Surg. Oncol.* **2021**, *28*, 3532–3544. [CrossRef]
22. Chen, K.; Pan, Y.; Zhang, B.; Maher, H.; Wang, X.F.; Cai, X.J. Robotic versus laparoscopic Gastrectomy for gastric cancer: A system-atic review and updated meta-analysis. *BMC Surg.* **2017**, *17*, 93. [CrossRef]
23. Pan, H.F.; Wang, G.; Liu, J.; Liu, X.X.; Zhao, K.; Tang, X.F.; Jiang, Z.W. Robotic versus laparoscopic gastrectomy for locally advanced gastric cancer. *Surg. Laparosc. Endosc. Percutan. Tech.* **2017**, *27*, 428–433. [CrossRef]
24. Lu, J.; Wu, D.; Wang, H.-G.; Zheng, C.-H.; Li, P.; Xie, J.-W.; Wang, J.-B.; Lin, J.-X.; Chen, Q.-Y.; Cao, L.-L.; et al. 114O Assessment of robotic versus laparoscopic distal gastrectomy for gastric cancer: A randomized controlled trial. *Ann. Oncol.* **2020**, *31*, S1287. [CrossRef]
25. Tian, Y.; Cao, S.; Kong, Y.; Shen, S.; Niu, Z.; Zhang, J.; Chen, D.; Jiang, H.; Lv, L.; Liu, X.; et al. Short- and long-term comparison of robotic and laparoscopic gastrectomy for gastric cancer by the same surgical team: A propensity score matching analysis. *Surg. Endosc.* **2021**, 1–11. [CrossRef]
26. Kinoshita, T.; Sato, R.; Akimoto, E.; Tanaka, Y.; Okayama, T.; Habu, T. Reduction in postoperative complications by robotic surgery: A case–control study of robotic versus conventional laparoscopic surgery for gastric cancer. *Surg. Endosc.* **2021**, 1–10. [CrossRef]
27. Li, Z.-Y.; Zhao, Y.-L.; Qian, F.; Tang, B.; Chen, J.; He, T.; Luo, Z.-Y.; Li, P.-A.; Shi, Y.; Yu, P.-W. Long-term oncologic outcomes of robotic versus laparoscopic gastrectomy for locally advanced gastric cancer: A propensity score-matched analysis of 1170 patients. *Surg. Endosc.* **2021**, 1–10. [CrossRef]
28. Alhossaini, R.M.; Altamran, A.A.; Cho, M.; Roh, C.K.; Seo, W.J.; Choi, S.; Son, T.; Kim, H.; Hyung, W.J. Lower rate of conversion using robotic-assisted surgery compared to lapa-roscopy in completion total gastrectomy for remnant gastric cancer. *Surg. Endosc.* **2020**, *34*, 847–852. [CrossRef] [PubMed]

29. Wang, W.-J.; Li, H.-T.; Yu, J.-P.; Su, L.; Guo, C.; Chen, P.; Yan, L.; Li, K.; Ma, Y.-W.; Wang, L.; et al. Severity and incidence of complications assessed by the Clavien–Dindo classification following robotic and laparoscopic gastrectomy for advanced gastric cancer: A retrospective and propensity score-matched study. *Surg. Endosc.* **2018**, *33*, 3341–3354. [CrossRef]
30. Choi, S.; Song, J.H.; Lee, S.; Cho, M.; Kim, Y.M.; Hyung, W.J.; Kim, H.-I. Surgical Merits of Open, Laparoscopic, and Robotic Gastrectomy Techniques with D2 Lymphadenectomy in Obese Patients with Gastric Cancer. *Ann. Surg. Oncol.* **2021**, 1–10. [CrossRef]
31. Uyama, I.; Suda, K.; Nakauchi, M.; Kinoshita, T.; Noshiro, H.; Takiguchi, S.; Ehara, K.; Obama, K.; Kuwabara, S.; Okabe, H.; et al. Clinical advantages of robotic gastrectomy for clinical stage I/II gastric cancer: A multi-institutional prospective sin-gle-arm study. *Gastric Cancer* **2019**, *22*, 377–385. [CrossRef]
32. Kim, H.I.; Han, S.U.; Yang, H.K.; Kim, Y.W.; Lee, H.J.; Ryu, K.W.; Park, J.M.; An, J.Y.; Kim, M.C.; Park, S.; et al. Multicenter Prospective Comparative Study of Robotic Versus Laparoscopic Gas-trectomy for Gastric Adenocarcinoma. *Ann. Surg.* **2016**, *263*, 103–109. [CrossRef]
33. Xie, F.-N.; Chen, J.; Li, Z.-Y.; Bai, B.; Song, D.; Xu, S.; Song, X.-T.; Ji, G. Impact of Laparoscopic Converted to Open Gastrectomy on Short- and Long-Term Outcomes of Patients with Locally Advanced Gastric Cancer: A Propensity Score-Matched Analysis. *J. Gastrointest. Surg.* **2021**, 1–11. [CrossRef]
34. Guerra, F.; Giuliani, G.; Coletta, D. The risk of conversion in minimally invasive oncological abdominal surgery. Me-ta-analysis of randomized evidence comparing traditional laparoscopic versus robot-assisted techniques. *Langenbecks Arch. Surg.* **2021**, *406*, 607–612. [CrossRef]
35. Dindo, D.; Demartines, N.; Clavien, P.-A. Classification of Surgical Complications: A new proposal with evaluation in a cohort of 6336 patients and results of a survey. *Ann. Surg.* **2004**, *240*, 205–213. [CrossRef] [PubMed]
36. Coletta, D.; Sandri, G.B.L.; Giuliani, G.; Guerra, F. Robot-assisted versus conventional laparoscopic major hepatectomies: Systematic review with meta-analysis. *Int. J. Med Robot. Comput. Assist. Surg.* **2021**, *17*. [CrossRef] [PubMed]
37. Cortolillo, N.; Patel, C.; Parreco, J.; Kaza, S.; Castillo, A. Nationwide outcomes and costs of laparoscopic and robotic vs. open hepatectomy. *J. Robot. Surg.* **2018**, *13*, 557–565. [CrossRef]
38. Park, S.H.; Hyung, W.J. Current perspectives on the safety and efficacy of robot-assisted surgery for gastric cancer. *Expert Rev. Gastroenterol. Hepatol.* **2020**, *14*, 1181–1186. [CrossRef] [PubMed]
39. Amore Bonapasta, S.; Checcacci, P.; Guerra, F.; Mirasolo, V.M.; Moraldi, L.; Ferrara, A.; Annecchiarico, M.; Coratti, A. Time-to-administration in postoperative chemotherapy for colorectal cancer: Does minimally-invasive surgery help? *Minerva Chir.* **2016**, *71*, 173–179. [PubMed]
40. van Boxel, G.I.; Ruurda, J.P.; van Hillegersberg, R. Robotic-assisted gastrectomy for gastric cancer: A European perspective. *Gastric Cancer* **2019**, *22*, 909–919. [CrossRef] [PubMed]
41. Guerra, F.; Giuliani, G.; Formisano, G.; Bianchi, P.P.; Patriti, A.; Coratti, A. Pancreatic Complications After Conventional Laparo-scopic Radical Gastrectomy Versus Robotic Radical Gastrectomy: Systematic Review and Meta-Analysis. *J. Laparoendosc Adv. Surg. Tech. A* **2018**, *28*, 1207–1215. [CrossRef]
42. Seo, H.S.; Shim, J.H.; Jeon, H.M.; Park, C.H.; Song, K.Y. Postoperative pancreatic fistula after robot distal gastrectomy. *J. Surg. Res.* **2015**, *194*, 361–366. [CrossRef] [PubMed]
43. Kwon, I.G.; Son, T.; Kim, H.I.; Hyung, W.J. Fluorescent lymphography-guided lymphadenectomy during robotic radical gastrec-tomy for gastric cancer. *JAMA Surg.* **2019**, *154*, 150–158. [CrossRef] [PubMed]

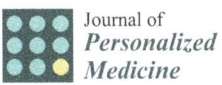

Systematic Review

Robotic Esophagectomy. A Systematic Review with Meta-Analysis of Clinical Outcomes

Michele Manigrasso [1], Sara Vertaldi [2], Alessandra Marello [2], Stavros Athanasios Antoniou [3,4], Nader Kamal Francis [5], Giovanni Domenico De Palma [2] and Marco Milone [2,*]

1 Department of Advanced Biomedical Sciences, University of Naples "Federico II", Via Pansini 5, 80131 Naples, Italy; michele.manigrasso@unina.it
2 Department of Clinical Medicine and Surgery, University of Naples "Federico II", Via Pansini 5, 80131 Naples, Italy; vertaldisara@gmail.com (S.V.); alessandramarello@gmail.com (A.M.); giovanni.depalma@unina.it (G.D.D.P.)
3 Medical School, European University Cyprus, 2404 Nicosia, Cyprus; stavros.antoniou@hotmail.com
4 Department of Surgery, Mediterranean Hospital of Cyprus, 3117 Limassol, Cyprus
5 Yeovil District Hospital, Somerset BA21 4AT, UK; nader.francis@ydh.nhs.uk
* Correspondence: milone.marco.md@gmail.com; Tel.: +39-333-299-36-37

Abstract: Background: Robot-Assisted Minimally Invasive Esophagectomy is demonstrated to be related with a facilitation in thoracoscopic procedure. To give an update on the state of art of robotic esophagectomy for cancr a systematic review with meta-analysis has been performed. **Methods:** a search of the studies comparing robotic and laparoscopic or open esophagectomy was performed trough the medical libraries, with the search string "robotic and (oesophagus OR esophagus OR esophagectomy OR oesophagectomy)". Outcomes were: postoperative complications rate (anastomotic leakage, bleeding, wound infection, pneumonia, recurrent laryngeal nerves paralysis, chylotorax, mortality), intraoperative outcomes (mean blood loss, operative time and conversion), oncologic outcomes (harvested nodes, R0 resection, recurrence) and recovery outcomes (length of hospital stay). **Results:** Robotic approach is superior to open surgery in terms of blood loss $p = 0.001$, wound infection rate, $p = 0.002$, pneumonia rate, $p = 0.030$ and mean number of harvested nodes, $p < 0.0001$ and R0 resection rate, $p = 0.043$. Similarly, robotic approach is superior to conventional laparoscopy in terms of mean number of harvested nodes, $p = 0.001$ pneumonia rate, $p = 0.003$. **Conclusions:** robotic surgery could be considered superior to both open surgery and conventional laparoscopy. These encouraging results should promote the diffusion of the robotic surgery, with the creation of randomized trials to overcome selection bias.

Keywords: robotic; esophagectomy; esophageal cancer; laparoscopic; open surgery

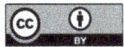

1. Introduction

Esophageal cancer represents the seventh most common cause of cancer morbidity and the sixth cause of cancer-related death [1].

Radical esophagectomy with lymphadenectomy represents nowadays the milestone for the treatment of esophageal cancer [2]. Since its introduction in the late 1940s, open esophagectomy has been adopted for a long time, obtaining considerable oncologic results [3]. In the new era of minimally invasive laparoscopic surgery, minimally invasive esophagectomy started to be performed in the 2000s, providing the well-known advantages on recovery of the minimally invasive procedures. Safety and efficacy of minimally invasive esophagectomy has been reported in several experiences [4–7], further providing similar oncologic results and long term recurrence rate [8–10]. However, on a clinical point of view, the introduction of minimally invasive esophagectomy in the clinical practice is far to be considered as a standard of care. Major reason for that should be considered technical challenges in performing minimally invasive esophagectomy.

Since its introduction in 2000s, robotic surgery has been adopted to overcome technical difficulties of laparoscopic surgery. The facilities of the robotic approach lay in the intrinsic characteristics of the robotic platforms. In fact, the three-dimensional view allowed a better visualization of the operative field and the EndoWrist® technology with the seven-degrees movement of the robotic arms allows to perform more accurate movements in narrow space [11,12]. Even if robotic approach could be considered the gold standard only for the treatment of the prostate cancer, it has accumulated consensus in many surgical fields [13–16]. In the setting of minimally invasive esophagectomy, it was first introduced in 2003 by Kernstine et al. [17], but controversies about the advantages of robotic approach have to be considered still an open issue.

Interest about the results of robotic surgery, also in comparison with open and laparoscopic approach, is fervent worldwide. Results on robotic esophagectomy were accumulated exponentially in the last years providing advantages of robot-assisted surgery.

To delineate the state of art of robotic approach to treat esophageal cancer, we have designed a systematic review and meta- analysis comparing robotic with both open and laparoscopic surgery, toward to the identification of a gold standard treatment.

2. Materials and Methods

2.1. Literature Search and Study Selection

This systematic review complied with PRISMA (Preferred Reporting Items for Systematic reviews and Meta-Analyses) reporting standards [18] and was developed in line with Meta-Analysis of Observational Studies Epidemiology (MOOSE) guidelines [19].

Cochrane Library, EMBASE, PubMed, SCOPUS, and Web of Science were interrogated. The search string "robotic and (oesophagus OR esophagus OR esophagectomy OR oesophagectomy)" was used. Only articles published in English were considered.

Indexed abstract of posters and podium presentations at international meetings were not included. We did not consider systematic reviews and meta-analyses. However, the latter were consulted to identify additional studies of interest. The reference lists of retrieved studies were reviewed. In case of overlapping series in different studies, only the most recent article was included.

The research question was structured within a PICO (Problem/Population, Intervention, Comparison and Outcome) framework. Population of interest included patients affected by histologically proven esophageal adenocarcinoma/squamous cells cancer. The intervention was robotic transthoracic esophagectomy, and the comparator was open esophagectomy and laparoscopic esophagectomy, respectively.

Outcome measures were divided in short- and long-term outcomes. Short-term outcomes encompassed postoperative complications rate, in terms of anastomotic leakage, postoperative bleeding, wound infection, pneumonia, recurrent laryngeal nerves (RLN) paralysis, chylotorax, reoperation rate and overall mortality, intraoperative outcomes (mean blood loss, operative time and conversion), oncologic outcomes (harvested nodes, R0 resection rate) and recovery outcomes (length of hospital stay). Long-term outcomes included recurrences and 5-year overall survival.

The literature search and study selection were performed independently by two reviewers. In case of disagreement, a third investigator was consulted and an agreement was reached by consensus.

2.2. Data Extraction and Risk of Bias Assessment

The following data were extracted from each study: first author, year of publication, study design, sample size, demographic characteristics, number of patients in each surgical group, gender, mean age, mean BMI (Body Mass Index), ASA (American Society of Anesthesiologists) Score, tumor stage according to UICC (Union for International Cancer Control), preoperative radio-chemotherapy rate, mean blood loss, operative time, conversion, anastomotic leakage, postoperative bleeding, wound infection, pneumonia, recurrent laryngeal nerves (RLN) paralysis, chylotorax, reoperation rate and overall mortality, harvested nodes, R0 resection rate, length of hospital stay, recurrence rate and 5-years overall survival. In order to assess overall mortality, we considered in-hospital mortality and 30-days and 90-days mortality, performing a sum of these data in each group.

Study quality assessment of the included studies was performed with the Newcastle Ottawa Scale (NOS) [20]. This scoring system encompasses three major domains (selection, comparability and exposure), with scores between 0 (lowest quality) to 9 (highest quality). In case of Randomized Controlled Trial (RCTs), the risk of bias was evaluated according to the Cochrane Collaboration Tool for assessing risk of bias [21]. According to this scoring system, seven domains were evaluated as "Low risk of bias" or "High risk of bias" or "Unclear" according to reporting on sequence generation, allocation concealment, blinding of participants, blinding of outcome assessment, incomplete outcome data, selective outcome reporting, and other potential threats to validity.

2.3. Statistical Analysis

Statistical analysis was performed using Comprehensive Meta-Analysis (Version 2.2, Biostat Inc, Englewood, NJ, USA, 2005). In order to provide a complete update on robotic surgery for esophageal cancer, two different group analyses were performed: robotic vs. laparoscopic and robotic vs. open approach.

Furthermore, for each meta-analysis, two subgroup analyses were performed dividing the studies according to the surgical procedure (Ivor-Lewis esophagectomy or McKeown esophagectomy). Finally, a sensitivity analysis excluded studies applying a hybrid approach (robotic abdominal phase and laparoscopic/open thoracic phase) and studies which did not specify the surgical procedure.

The odds ratio (OR) along with 95% confidence interval was used as effect estimate for dichotomous outcomes. In case of rare events, the risk difference (RD) with corresponding 95%CI were calculated, maintaining analytic consistency and including all available data, in accordance with Messori et al. [22]. In case studies reporting median, range and sample size, or studies reporting median and quartile ranges, the means and standard deviations were estimated according to Shi, Luo and Wan [23–25]. In studies reporting mean values without standard deviation, the latter was imputed, according to Furukawa et al. [26]. The overall effect was tested using Z scores and significance was set at $p < 0.05$. The summary estimate was computed under a random effects assumption as per DerSimonian and Laird [27]. A conservative random effect model was chosen a priori in consideration of foreseen heterogeneity among the included studies. The heterogeneity among the studies was quantified by the I^2 statistic, with I^2 values < 25%, between 25–50%, and >50% indicating respectively low, moderate, and high heterogeneity [28,29]. The presence of publication bias was investigated through a funnel plot where the summary estimate of each study (OR) was plotted against the standard error as a measure of study precision. In addition to visual inspection, funnel plot symmetry was tested using the Egger's linear regression method [30]. p values ≤ 0.05 were considered statistically significant.

3. Results

Study Selection

The electronic search returned a total of 2113 results. After duplicates removal, 543 studies entered first-level screening. A total of 507 studies were excluded for the following reasons: 44 were written in a language other than English, 10 were case reports/case series, 97 were reviews, 46 were non-comparative studies, 293 were off-topic and 18 did not provide any usable data. Thus, 35 studies were included in the final analysis, out of which 20 compared robotic vs. laparoscopic surgery, 11 compared robotic vs. open esophagectomy and 4 reported on a three-arms comparison (robotic vs. laparoscopic vs. open) [20–54]. From the latter [54], it was possible to extract only data about the comparison between robotic and laparoscopic esophagectomy. Record selection is illustrated in the PRISMA flowchart (Figure 1). Inter-rater agreement was perfect (κ = 1).

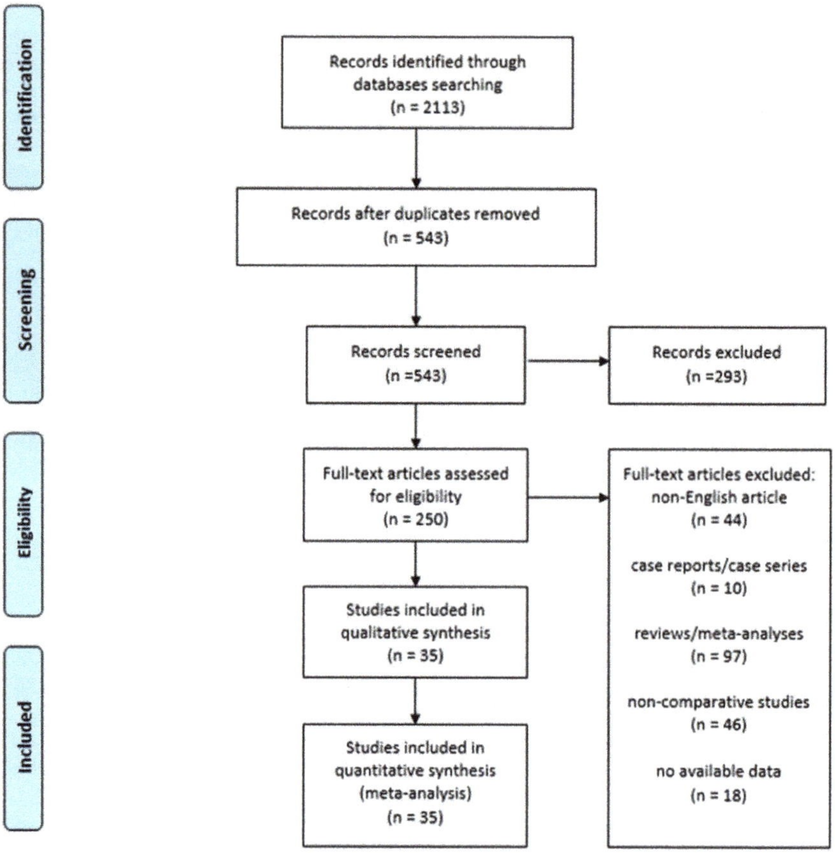

Figure 1. PRISMA Flowchart.

4. Robotic Versus Laparoscopic Esophagectomy

4.1. Study Characteristics

All were prospective ($n = 5$) or retrospective studies ($n = 18$) [20–23,29,32,33,37,40,42–46,48,51,53], reporting on 11,779 patients, of whom 3832 underwent robotic esophagectomy and 7947 laparoscopic esophagectomy. The characteristics of the included studies are summarized in Table 1.

Table 1. Characteristics of the included studies comparing robotic and laparoscopic approach.

Study	Study Design	N. of Enrolled Patients		Mean Age	Mean BMI	ASA Score (%)				Tumor Stage (%)					Tumor Localization (%)			
		RAMIE	MIE			I	II	III	IV	0	I	II	III	IV				
Ali et al., 2020	retro	1543	5118	63.71	NR	NR	NR	NR	NR	NR	NR	NR	NR	NR	NR	NR	NR	NR
Chao et al., 2018	retro	34	34	55.12	NR	NR	NR	NR	NR	0.00	47.10	0.00	52.90	0.00	29.40	50.00	20.60	0.00
Chao et al., 2020	retro	39	67	55.60	22.34	NR	NR	NR	NR	0.00	0.00	7.55	92.45	0.00	22.65	48.08	29.27	0.00
Chen et al., 2019	retro	54	54	61.80	22.85	NR	NR	NR	NR	NR	NR	NR	NR	NR	NR	NR	NR	NR
Deng et al., 2018	prosp	52	52	60.95	NR	NR	NR	NR	NR	0.00	12.50	45.15	37.50	0.00	16.35	60.60	22.10	0.95
Duan et al., 2020	retro	109	75	60.45	NR	NR	NR	NR	NR	NR	NR	NR	NR	NR	NR	NR	NR	NR
Gong et al., 2020	retro	91	144	NR	NR	NR	NR	NR	NR	0.00	18.59	33.33	20.83	2.57	3.53	33.01	38.78	0.00
Grimminger et al., 2019	prosp	25	25	62.05	25.55	NR	NR	NR	NR	0.00	0.00	0.00	0.00	0.00	0.00	14.00	89.00	0.00
Harbison et al., 2019	retro	100	625	64.00	27.63	17.38	0.00	77.66	4.97	0.00	NR	NR	NR	NR	NR	61.10	31.45	0.00
He et al., 2018	retro	27	27	61.30	21.70	NR	NR	NR	NR	0.00	0.00	0.00	0.00	0.00	7.40	NR	NR	NR
Meredith et al., 2020	prosp	144	95	50.97	21.84	0.35	35.94	42.15	0.67	0.00	15.70	25.11	35.37	2.22	NR	38.80	35.42	0.00
Motoyama et al., 2019	retro	21	38	64.10	NR	NR	NR	NR	NR	0.00	38.80	15.14	45.71	0.00	25.78	22.85	62.86	0.00
Park et al., 2016	retro	62	43	65.08	23.42	30.50	65.72	3.84	0.00	0.00	58.08	25.79	15.24	0.94	14.29	46.10	25.50	3.90
Shirakawa et al., 2020	retro	51	51	68.00	21.95	21.60	64.70	13.70	NR	NR	NR	NR	NR	NR	18.60	52.78	36.11	0.00
Suda et al., 2012	prosp	16	20	65.39	20.78	NR	NR	NR	NR	2.78	33.33	11.11	50.00	2.78	11.11	NR	NR	NR
Tagkalos et al., 2020	prosp	40	40	62.50	26.00	NR	NR	NR	NR	NR	NR	NR	NR	NR	NR	28.00	57.50	0.00
Tsunoda et al., 2021	retro	45	45	NR	NR	9.00	89.00	2.00	0.00	0.00	51.00	19.00	23.00	7.00	14.50	NR	NR	NR
Weksler et al., 2012	retro	11	26	62.64	27.66	NR	NR	NR	NR	27.02	32.39	16.23	24.35	0.00	NR	NR	NR	NR
Weksler et al., 2017	retro	569	569	41.90	NR	NR	NR	NR	NR	4.70	22.73	19.33	17.53	2.40	NR	NR	NR	NR
Xu et al., 2020	retro	292	292	64.63	23.09	17.50	76.05	6.50	0.00	0.00	38.90	20.90	39.05	1.15	7.50	73.30	19.20	0.00
Yang et al., 2020	retro	271	271	63.45	23.20	1.50	89.50	9.05	0.00	0.00	28.20	33.75	26.95	11.05	12.70	62.75	24.55	0.00
Yerokun et al., 2016	retro	170	170	62.95	NR	NR	NR	NR	NR	0.00	0.00	0.00	0.00	0.00	2.95	51.15	45.90	0.00
Zhang et al., 2019	retro	66	66	62.15	23.00	42.45	52.25	5.30	0.00	6.10	27.25	43.20	23.45	0.00	0.00	21.95	28.05	0.00

BMI: Body Mass Index; RAMIE: Robot-Assisted Minimally Invasive Esophagectomy; MIE: Minimally Invasive Esophagectomy; RCT: Randomized Controlled Trial; NR: not reported. All studies reported on the surgical approach, adopting totally robotic or totally laparoscopic approach, except for the study by Yerokun et al. [55] and Harbison et al. [33], in which a hybrid approach was used and for the study by Weksler et al. [52], in which information on surgical procedures was insufficiently provided.

Ivor-Lewis procedure was performed in four studies [39,49,51,56], McKeown esophagectomy in ten studies [34,42,43,53,54,57–61] while nine studies did not specify the intervention [31–33,40,47,48,50,52,55].

4.2. Risk of Bias Assessment

All studies had NOS quality scores greater than 6, indicating fair methodological quality. Specifically, thirteen studies had NOS quality score = 7; ten studies had NOS quality score = 8. The NOS quality score is represented in Supplementary Table S1. No RCTs comparing robotic and laparoscopic transthoracic esophagectomy were published.

4.3. Short Term-Outcomes

Intraoperative outcomes are shown in Figure 2. Operative time was reported by 15 Authors [23,25,26,28–31,35,37,40,45,46,49,54,57] on 2690 procedures (which of 1089 robotic and 1601 laparoscopic), demonstrating a lower operative time in the laparoscopic group (MD = 31, p = 0.003, 95%CI 10.743; 52.478), with a significant heterogeneity among the studies (I^2 = 93.720%, p < 0.0001). Estimated blood loss was analysed by 14 Authors [21,23,28,29,33,37–39,42,48,50,51,53,57], on 1977 procedures (which of 995 robotic and 982 laparoscopic), demonstrating no significant differences between the two approaches (MD = 1.673, p = 0.805, 95%CI −11.638; 14.985), with no heterogeneity among the studies (I^2 = 0%, p = 0.760). Number of conversion was reported by 5 Authors [33,47,50,56,57] on 1591 procedures (which of 533 robotic and 1058 laparoscopic), with no significant difference between the two groups (RD = −0.007, p = 0.662, 95%CI −0.036; 0.023), but with a significant heterogeneity among the studies (I^2 = 61.532%, p = 0.034).

Statistical analysis for postoperative complications are shown in Figure 3. Anastomotic leakage was analysed by 18 Authors [22,23,28,29,32,33,37–39,42,43,45,48,50,51,53,54,57] on 3482 procedures (1471 robotic and 2011 laparoscopic), with no statistical differences between the two approaches (OR = 0.936, p = 0.612, 95%CI 0.724, 1.210) and no significant heterogeneity among the studies (I^2 = 0%, p = 0.871). Postoperative bleeding was reported by 4 Authors [33,34,57,61] on 1556 procedures (489 robotic and 1067 laparoscopic), demonstrating no significant differences between the two groups (OR = 0.952, p = 0.882, 95%CI 0.494, 1.831) and no significant heterogeneity among the studies (I^2 = 0%, p = 0.898). Postoperative wound infection was analysed by 10 Authors [32,38,49,51,53,54,56,57,60,61] on 2189 procedures (1088 robotic and 1101 laparoscopic), with no significant differences between the two approaches (RD = −0.001, p = 0.885, 95%CI −0.010; 0.009) and no significant heterogeneity among the studies (I^2 = 7.881%, p = 0.370). Pneumonia was reported by 15 Authors [27,29,32,38–40,42,43,45,48,50,51,53,54,57] on 2586 procedures (1276 robotic and 1310 laparoscopic), with a lower number of pneumonias in the robotic group (RD = −0.038, p = 0.003, 95%CI −0.064; −0.013) and no significant heterogeneity among the studies (I^2 = 0%, p = 0.726).

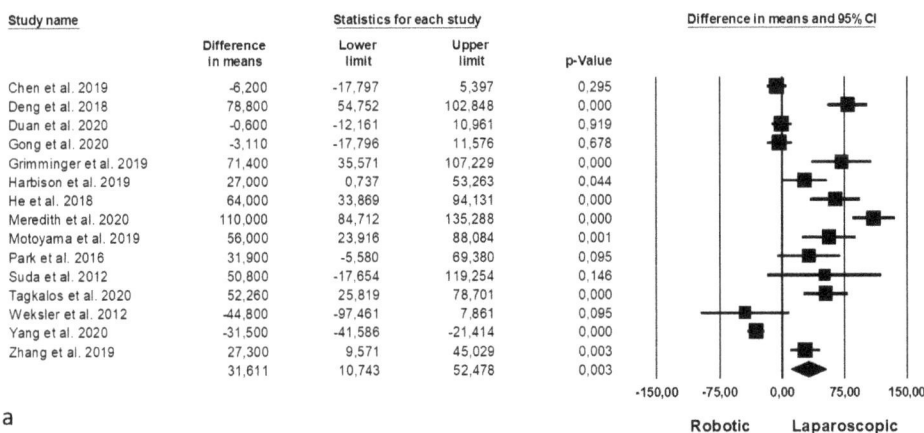

Figure 2. Robotic versus laparoscopic surgery: intraoperative outcomes. (**a**) operative time; (**b**) estimated blood loss; (**c**) conversion.

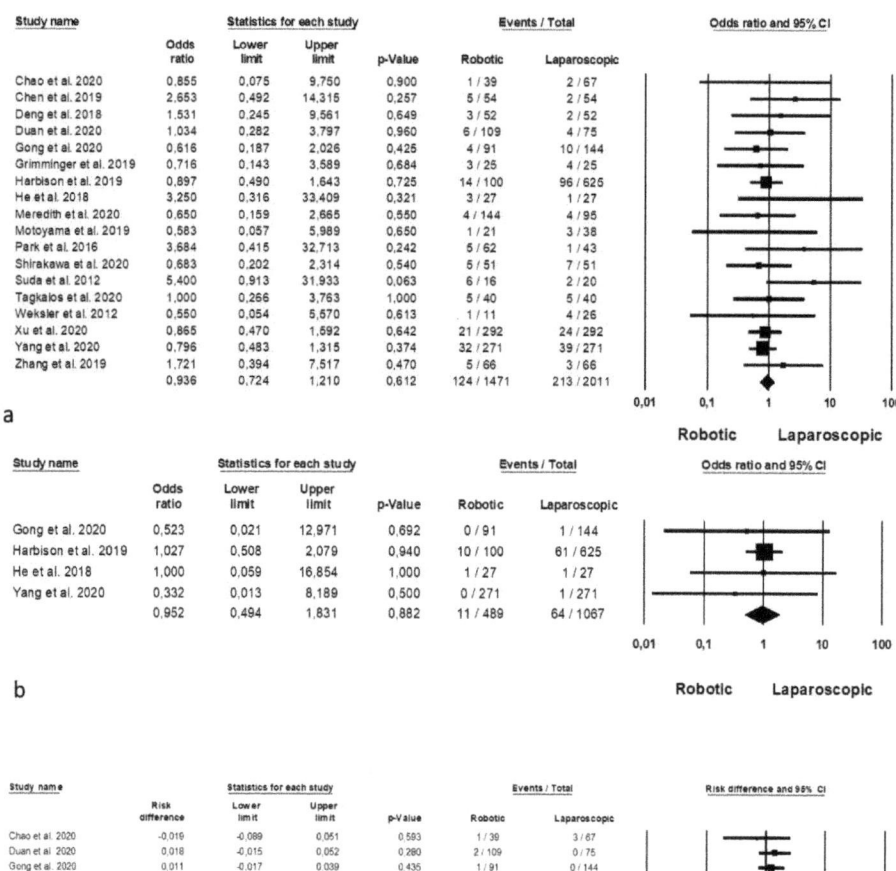

Figure 3. Cont.

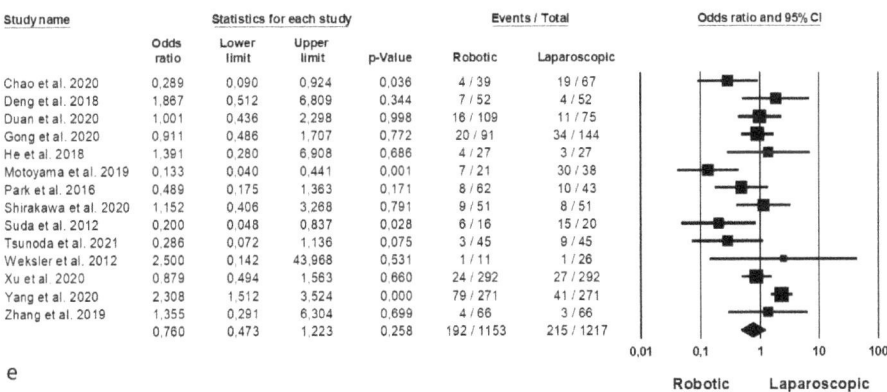

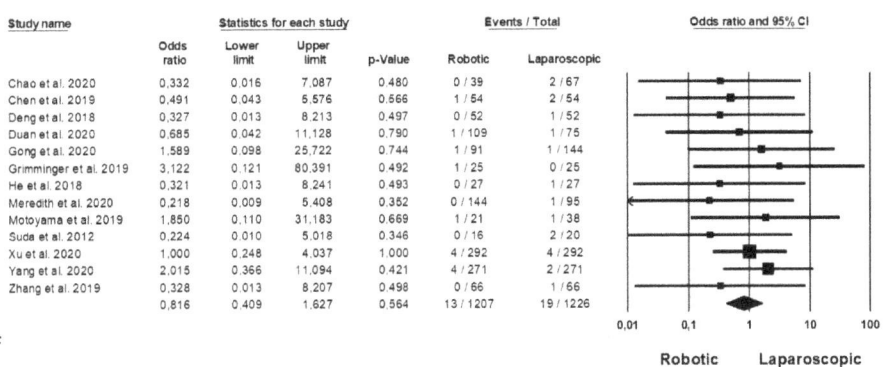

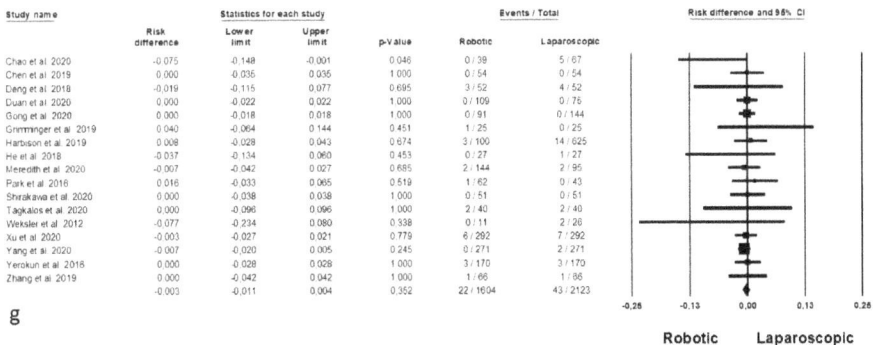

Figure 3. Robotic versus laparoscopic surgery: postoperative complications. (**a**) anastomotic leakage; (**b**) postoperative bleeding; (**c**) wound infection; (**d**) pneumonia; (**e**) RLN paralysis; (**f**) chylothorax; (**g**) mortality.

RLN paralysis was reported by 14 Authors [23,29,32,33,37,38,40,42,45,48,50,51,53,57] on 2370 procedures (1153 robotic and 1217 laparoscopic), with no significant differences between the two approaches (OR = 0.760, p = 0.258, 95%CI 0.473, 1.223), but with a significant heterogeneity among the studies (I^2 = 69.109%, p < 0.0001). Chylothorax was analysed by 13 Authors [23,27,29,32,38,43,45,48,50,51,53,54,57] on 2433 procedures (1207 robotic and 1226 laparoscopic), with no significant differences between the two groups (OR = 0.816, p = 0.564, 95%CI 0.409, 1.627), and no significant heterogeneity among the studies (I^2 = 0%, p = 0.954). Mortality was analysed by 17 Authors [22,23,28,31,32,36,38,41,43–46,48,50,51,53,54] including 3727 patients (1604 robotic and 2123 laparoscopic) with no differences between the two groups (RD = −0.003, p = 0.352, 95%CI −0.011; 0.004) and no significant heterogeneity among the studies (I^2 = 0%, p = 0.962). It was not possible to assess the reoperation rate because no studies reported this data.

Oncologic outcomes are shown in Figure 4. Mean number of harvested nodes was reported by 17 Authors [31,34,38,40,43,48,49,52–61] on 10,707 procedures (which of 3566 robotic and 7141 laparoscopic), demonstrating a higher number in the harvested nodes during the robotic approach (MD = 1.307, p = 0.001, 95%CI 0.553; 2.060), with a significant heterogeneity among the studies (I^2 = 74.857%, p < 0.0001). The number of complete resection (R0 resection) was reported by 12 Authors [32,38,48–50,52,53,56–58,60,61] on 2940 procedures (which of 1469 robotic and 1471 laparoscopic), with no significant differences between the two procedures (RD = 0.005, p = 0.473, 95%CI −0.009; 0.019), and no significant heterogeneity among the studies (I^2 = 20.790%, p = 0.258).

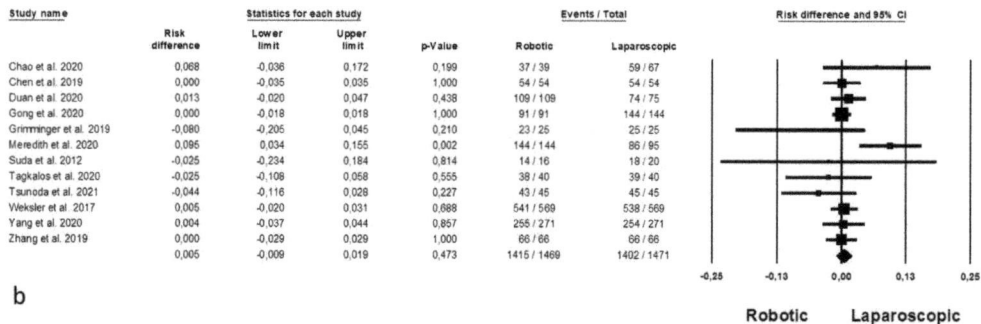

Figure 4. Robotic versus laparoscopic surgery: oncologic outcomes. (a) Number of harvested nodes; (b) R0 resection.

Length of hospital stay was represented in Figure 5. This data was reported by 16 Authors [20–23,28,36–38,41,43,45,46,48,50,51,54], on 9642 patients (2713 robotic and 6749 laparoscopic), demonstrating no differences between the two approaches (MD = −0.476, p = 0.289, 95%CI −1.241; 0.289), with a significant heterogeneity among the studies (I^2 = 72.303%, p < 0.0001).

Study name	Difference in means	Lower limit	Upper limit	p-Value
Ali et al. 2020	-0,720	-1,346	-0,094	0,024
Chao et al. 2018	-1,460	-4,205	1,285	0,297
Chen et al. 2019	1,900	-1,854	5,654	0,321
Deng et al. 2018	1,600	-1,210	4,410	0,264
Duan et al. 2020	-0,900	-2,881	1,081	0,373
Grimminger et al. 2019	4,600	-3,891	13,091	0,288
Harbison et al. 2019	-2,000	-3,818	-0,182	0,031
He et al. 2018	-5,200	-7,231	-3,169	0,000
Meredith et al. 2020	0,400	-2,567	3,367	0,792
Shirakawa et al. 2020	2,000	0,545	3,455	0,007
Suda et al. 2012	-21,000	-37,839	-4,161	0,015
Tagkalos et al. 2020	-0,100	-5,021	4,821	0,968
Weksler et al. 2012	-1,300	-6,063	3,463	0,593
Yang et al. 2020	-1,080	-3,225	1,065	0,324
Yerokun et al. 2016	0,400	-0,476	1,276	0,371
Zhang et al. 2019	0,000	-0,275	0,275	1,000
	-0,476	-1,241	0,289	0,222

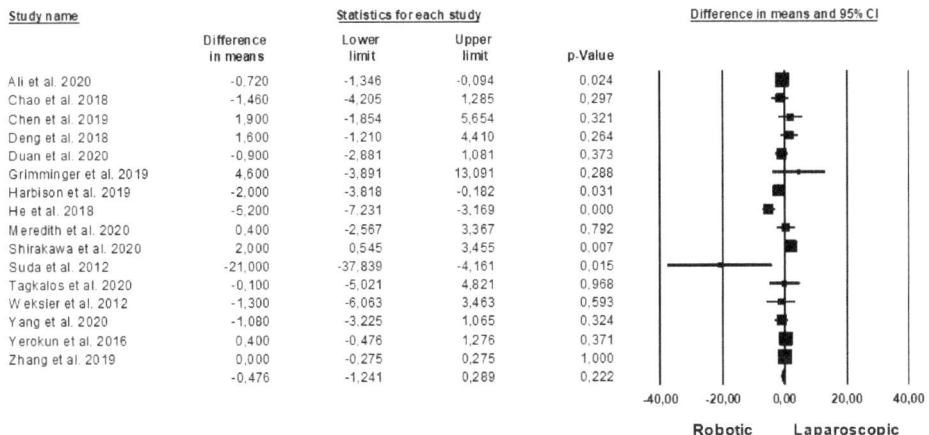

Figure 5. Robotic versus laparoscopic surgery: length of hospital stay.

5. Long-Term Outcomes

Long-term outcomes are summarized in Figure 6. Recurrences were analysed by 3 Authors [32,54,57] on 1176 patients (588 in each arm), with no significant differences between the two groups (OR = 1.035, p = 0.855, 95%CI 0.720, 1.487) and no significant heterogeneity among the studies (I^2 = 0%, p = 0.742). The 5-years overall survival was reported by 2 Authors [43,54], with no significant differences between the two groups (OR = 1.105, p = 0.527, 95%CI 0.811, 1.506) and no significant differences among the studies (I^2 = 0%, p = 0.380).

Study name	Odds ratio	Lower limit	Upper limit	p-Value	Events / Total: Robotic	Events / Total: Laparoscopic
Grimminger et al. 2019	1,397	0,279	7,002	0,684	4 / 25	3 / 25
Xu et al. 2020	0,906	0,548	1,498	0,701	33 / 292	36 / 292
Yang et al. 2020	1,173	0,674	2,042	0,573	30 / 271	26 / 271
	1,035	0,720	1,487	0,855	67 / 588	65 / 588

a

Study name	Odds ratio	Lower limit	Upper limit	p-Value	Events / Total: Robotic	Events / Total: Laparoscopic
Park et al. 2016	1,547	0,687	3,483	0,292	43 / 62	25 / 43
Xu et al. 2020	1,044	0,746	1,459	0,803	184 / 292	181 / 292
	1,105	0,811	1,506	0,527	227 / 354	206 / 335

b

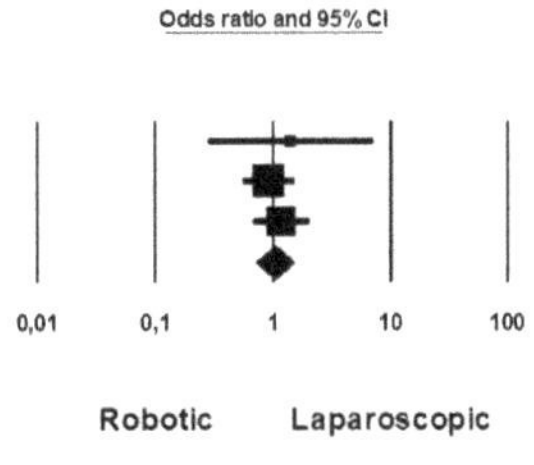

Figure 6. Robotic versus laparoscopic surgery: long-term outcomes. (**a**) recurrences; (**b**) 5-years overall survival.

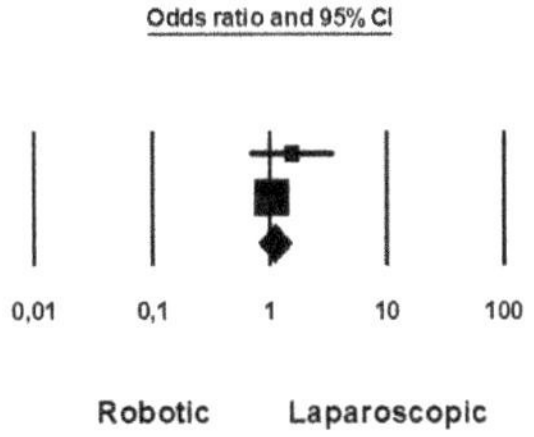

6. Subgroup Analysis

6.1. Fully Robotic vs. Fully Laparoscopic Procedures

Excluding the two studies in which the surgical procedures was not clearly described [52] or in which a hybrid approach was adopted [33,55], this subgroup analysis included 21 studies [31–34,38,40,42,43,47–51,53,54,56–61].

It was not possible to obtain data about blood loss, wound infection, postoperative pneumonia, RLN paralysis and chylothorax because the above-mentioned study did not report these data.

Of the remaining outcomes, the subgroup analysis confirmed the results of the main analysis in terms of operative time (lower in the laparoscopic group, MD = 32, $p = 0.004$, 95%CI 9.983; 53.978), conversion (RD = -0.011, $p = 0.495$, 95%CI -0.043; 0.021), anastomotic leakage (OR = 0.945, $p = 0.693$, 95%CI 0.711; 1.254), bleeding (OR = 0.587, $p = 0.555$, 95%CI 0.100; 3.443), mortality (RD = -0.004, $p = 0.283$, 95%CI -0.012; 0.003), harvested nodes (MD = 1.748, $p < 0.0001$, 95%CI 0.795; 2.701), R0 resection (RD = 0.005, $p = 0.528$, 95%CI -0.011; 0.022) and hospital stay (MD = -0.462, $p = 0.318$, 95%CI -1.369; 0.444).

6.2. McKeown Esophagectomy

After excluding four studies about Ivor-Lewis procedure [38,49,51,56] and other nine in which Ivor-Lewis and Mckeown were not separately analysed [31–33,40,47,48,50,52,55], ten studies [34,42,43,53,54,57–61] were included in the subgroup analysis according to Mckeown procedure.

Of intraoperative data, no difference was found between robotic and laparoscopic approach in terms of estimated blood loss (MD = -1.370, $p = 0.876$, 95%CI -18.547; 15.808, respectively). Interestingly, in this subgroup analysis there was no difference in term of operative time (MD = 11.262, $p = 0.334$, 95%CI -11.595; 34.118), conversely to the main analysis. It was not possible to extract data about conversion because only one study was about McKeown esophagectomy.

Of postoperative complications, the subgroups analysis confirmed no significant differences were between the two approaches in terms of anastomotic leakage (OR = 0.928, $p = 0.659$, 95%CI 0.667, 1.291), bleeding (OR = 0.587, $p = 0.555$, 95%CI 0.100; 3.443), wound infection (RD = -0.001, $p = 0.878$, 95%CI -0.009; 0.011), RLN paralysis (OR = 0.994, $p = 0.981$, 95%CI 0.609; 1.623), chylothorax (OR = 0.880, $p = 0.753$, 95%CI 0.397; 1.949) and mortality (RD = -0.004, $p = 0.285$, 95%CI -0.013; 0.004). Similarly, a significant difference was confirmed in terms of postoperative pneumonia between the two groups in favour of robotic surgery (RD = -0.035, $p = 0.028$, 95%CI -0.066; -0.004).

Confirming the data of the main analysis, robotic surgery was associated with a higher number of harvested nodes (MD = 1.445, $p = 0.001$, 95%CI 0.572; 2.318), while no differences were found in terms of R0 resection and recurrences (RD = 0.004, $p = 0.593$, 95%CI -0.010; 0.017 and OR = 1.018, $p = 0.925$, 95%CI 0.701; 1.478, respectively).

Finally, no significant differences were found in terms of length of hospital stay between the two approaches (MD = -1.058, $p = 0.316$, 95%CI -3.125; 1.009).

6.3. Ivor-Lewis Esophagectomy

The subgroup analysis on Ivor-Lewis esophagectomy included four studies [38,49,51,56].

The sub-analysis of intraoperative data confirmed that there was no difference between the two approaches in terms of estimated blood loss (MD = 11.916, $p = 0.513$, 95%CI -23.794; 47.626, respectively). On the contrary, subgroup analysis showed no difference in terms of operative time (MD = 39.990, $p = 0.112$, 95%CI -9.367; 89.347) between the two approaches. It was not possible to extract data about conversions because only one study was about the Ivor-Lewis procedure.

Of postoperative complications, no significant differences were found in terms of anastomotic leakage (OR = 0.956, $p = 0.907$, 95%CI 0.446; 2.049), wound infection (RD = -0.014, $p = 0.531$, 95%CI -0.059; 0.030), RLN paralysis (OR = 1.553, $p = 0.524$, 95%CI 0.401; 6.022), chylothorax (OR = 0.267, $p = 0.255$, 95%CI 0.028; 2.597) and mortality (RD = -0.006,

$p = 0.652$, 95%CI -0.031; 0.019), confirming the data of the main analysis. Interestingly, rate of postoperative pneumonia (RD = -0.042, $p = 0.123$, 95%CI -0.096; 0.011) did not differ between the two approaches. No data were extracted about postoperative bleeding because no studies about Ivor-Lewis esophagectomy reported this data.

About oncologic outcomes, no difference was found in terms of R0 resection (RD = 0.024, $p = 0.473$, 95%CI -0.042; 0.091) and differently to the main analysis, no difference was found on number of harvested nodes (MD = 4.091, $p = 0.077$, 95%CI -0.450; 8.631). No data were extracted about recurrence because of the absence of studies about Ivor-Lewis esophagectomy analysing this aspect.

No differences in terms of length of hospital stay was found between the two approaches (MD = -0.001, $p = 0.993$, 95%CI -0.274; 0.272).

6.4. Publication Bias

Forest plots were symmetrical across outcomes and the Egger's test was not suggestive of publication bias, except for the mean number of harvested nodes and operative time, in which visual inspection suggested an asymmetric distribution of studies around the mean and the Egger's test confirmed significant publication bias ($p = 0.01$ and $p = 0.006$, respectively). Funnel plots are provided in Supplementary Figures S1–S4.

7. Robotic Versus Open Esophagectomy

7.1. Study Characteristics

Seven retrospective [35,41,44,45,52,61,62] and four prospective cohort studies [37,39,46,63], and two RCTs were identified [11,64], reporting on 4485 patients, out of whom 1919 underwent robotic esophagectomy and 2566 open esophagectomy. The characteristics of the included studies are detailed in Table 2.

About surgical intervention, all the surgical interventions of the included studies were performed with a fully robotic approach, except for the study by Rolff et al. [45], in which an hybrid procedure (robotic approach to the abdomen and open approach to the thorax) was used. Two articles reported on Ivor-Lewis procedure [37,39], one on McKeown esophagectomy [61] while ten did not provide relevant data to allow subgroup analysis [11,35,41,44–46,52,62–64].

Table 2. Characteristics of the included studies comparing robotic and open approach.

Study	Study Design	N. of Enrolled Patients		Mean Age	Mean BMI	ASA Score (%)					Tumor Stage (%)				Tumor Localization (%)			
		RAMIE	OPEN			I	II	III	IV	0	I	II	III	IV				
Espinoza-Mercado et al., 2019	retro	406	406	64	NR	NR	NR	NR	NR	14.65	25.75	37.8	21.3	0	NR	NR	NR	NR
Gong et al., 2020	retro	91	77	NR	NR	NR	NR	NR	NR	2.974	33.33	39.88	21.42	2.38	26.18	37.50	31.54	0.91
Jeong et al., 2016	retro	88	159	NR	22.66	NR	NR	NR	NR	41.19838	42.53	13.12	2.78	0.35	NR	NR	NR	NR
Mehdorn et al., 2020	prosp	11	11	63.8	27.4	0	31.85	68.15	0	13.65	9.1	36.4	27.3	4.55	NR	NR	NR	NR
Meredith et al., 2020	prosp	144	475	64.46	28	0.38	49.62	49.20	0.70	9.66	34.78	41.24	12.27	44.43	NR	NR	NR	NR
Osaka et al., 2018	retro	30	30	62.5	NR	NR	NR	NR	NR	26.65	45	18.3	10	0	26.65	48.35	26.35	0
Fointer et al., 2020	retro	222	222	NR	NR	NR	NR	NR	NR	NR	NR	NR	NR	NR	NR	NR	NR	NR
Rolff et al., 2017	retro	56	160	64.65	26.51	27.03	50	23.22	0.51	NR	NR	NR	NR	NR	NR	NR	NR	NR
Sarkaria et al., 2019	prosp	64	106	61.89	29.12	0	14.16	79.38	6.48	22.48	32.52	24.83	8.24	0	0	1.18	63.54	41.54
Weksler et al., 2017	retro	569	569	63	NR	NR	NR	NR	NR	20.4	32.15	27.7	14.35	35.55	NR	NR	NR	NR
Yun et al., 2020	prosp	130	241	62.92	23.21	NR	NR	NR	NR	20.74	19.16	20.51	3.78	0	43.62	31.80	5.92	4.54

BMI: Body Mass Index; RAMIE: Robot-Assisted Minimally Invasive Esophagectomy; RCT: Randomized Controlled Trial; NR: not reported.

7.2. Risk of Bias Assessment

All studies had NOS quality scores greater than 6, indicating that all these studies had fair methodological quality. Specifically, seven studies had NOS quality score = 8; six had NOS quality score = 7. The NOS quality score is represented in Table 2. The two included RCTs [11,64] had low risk of bias.

7.3. Short-Term Outcomes

Intraoperative outcomes are shown in Figure 7. Operative time was reported by 9 Authors [11,35,37,38,41,45,46,61,63] on 1982 procedure (which of 668 robotic and 1314 open), demonstrating a lower operative time in the open group (MD = 57, $p < 0.0001$, 95%CI 27.597; 87.684), with a significant heterogeneity among the studies ($I^2 = 97.190\%$, $p < 0.0001$). Estimated blood loss was analysed by 8 Authors [11,35,39,41,45,46,61,63], on 1960 procedures (which of 657 robotic and 1303 open), demonstrating a significantly lower blood loss in the robotic group (MD = -118.783, $p = 0.001$, 95%CI -187.492; -50.073), with a significant heterogeneity among the studies ($I^2 = 96.086\%$, $p < 0.0001$).

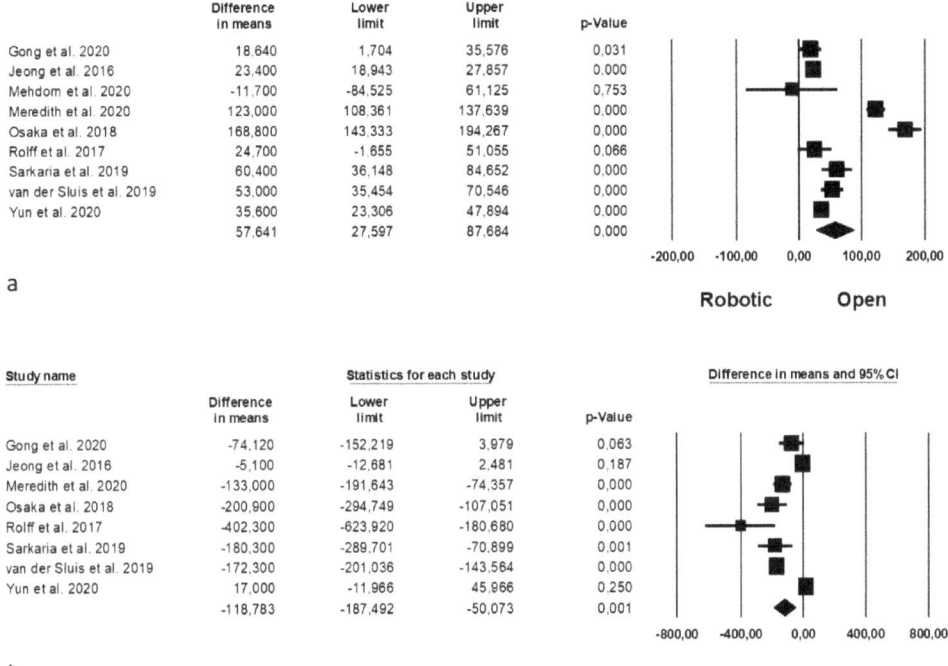

Figure 7. Robotic versus open surgery: intraoperative outcomes. (a) operative time; (b) estimated blood loss.

Postoperative complications are shown in Figure 8. Anastomotic leakage was analysed by 8 Authors [11,35,39,41,44,46,61,63] on 2188 procedures (823 robotic and 1365 open), with no statistical differences between the two approaches (OR = 0.953, $p = 0.799$, 95%CI 0.655; 1.385) and no significant heterogeneity among the studies ($I^2 = 0\%$, $p = 0.556$). Postoperative bleeding was reported by 4 Authors [11,46,61,63] on 818 procedures (339 robotic and 479 open), demonstrating no significant differences between the two groups (RD = -0.007, $p = 0.372$, 95%CI -0.022; 0.008) and no significant heterogeneity among the studies ($I^2 = 0\%$, $p = 0.439$). Postoperative wound infection was analysed by 6 Authors [11,39,41,44,46,61] on 1570 procedures (605 robotic and 965 open), with a significant differences between the two approaches in favour of robotic surgery (OR = 0.425, p = 0.002, 95%CI 0.245; 0.737) and no significant heterogeneity among the studies (I^2 = 11.051%, p = 0.345). Pneumonia was reported by 6 Authors [11,35,39,44,61,63] on 1958 procedures (729 robotic and 1229 open), with a lower number of pneumonias in the robotic group (OR = 0.548, p = 0.03, 95%CI 0.318; 0.944), but with a significant heterogeneity among the studies (I^2 = 61.247%, p = 0.024). Pneumonia rate are expressed in percentage and are available in Supplementary Table S3.

RLN paralysis was reported by 6 Authors [11,35,41,46,61,63] on 1125 procedures (457 robotic and 668 open), with no significant differences between the two approaches (OR = 1.352, p = 0.120, 95%CI 0.925, 1.978) and no significant heterogeneity among the studies (I^2 = 0%, p = 0.807). Chylothorax was analysed by 4 Authors [11,46,61,63] on 818 procedures (339 robotic and 479 open), with no significant differences between the two groups (OR = 1.407, p = 0.273, 95%CI 0.764; 2.589), and no significant heterogeneity among the studies (I^2 = 0%, p =.0.463). Re-operations were reported by 3 Authors [11,38,44] on 1172 procedures (420 robotic and 752 open), with a significant differences in favour of robotic surgery approaches (OR = 0.300, p = 0.035, 95%CI 0.098, 0.919) with no significant heterogeneity among the studies (I^2 = 58.531%, p = 0.09). Mortality was analysed by 9 Authors [11,39,44–46,52,61–63] including 4047 patients (1736 robotic and 2311 open) with no differences between the two groups (OR = 0.971, p = 0.917, 95%CI 0.555; 1.699) and no significant heterogeneity among the studies (I^2 = 72.556%, p < 0.0001).

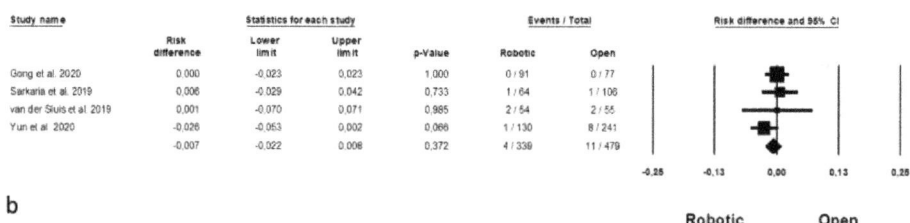

Figure 8. *Cont.*

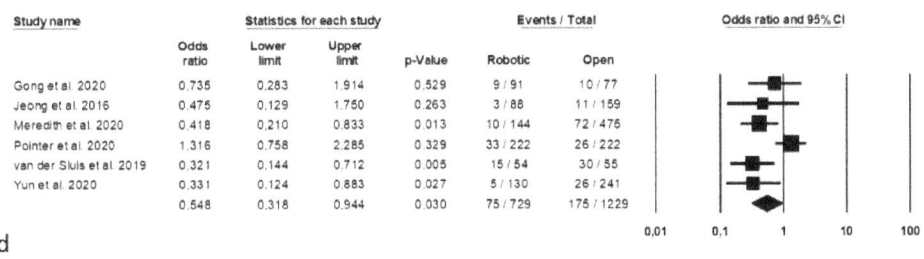

Figure 8. Cont.

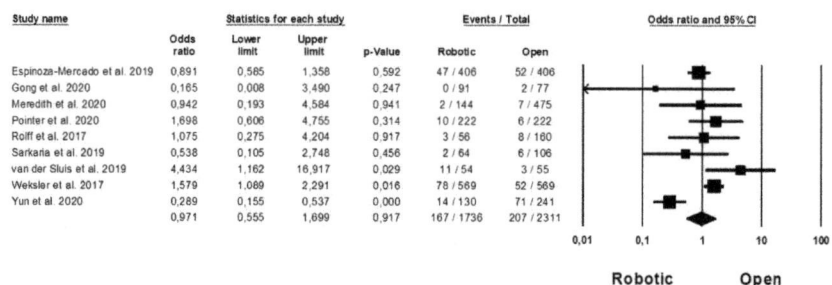

Figure 8. Robotic versus open surgery: postoperative complications. (**a**) anastomotic leakage; (**b**) postoperative bleeding; (**c**) wound infection; (**d**) pneumonia; (**e**) RLN paralysis; (**f**) chylothorax; (**g**) re-operation rate; (**h**) mortality.

Oncologic outcomes are shown in Figure 9. Mean number of harvested nodes was reported by 10 Authors [11,37,38,41,45,46,52,61–63] on 3685 procedures (which of 1555 robotic and 2130 open), demonstrating a higher number of the harvested nodes during the robotic approach (MD = -4, $p < 0.0001$, 95%CI -5.299; -2.888), with a significant heterogeneity among the studies ($I^2 = 94.059\%$, $p < 0.0001$). The number of complete resection (R0 resection) was reported by 7 Authors [11,39,46,52,61–63] on 3387 procedures (which of 1458 robotic and 1929 open), with a significantly higher number of R0 resection in the robotic group (OR = 1.420, $p = 0.043$, 95%CI 1.011; 1.994), and no significant heterogeneity among the studies ($I^2 = 0\%$, $p = 0.462$). Oncologic outcomes are expressed as means and standard deviation (harvested nodes) and percentage (R0 resection rate) in Supplementary Tables S4 and S5, respectively.

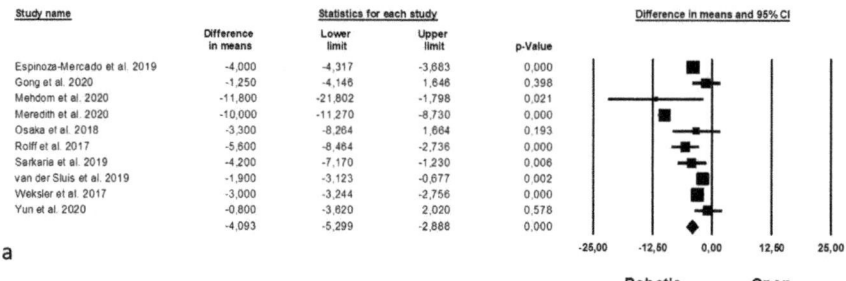

Figure 9. Robotic versus open surgery: oncologic outcomes. (**a**) number of harvested nodes; (**b**) R0 resection.

Length of hospital stay was represented in Figure 10. This data was reported by 9 Authors [11,35,37,41,44–46,62,63], on 2549 patients (1110 robotic and 1439 open), demonstrating a shorter length of hospital stay in the robotic group (MD = -1.341, $p < 0.0001$, 95%CI -1.797; -0.885), with a significant heterogeneity among the studies ($I^2 = 87.169\%$, $p < 0.0001$).

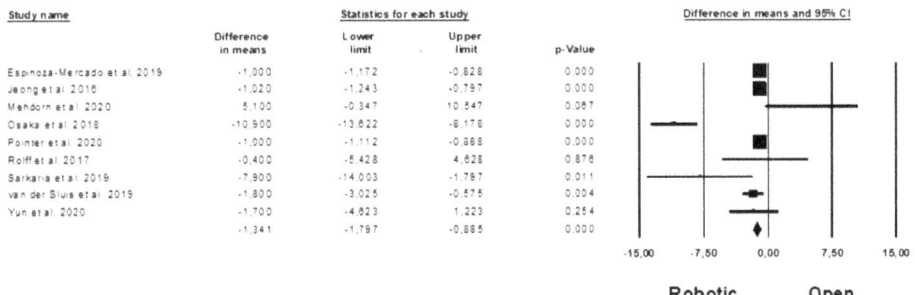

Figure 10. Robotic versus open surgery: length of hospital stay.

8. Long-Term Outcomes

Long-term outcomes are represented in Figure 11. Recurrences was analysed by 2 Authors [63,64] on 480 patients (184 robotic and 296 open), with no significant differences between the two groups (OR = 0.955, p = 0.853, 95%CI 0.590; 1.547) and no significant heterogeneity among the studies (I^2 = 0%, p = 0.971). The 5-years overall survival was reported by 4 Authors [11,36,44,64] on 1670 procedures (834 robotic and 836 open), with no significant differences (OR = 1.018, p = 0.861, 95%CI 0.837; 1.237) and no significant heterogeneity among the studies (I^2 = 0%, p = 0.562).

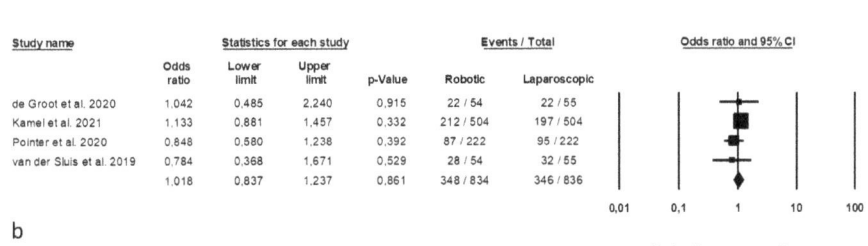

Figure 11. Robotic versus open surgery: long-term outcomes. (**a**) recurrences; (**b**) 5-years overall survival.

9. Subgroup Analysis

9.1. Fully Robotic vs. Open Procedures

To perform this subgroup analysis only the study by Rolff et al. [45] and Weksler et al. [52] were excluded. Thus, the subgroup analysis included eleven studies [11,35,37,38,41,44,46,61–64].

About intraoperative outcomes, subgroup analysis confirmed a significantly lower operative time (MD = 61.676, p < 0.0001, 95%CI 28.905; 94.448) in the open surgery group and lower estimated blood estimated blood loss (MD = −100.742, p = 0.004, 95%CI −169.793; −31.692) in the robotic group.

About postoperative complications, only data about mortality could be extracted, without a significant difference between the two approaches (OR = 0.855, p = 0.668, 95%CI 0.418; 1.748).

Only data regarding harvested nodes could be extracted in terms of oncologic outcomes in the subgroup analysis, confirming a significant difference between the two approaches in favour of robotic approach (MD = 3.783, p = 0.002, 95%CI 1.385; 6.180).

Hospital stay was confirmed to be shorter in the robotic group (MD = -1.353, $p < 0.0001$, 95%CI -1.814; -0.892).

9.2. McKeown Esophagectomy

It was not possible to perform a subgroup analysis because only one study [61] reported data about the comparison between robotic and open McKeown esophagectomy.

9.3. Ivor-Lewis Esophagectomy

Ivor-Lewis esophagectomy was described by only two studies [37,38]. It was possible to perform a subgroup analysis about operative time and harvested nodes. Analysis of operative time showed no significant differences between the two approaches (MD = 60.568, p = 0.367, 95%CI -71.084; 192.219). On the contrary, the analysis on harvested nodes confirmed the higher number of this parameter in the robotic group (MD = 10.029, $p < 0.0001$, 95%CI 8.768; 11.289).

9.4. Publication Bias

Plot analysis showed a symmetrical distribution of the studies evaluating all the analysed outcomes, without evidence of publication bias by the Egger's test. Funnel plots are shown in Supplementary Figures S5–S8.

10. Discussion

The standard treatment of the esophageal cancer is nowadays considered radical esophagectomy with a complete lymphadenectomy whenever this is feasible [65]. Minimally invasive approaches have emerged over the last decades, with the objective to minimize surgical trauma and optimize postoperative outcomes [65].

Minimally invasive esophagectomy (MIE) has gained momentum because of evidence suggesting lower postoperative complication rate and similar oncologic results compared to conventional thoracotomy approaches [66–68].

More recently, Robot-Assisted Minimally Invasive Esophagectomy (RAMIE) was introduced as an alternative minimally invasive method which may allow improved view of thoracic structures and increased precision [69]. Nevertheless, the presumed advantages of the robotic surgery are still under debate [69–71]. In this setting, three meta-analysis tried to assess if the robotic approach could be considered the best treatment to the esophageal cancer [70–72]. In a network meta-analysis on 98 studies and 32,315 patients, Siaw-Acheampong et al. [70] compared all combinations of open, laparoscopic and robotic approaches to transthoracic esophagectomy. Their results demonstrated that compared with open surgery, both laparoscopic and robotic approaches were associated with less blood loss, significantly lower rates of pulmonary complications, shorter hospital stay and higher mean of harvested nodes, concluding that minimally invasive approaches were related with better postoperative outcomes with no compromise in oncologic results. Regarding the comparison between laparoscopic and robot-assisted approach, Zheng et al. [71] identified fourteen studies with a total of 2887 patients included in the final an analysis. The Authors demonstrated that RAMIE was associated with a lower incidence of pneumonia and vocal cord palsy than MIE, but still be associated with longer operative time. Additionally, Li et al. [72] demonstrated in a meta-analytic comparison between 866 patients in the RAMIE group and 883 patients in the MIE group that RAMIE yielded significantly higher number of lymph nodes. Both Authors independently concluded that RAMIE could be a standard treatment for transthoracic approach to esophageal cancer. From that knowledge, in the last two years fifteen new studies have been published comparing robotic approach with the other surgical techniques, confirming the fervid interest in this topic.

By pooling respectively 11,779 comparing robotic versus laparoscopic and 4485 robotic versus open esophagectomy we are able to provide pros and cons of the robotic approach.

Robotic approach appears to provide some advantages over open approach. In fact, our results showed that robotic approach is clearly superior over open surgery in terms of intraoperative outcomes (less blood loss $p = 0.001$), postoperative complications (lower wound infection rate, $p = 0.002$; pneumonia rate, $p = 0.03$; re-operation rate $p = 0.03$) and oncologic outcomes (mean number of harvested nodes, $p < 0.0001$; R0 resection rate, $p = 0.043$). The possible explanation of these better oncologic results could lay in the magnification of the images and in the finer dissection movements properly related to the robotic technology. Considering the current literature, these results are completely in accordance with the previous network meta-analysis by Siaw-Acheampong et al. [70], confirming the advantages of the robotic approach over open technique. On the contrary, no disadvantages were associated with the robotic surgery, except for operative time (longer in the robotic group, $p < 0.0001$), but with no association with non-surgical postoperative complications. Finally, we can assess the safety of robotic approach, guaranteed by the absence of significant differences over open surgery in terms of postoperative complications. Additional conclusion could be provided by the comparison between robotic and conventional laparoscopic approach. Robotic approach seemed to be superior to conventional laparoscopy in terms of oncologic outcomes (mean number of harvested nodes obtained, $p = 0.001$) and postoperative complications (incidence of pneumonia after surgery, $p = 0.003$). Even in this case robotic surgery has the only disadvantage of operative time (shorter in the laparoscopic group, $p = 0.003$), but this data was not associated with increased postoperative morbidities. Our results are in accordance with the results of the meta-analysis by Zheng et al. [71] in terms of longer operative time in the robotic group. Similarly pneumonia rate was lower in the robotic group, and this data has been confirmed by our analysis. Comparing our results with the results obtained by the meta-analysis by Li et al. [72], it is easy to notice an accordance in the setting of number of yielded lymph nodes, significantly higher in the robotic group. On the contrary, Li et al. [72] demonstrated a lower blood loss in the robotic group, in our meta-analysis there was no significant differences between the two groups.

Finally, it is important to highlight that our results were confirmed by the subgroups analyses both for robotic versus laparoscopic and robotic versus open comparison.

In fact, excluding hybrid procedures in both main comparisons, and organizing the studies according to Ivor-Lewis or McKeown procedures, we could confirm the superiority of robotic approach.

Despite these results, major limitation of this study has to be addressed. As known, meta-analysis has to be considered the mirror of the current literature and, thus, the major limitation of our report is that most studies are on a retrospective manner, foreclosing the possibility to exclude patients selection bias.

We cannot exclude that patients' allocation into robotic, laparoscopic or open group would be related to surgeons' preference and experience, patients' and tumors' characteristics.

11. Conclusions

Even if further randomized clinical trials are needed to give definitive conclusions to include the robotic esophagectomy as the gold standard treatment for esophageal cancer, we can assess that robotic surgery could be considered associated with several advantages over both open and laparoscopic surgery.

Take home messages from our analysis are:

- robotic surgery could be considered absolutely safe, being the results about postoperative complications comparable to open and laparoscopic surgery;
- robotic surgery could be considered superior to open approach, being guaranteed less postoperative complications and superior oncologic results;
- robotic approach appeared to be slightly superor to laparoscopic surgery, providing less postoperative pneumonia and higher number of harvested nodes;

- being by our results safety and effectiveness of robotic surgery to treat esophageal cancer, future perspective is the call to perform randomized clinical trial to confirm the advantages of robotic surgery. Definitive conclusions cannot be drawn, due to limitations of the current literature.

Supplementary Materials: The following are available online at https://www.mdpi.com/article/10.3390/jpm11070640/s1, Supplementary Figure S1. Funnel plot analysis of the comparison between robotic and laparoscopic surgery about intraoperative outcomes. (a) operative time; (b) estimated blood loss; (c) conversion. Supplementary Figure S2. Funnel plot analysis of the comparison between robotic and laparoscopic surgery about postoperative complications. (a) anastomotic leakage; (b) postoperative bleeding; (c) wound infection; (d) pneumonia; (e) RLN paralysis; (f) chylothorax; (g) mortality. Supplementary Figure S3. Funnel plot analysis of the comparison between robotic and laparoscopic surgery about oncologic outcomes. (a) number of harvested nodes; (b) R0 resection. Supplementary Figure S4. Funnel plot analysis of the comparison between robotic and laparoscopic surgery about length of hospital stay. Supplementary Figure S5. Funnel plot analysis of the comparison between robotic and laparoscopic surgery about long-term outcomes. (a) recurrences; (b) 5-years overall survival. Supplementary Figure S6. Funnel plot analysis of the comparison between robotic and open surgery about intraoperative outcomes. (a) operative time; (b) estimated blood loss. Supplementary Figure S7. Funnel plot analysis of the comparison between robotic and open surgery about postoperative complications. (a) anastomotic leakage; (b) postoperative bleeding; (c) wound infection; (d) pneumonia; (e) RLN paralysis; (f) chylothorax; (g) re-operation rate; (h) mortality. Supplementary Figure S8. Funnel plot analysis of the comparison between robotic and open surgery about oncologic outcomes. (a) number of harvested nodes; (b) R0 resection. Supplementary Figure S9. Funnel plot analysis of the comparison between robotic and open surgery about length of hospital stay. Supplementary Figure S10. Funnel plot analysis of the comparison between robotic and open surgery about 5-years overall survival. Supplementary Table S1. NOS quality assessment of the included studies comparing robotic and laparoscopic approach. Supplementary Table S2. NOS quality assessment of the included studies comparing robotic and open approach. Supplementary Table S3. Comparison between robotic and open surgery in terms of pneumonia rate.

Author Contributions: M.M. (Marco Milone): design of the study; S.V., A.M., S.A.A., N.K.F.: Acquisition, analysis and interpretation of the data; G.D.D.P. and M.M. (Michele Manigrasso): Interpretation of the data and critical revisions; M.M. (Michele Manigrasso): Conception of the study, critical revisions and final approval. All authors have read and agreed to the published version of the manuscript.

Funding: This research received no external funding.

Institutional Review Board Statement: Not applicable.

Informed Consent Statement: Not applicable.

Data Availability Statement: Not applicable.

Conflicts of Interest: The authors have no conflict of interest to declare.

References

1. Arnold, M.; Abnet, C.C.; Neale, R.E.; Vignat, J.; Giovannucci, E.L.; McGlynn, K.A.; Bray, F. Global Burden of 5 Major Types of Gastrointestinal Cancer. *Gastroenterology* **2020**. [CrossRef] [PubMed]
2. Chen, M.F.; Yang, Y.H.; Lai, C.H.; Chen, P.C.; Chen, W.C. Outcome of patients with esophageal cancer: A nationwide analysis. *Ann. Surg. Oncol.* **2013**. [CrossRef]
3. Lewis, I. The surgical treatment of carcinoma of the oesophagus with special reference to a new operation for growths of the middle third. *Br. J. Surg.* **1946**. [CrossRef] [PubMed]
4. Wang, B.; Zuo, Z.; Chen, H.; Qiu, B.; Du, M.; Gao, Y. The comparison of thoracoscopic-laparoscopic esophagectomy and open esophagectomy: A meta-analysis. *Indian J. Cancer* **2017**. [CrossRef]
5. Guo, W.; Ma, X.; Yang, S.; Zhu, X.; Qin, W.; Xiang, J.; Lerut, T.; Li, H. Combined thoracoscopic-laparoscopic esophagectomy versus open esophagectomy: A meta-analysis of outcomes. *Surg. Endosc.* **2016**. [CrossRef]
6. Wang, K.; Zhong, J.; Liu, Q.; Lin, P.; Fu, J. A Propensity Score-matched Analysis of Thoraco-laparoscopic versus Open McKeown's Esophagectomy. *Ann. Thorac. Surg.* **2021**. [CrossRef] [PubMed]

7. Nuytens, F.; Dabakuyo-Yonli, T.S.; Meunier, B.; Gagnière, J.; Collet, D.; D'Journo, X.B.; Brigand, C.; Perniceni, T.; Carrère, N.; Mabrut, J.Y.; et al. Five-Year Survival Outcomes of Hybrid Minimally Invasive Esophagectomy in Esophageal Cancer: Results of the MIRO Randomized Clinical Trial. *JAMA Surg.* **2021**. [CrossRef] [PubMed]
8. Mariette, C.; Markar, S.; Dabakuyo-Yonli, T.S.; Meunier, B.; Pezet, D.; Collet, D.; D'Journo, X.B.; Brigand, C.; Perniceni, T.; Carrere, N.; et al. Health-related quality of life following hybrid minimally invasive versus open esophagectomy for patients with esophageal cancer, analysis of a multicenter, open-label, randomized phase III controlled trial: The MIRO trial. *Ann. Surg.* **2020**. [CrossRef]
9. Yoshida, N.; Yamamoto, H.; Baba, H.; Miyata, H.; Watanabe, M.; Toh, Y.; Matsubara, H.; Kakeji, Y.; Seto, Y. Can Minimally Invasive Esophagectomy Replace Open Esophagectomy for Esophageal Cancer? Latest Analysis of 24,233 Esophagectomies from the Japanese National Clinical Database. *Ann. Surg.* **2020**. [CrossRef]
10. Maas, K.W.; Cuesta, M.A.; Van Berge Henegouwen, M.I.; Roig, J.; Bonavina, L.; Rosman, C.; Gisbertz, S.S.; Biere, S.S.A.Y.; Van Der Peet, D.L. Quality of Life and Late Complications After Minimally Invasive Compared to Open Esophagectomy: Results of a Randomized Trial. *World J. Surg.* **2015**. [CrossRef]
11. van der Sluis, P.C.; van der Horst, S.; May, A.M.; Schippers, C.; Brosens, L.A.A.; Joore, H.C.A.; Kroese, C.C.; Haj Mohammad, N.; Mook, S.; Vleggaar, F.P.; et al. Robot-assisted Minimally Invasive Thoracolaparoscopic Esophagectomy Versus Open Transthoracic Esophagectomy for Resectable Esophageal Cancer: A Randomized Controlled Trial. *Ann. Surg.* **2019**. [CrossRef] [PubMed]
12. Egberts, J.H.; Stein, H.; Aselmann, H.; Jan-Hendrik, A.; Becker, T. Fully robotic da Vinci Ivor-Lewis esophagectomy in four-arm technique-problems and solutions. *Dis. Esophagus* **2017**. [CrossRef] [PubMed]
13. Milone, M.; Manigrasso, M.; Velotti, N.; Torino, S.; Vozza, A.; Sarnelli, G.; Aprea, G.; Maione, F.; Gennarelli, N.; Musella, M.; et al. Completeness of total mesorectum excision of laparoscopic versus robotic surgery: A review with a meta-analysis. *Int. J. Colorectal Dis.* **2019**, *34*, 983–991. [CrossRef] [PubMed]
14. Ceccarelli, G.; Andolfi, E.; Biancafarina, A.; Rocca, A.; Amato, M.; Milone, M.; Scricciolo, M.; Frezza, B.; Miranda, E.; De Prizio, M.; et al. Robot-assisted surgery in elderly and very elderly population: Our experience in oncologic and general surgery with literature review. *Aging Clin. Exp. Res.* **2017**. [CrossRef] [PubMed]
15. Moon, A.S.; Garofalo, J.; Koirala, P.; Vu, M.L.T.; Chuang, L. Robotic Surgery in Gynecology. *Surg. Clin. N. Am.* **2020**, *82*, 96–109. [CrossRef]
16. Tang, A.B.; Lamaina, M.; Childers, C.P.; Mak, S.S.; Ruan, Q.; Begashaw, M.M.; Bergman, J.; Booth, M.S.; Shekelle, P.G.; Wilson, M.; et al. Perioperative and Long-Term Outcomes of Robot-Assisted Partial Nephrectomy: A Systematic Review. *Am. Surg.* **2021**. [CrossRef] [PubMed]
17. Kernstine, K.H.; DeArmond, D.T.; Karimi, M.; Van Natta, T.L.; Campos, J.C.; Yoder, M.R.; Everett, J.E. The robotic, 2-stage, 3-field esophagolymphadenectomy. *J. Thorac. Cardiovasc. Surg.* **2004**. [CrossRef]
18. Moher, D.; Liberati, A.; Tetzlaff, J.; Altman, D.G.; Altman, D.; Antes, G.; Atkins, D.; Barbour, V.; Barrowman, N.; Berlin, J.A.; et al. Preferred reporting items for systematic reviews and meta-analyses: The PRISMA statement. *PLoS Med.* **2009**, *6*, e1000097. [CrossRef]
19. Brooke, B.S.; Schwartz, T.A.; Pawlik, T.M. MOOSE Reporting Guidelines for Meta-analyses of Observational Studies. *JAMA Surg.* **2021**. [CrossRef]
20. Wells, G.A.; Shea, B.; O'connell, D.; Petersen, J.; Welch, V.; Losos, M.; Tugwell, P.; The Newcastle-Ottawa Scale (NOS) for Assessing the Quality of Nonrandomized Studies in Meta-Analyses. Department of Epidemiology and Community Medicine, University of Ottawa: ottawa, ON, Canada, 2012. Available online: www.ohri.ca/programs/clinical_epidemiology/oxford.asp (accessed on 12 May 2021).
21. Higgins, J.P.T.; Altman, D.G.; Gøtzsche, P.C.; Jüni, P.; Moher, D.; Oxman, A.D.; Savović, J.; Schulz, K.F.; Weeks, L.; Sterne, J.A.C. The Cochrane Collaboration's tool for assessing risk of bias in randomised trials. *BMJ* **2011**. [CrossRef]
22. Messori, A.; Maratea, D.; Fadda, V.; Trippoli, S. Using risk difference as opposed to odds-ratio in meta-analysis. *Int. J. Cardiol.* **2013**. [CrossRef] [PubMed]
23. Shi, J.; Luo, D.; Weng, H.; Zeng, X.T.; Lin, L.; Chu, H.; Tong, T. Optimally estimating the sample standard deviation from the five-number summary. *Res. Synth. Methods* **2020**. [CrossRef] [PubMed]
24. Luo, D.; Wan, X.; Liu, J.; Tong, T. Optimally estimating the sample mean from the sample size, median, mid-range, and/or mid-quartile range. *Stat. Methods Med. Res.* **2018**. [CrossRef] [PubMed]
25. Wan, X.; Wang, W.; Liu, J.; Tong, T. Estimating the sample mean and standard deviation from the sample size, median, range and/or interquartile range. *BMC Med. Res. Methodol.* **2014**. [CrossRef]
26. Furukawa, T.A.; Barbui, C.; Cipriani, A.; Brambilla, P.; Watanabe, N. Imputing missing standard deviations in meta-analyses can provide accurate results. *J. Clin. Epidemiol.* **2006**. [CrossRef] [PubMed]
27. DerSimonian, R.; Laird, N. Meta-analysis in clinical trials revisited. *Contemp. Clin. Trials* **2015**. [CrossRef] [PubMed]
28. Higgins, J.P.T.; Thompson, S.G.; Deeks, J.J.; Altman, D.G. Measuring inconsistency in meta-analyses. *Br. Med. J.* **2003**, *327*, 557–560. [CrossRef]
29. Thompson, S.G.; Sharp, S.J. Explaining heterogeneity in meta-analysis: A comparison of methods. *Stat. Med.* **1999**, *18*, 2693–2708. [CrossRef]
30. Egger, M.; Smith, G.D.; Schneider, M.; Minder, C. Bias in meta-analysis detected by a simple, graphical test. *Br. Med. J.* **1997**. [CrossRef]

31. Ali, A.M.; Bachman, K.C.; Worrell, S.G.; Gray, K.E.; Perry, Y.; Linden, P.A.; Towe, C.W. Robotic minimally invasive esophagectomy provides superior surgical resection. *Surg. Endosc.* **2020**. [CrossRef]
32. Grimminger, P.P.; Tagkalos, E.; Hadzijusufovic, E.; Corvinus, F.; Babic, B.; Lang, H. Change from Hybrid to Fully Minimally Invasive and Robotic Esophagectomy is Possible without Compromises. *Thorac. Cardiovasc. Surg.* **2019**. [CrossRef]
33. Harbison, G.J.; Vossler, J.D.; Yim, N.H.; Murayama, K.M. Outcomes of robotic versus non-robotic minimally-invasive esophagectomy for esophageal cancer: An American College of Surgeons NSQIP database analysis. *Am. J. Surg.* **2019**. [CrossRef]
34. He, H.; Wu, Q.; Wang, Z.; Zhang, Y.; Chen, N.; Fu, J.; Zhang, G. Short-term outcomes of robot-assisted minimally invasive esophagectomy for esophageal cancer: A propensity score matched analysis. *J. Cardiothorac. Surg.* **2018**. [CrossRef]
35. Jeong, D.M.; Kim, J.A.; Ahn, H.J.; Yang, M.; Heo, B.Y.; Lee, S.H. Decreased Incidence of Postoperative Delirium in Robot-assisted Thoracoscopic Esophagectomy Compared with Open Transthoracic Esophagectomy. *Surg. Laparosc. Endosc. Percutaneous Tech.* **2016**, *26*, 516–522. [CrossRef] [PubMed]
36. Kamel, M.K.; Sholi, A.N.; Rahouma, M.; Harrison, S.W.; Lee, B.; Stiles, B.M.; Altorki, N.K.; Port, J.L. National trends and perioperative outcomes of robotic oesophagectomy following induction chemoradiation therapy: A National Cancer Database propensity-matched analysis. *Eur. J. Cardio-Thoracic Surg.* **2021**. [CrossRef]
37. Mehdorn, A.-S.; Möller, T.; Franke, F.; Richter, F.; Kersebaum, J.-N.; Becker, T.; Egberts, J.-H. Long-Term, Health-Related Quality of Life after Open and Robot-Assisted Ivor-Lewis Procedures—A Propensity Score-Matched Study. *J. Clin. Med.* **2020**. [CrossRef] [PubMed]
38. Meredith, K.L.; Maramara, T.; Blinn, P.; Lee, D.; Huston, J.; Shridhar, R. Comparative Perioperative Outcomes by Esophagectomy Surgical Technique. *J. Gastrointest. Surg.* **2020**. [CrossRef] [PubMed]
39. Meredith, K.; Blinn, P.; Maramara, T.; Takahashi, C.; Huston, J.; Shridhar, R. Comparative outcomes of minimally invasive and robotic-assisted esophagectomy. *Surg. Endosc.* **2020**. [CrossRef]
40. Motoyama, S.; Sato, Y.; Wakita, A.; Kawakita, Y.; Nagaki, Y.; Imai, K.; Minamiya, Y. Extensive lymph node dissection around the left laryngeal nerve achieved with robot-assisted thoracoscopic esophagectomy. *Anticancer Res.* **2019**. [CrossRef]
41. Osaka, Y.; Tachibana, S.; Ota, Y.; Suda, T.; Makuuti, Y.; Watanabe, T.; Iwasaki, K.; Katsumata, K.; Tsuchida, A. Usefulness of robot-assisted thoracoscopic esophagectomy. *Gen. Thorac. Cardiovasc. Surg.* **2018**. [CrossRef] [PubMed]
42. Chao, Y.K.; Hsieh, M.J.; Liu, Y.H.; Liu, H.P. Lymph Node Evaluation in Robot-Assisted Versus Video-Assisted Thoracoscopic Esophagectomy for Esophageal Squamous Cell Carcinoma: A Propensity-Matched Analysis. *World J. Surg.* **2018**. [CrossRef] [PubMed]
43. Park, S.; Hwang, Y.; Lee, H.J.; Park, I.K.; Kim, Y.T.; Kang, C.H. Comparison of robot-assisted esophagectomy and thoracoscopic esophagectomy in esophageal squamous cell carcinoma. *J. Thorac. Dis.* **2016**. [CrossRef]
44. Pointer, D.T.; Saeed, S.; Naffouje, S.A.; Mehta, R.; Hoffe, S.E.; Dineen, S.P.; Fleming, J.B.; Fontaine, J.P.; Pimiento, J.M. Outcomes of 350 Robotic-assisted Esophagectomies at a High-volume Cancer Center. *Ann. Surg.* **2020**. [CrossRef] [PubMed]
45. Rolff, H.C.; Ambrus, R.B.; Belmouhand, M.; Achiam, M.P.; Wegmann, M.; Siemsen, M.; Kofoed, S.C.; Svendsen, L.B. Robot-Assisted Hybrid Esophagectomy Is Associated with a Shorter Length of Stay Compared to Conventional Transthoracic Esophagectomy: A Retrospective Study. *Minim. Invasive Surg.* **2017**. [CrossRef] [PubMed]
46. Sarkaria, I.S.; Rizk, N.P.; Goldman, D.A.; Sima, C.; Tan, K.S.; Bains, M.S.; Adusumilli, P.S.; Molena, D.; Bott, M.; Atkinson, T.; et al. Early Quality of Life Outcomes After Robotic-Assisted Minimally Invasive and Open Esophagectomy. *Ann. Thorac. Surg.* **2019**. [CrossRef]
47. Shirakawa, Y.; Noma, K.; Kunitomo, T.; Hashimoto, M.; Maeda, N.; Tanabe, S.; Sakurama, K.; Fujiwara, T. Initial introduction of robot-assisted, minimally invasive esophagectomy using the microanatomy-based concept in the upper mediastinum. *Surg. Endosc.* **2020**. [CrossRef]
48. Suda, K.; Ishida, Y.; Kawamura, Y.; Inaba, K.; Kanaya, S.; Teramukai, S.; Satoh, S.; Uyama, I. Robot-assisted thoracoscopic lymphadenectomy along the left recurrent laryngeal nerve for esophageal squamous cell carcinoma in the prone position: Technical report and short-term outcomes. *World J. Surg.* **2012**. [CrossRef] [PubMed]
49. Tagkalos, E.; Goense, L.; Hoppe-Lotichius, M.; Ruurda, J.P.; Babic, B.; Hadzijusufovic, E.; Kneist, W.; Van Der Sluis, P.C.; Lang, H.; Van Hillegersberg, R.; et al. Robot-assisted minimally invasive esophagectomy (RAMIE) compared to conventional minimally invasive esophagectomy (MIE) for esophageal cancer: A propensity-matched analysis. *Dis. Esophagus* **2020**. [CrossRef] [PubMed]
50. Tsunoda, S.; Obama, K.; Hisamori, S.; Nishigori, T.; Okumura, R.; Maekawa, H.; Sakai, Y. Lower Incidence of Postoperative Pulmonary Complications Following Robot-Assisted Minimally Invasive Esophagectomy for Esophageal Cancer: Propensity Score-Matched Comparison to Conventional Minimally Invasive Esophagectomy. *Ann. Surg. Oncol.* **2021**. [CrossRef] [PubMed]
51. Weksler, B.; Sharma, P.; Moudgill, N.; Chojnacki, K.A.; Rosato, E.L. Robot-assisted minimally invasive esophagectomy is equivalent to thoracoscopic minimally invasive esophagectomy. *Dis. Esophagus* **2012**. [CrossRef]
52. Weksler, B.; Sullivan, J.L. Survival after Esophagectomy: A Propensity-Matched Study of Different Surgical Approaches. *Ann. Thorac. Surg.* **2017**. [CrossRef]
53. Chao, Y.K.; Wen, Y.W.; Chuang, W.Y.; Cerfolio, R.J. Transition from video-assisted thoracoscopic to robotic esophagectomy: A single surgeon's experience. *Dis. Esophagus* **2020**. [CrossRef] [PubMed]
54. Xu, Y.; Li, X.-K.; Cong, Z.-Z.; Zhou, H.; Wu, W.-J.; Qiang, Y.; Yi, J.; Shen, Y. Long-term outcomes of robotic-assisted versus thoraco-laparoscopic McKeown esophagectomy for esophageal cancer: A propensity score-matched study. *Dis. Esophagus* **2020**. [CrossRef] [PubMed]

55. Yerokun, B.A.; Sun, Z.; Jeffrey Yang, C.F.; Gulack, B.C.; Speicher, P.J.; Adam, M.A.; D'Amico, T.A.; Onaitis, M.W.; Harpole, D.H.; Berry, M.F.; et al. Minimally Invasive Versus Open Esophagectomy for Esophageal Cancer: A Population-Based Analysis. *Ann. Thorac. Surg.* **2016**. [CrossRef] [PubMed]
56. Zhang, Y.; Han, Y.; Gan, Q.; Xiang, J.; Jin, R.; Chen, K.; Che, J.; Hang, J.; Li, H. Early Outcomes of Robot-Assisted Versus Thoracoscopic-Assisted Ivor Lewis Esophagectomy for Esophageal Cancer: A Propensity Score-Matched Study. *Ann. Surg. Oncol.* **2019**. [CrossRef]
57. Yang, Y.; Zhang, X.; Li, B.; Hua, R.; Yang, Y.; He, Y.; Ye, B.; Guo, X.; Sun, Y.; Li, Z. Short- And mid-term outcomes of robotic versus thoraco-laparoscopic McKeown esophagectomy for squamous cell esophageal cancer: A propensity score-matched study. *Dis. Esophagus* **2020**. [CrossRef] [PubMed]
58. Chen, J.; Liu, Q.; Zhang, X.; Yang, H.; Tan, Z.; Lin, Y.; Fu, J. Comparisons of short-term outcomes between robot-assisted and thoraco-laparoscopic esophagectomy with extended two-field lymph node dissection for resectable thoracic esophageal squamous cell carcinoma. *J. Thorac. Dis.* **2019**. [CrossRef]
59. Deng, H.Y.; Luo, J.; Li, S.X.; Li, G.; Alai, G.; Wang, Y.; Liu, L.X.; Lin, Y.D. Does robot-assisted minimally invasive esophagectomy really have the advantage of lymphadenectomy over video-assisted minimally invasive esophagectomy in treating esophageal squamous cell carcinoma? A propensity score-matched analysis based on short-term. *Dis. Esophagus* **2019**. [CrossRef]
60. Duan, X.; Yue, J.; Chen, C.; Gong, L.; Ma, Z.; Shang, X.; Yu, Z.; Jiang, H. Lymph node dissection around left recurrent laryngeal nerve: Robot-assisted vs. video-assisted McKeown esophagectomy for esophageal squamous cell carcinoma. *Surg. Endosc.* **2020**. [CrossRef]
61. Gong, L.; Jiang, H.; Yue, J.; Duan, X.; Tang, P.; Ren, P.; Zhao, X.; Liu, X.; Zhang, X.; Yu, Z. Comparison of the short-term outcomes of robot-assisted minimally invasive, video-assisted minimally invasive, and open esophagectomy. *J. Thorac. Dis.* **2020**. [CrossRef]
62. Espinoza-Mercado, F.; Imai, T.A.; Borgella, J.D.; Sarkissian, A.; Serna-Gallegos, D.; Alban, R.F.; Soukiasian, H.J. Does the Approach Matter? Comparing Survival in Robotic, Minimally Invasive, and Open Esophagectomies. *Ann. Thorac. Surg.* **2019**. [CrossRef]
63. Yun, J.K.; Chong, B.K.; Kim, H.J.; Lee, I.S.; Gong, C.S.; Kim, B.S.; Lee, G.D.; Choi, S.; Kim, H.R.; Kim, D.K.; et al. Comparative outcomes of robot-assisted minimally invasive versus open esophagectomy in patients with esophageal squamous cell carcinoma: A propensity score-weighted analysis. *Dis. Esophagus* **2021**. [CrossRef] [PubMed]
64. de Groot, E.M.; van der Horst, S.; Feike Kingma, B.; Goense, L.; van der Sluis, P.C.; Ruurda, J.P.; van Hillegersberg, R. Robot-assisted minimally invasive thoracolaparoscopic esophagectomy versus open esophagectomy: Long-term follow-up of a randomized clinical trial. *Dis. Esophagus* **2020**. [CrossRef]
65. Gisbertz, S.S.; Hagens, E.R.C.; Ruurda, J.P.; Schneider, P.M.; Tan, L.J.; Domrachev, S.A.; Hoeppner, J.; van Berge Henegouwen, M.I. The evolution of surgical approach for esophageal cancer. *Ann. N. Y. Acad. Sci.* **2018**. [CrossRef] [PubMed]
66. Lv, L.; Hu, W.; Ren, Y.; Wei, X. Minimally invasive esophagectomy versus open esophagectomy for esophageal cancer: A meta-analysis. *OncoTargets Ther.* **2016**. [CrossRef] [PubMed]
67. Mariette, C.; Piessen, G.; Triboulet, J.P. Therapeutic strategies in oesophageal carcinoma: Role of surgery and other modalities. *Lancet Oncol.* **2007**, *8*, 545–553. [CrossRef]
68. Biere, S.S.A.Y.; Van Berge Henegouwen, M.I.; Maas, K.W.; Bonavina, L.; Rosman, C.; Garcia, J.R.; Gisbertz, S.S.; Klinkenbijl, J.H.G.; Hollmann, M.W.; De Lange, E.S.M.; et al. Minimally invasive versus open oesophagectomy for patients with oesophageal cancer: A multicentre, open-label, randomised controlled trial. *Lancet* **2012**. [CrossRef]
69. Jin, D.; Yao, L.; Yu, J.; Liu, R.; Guo, T.; Yang, K.; Gou, Y. Robotic-assisted minimally invasive esophagectomy versus the conventional minimally invasive one: A meta-analysis and systematic review. *Int. J. Med. Robot. Comput. Assist. Surg.* **2019**, *15*, e1988. [CrossRef]
70. Siaw-Acheampong, K.; Kamarajah, S.K.; Gujjuri, R.; Bundred, J.R.; Singh, P.; Griffiths, E.A. Minimally invasive techniques for transthoracic oesophagectomy for oesophageal cancer: Systematic review and network meta-analysis. *BJS Open* **2020**, *4*, 787–803. [CrossRef]
71. Zheng, C.; Li, X.K.; Zhang, C.; Zhou, H.; Ji, S.G.; Zhong, J.H.; Xu, Y.; Cong, Z.Z.; Wang, G.M.; Wu, W.J.; et al. Comparison of short-term clinical outcomes between robot-assisted minimally invasive esophagectomy and video-assisted minimally invasive esophagectomy: A systematic review and meta-analysis. *J. Thorac. Dis.* **2021**. [CrossRef]
72. Li, X.K.; Xu, Y.; Zhou, H.; Cong, Z.Z.; Wu, W.J.; Qiang, Y.; Shen, Y. Does robot-assisted minimally invasive oesophagectomy have superiority over thoraco-laparoscopic minimally invasive oesophagectomy in lymph node dissection? *Dis. esophagus Off. J. Int. Soc. Dis. Esophagus* **2021**. [CrossRef] [PubMed]

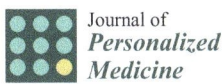

Article

Robotic Colorectal Cancer Surgery. How to Reach Expertise? A Single Surgeon-Experience

Michele Manigrasso [1,*], Sara Vertaldi [2], Pietro Anoldo [2], Anna D'Amore [2], Alessandra Marello [2], Carmen Sorrentino [2], Alessia Chini [2], Salvatore Aprea [3], Salvatore D'Angelo [3], Nicola D'Alesio [3], Mario Musella [1], Antonio Vitiello [1], Giovanni Domenico De Palma [2] and Marco Milone [2]

1. Department of Advanced Biomedical Sciences, University of Naples "Federico II", Via Pansini 5, 80131 Naples, Italy; mario.musella@unina.it (M.M.); antoniovitiello_@hotmail.it (A.V.)
2. Department of Clinical Medicine and Surgery, University of Naples "Federico II", Via Pansini 5, 80131 Naples, Italy; vertaldisara@gmail.com (S.V.); pietro.anoldo@gmail.com (P.A.); anna.damore1993@libero.it (A.D.); alessandramarello@gmail.com (A.M.); carmensor94@gmail.com (C.S.); dr.alessiachini@gmail.com (A.C.); giovanni.depalma@unina.it (G.D.D.P.); milone.marco.md@gmail.com (M.M.)
3. "Federico II" University Hospital, Via Pansini 5, 80131 Naples, Italy; sa.aprea@gmail.com (S.A.); salvatore220987@hotmail.it (S.D.); nicodale1987@hotmail.it (N.D.)
* Correspondence: michele.manigrasso@unina.it

Abstract: The complexity associated with laparoscopic colorectal surgery requires several skills to overcome the technical difficulties related to this procedure. To overcome the technical challenges of laparoscopic surgery, a robotic approach has been introduced. Our study reports the surgical outcomes obtained by the transition from laparoscopic to robotic approach in colorectal cancer surgery to establish in which type of approach the proficiency is easier to reach. Data about the first consecutive 15 laparoscopic and the first 15 consecutive robotic cases are extracted, adopting as a comparator of proficiency the last 15 laparoscopic colorectal resections for cancer. The variables studied are operative time, number of harvested nodes, conversion rate, postoperative complications, recovery outcomes. Our analysis includes 15 patients per group. Our results show that operative time is significantly longer in the first 15 laparoscopic cases ($p = 0.001$). A significantly lower number of harvested nodes was retrieved in the first 15 laparoscopic cases ($p = 0.003$). Clavien Dindo I complication rate was higher in the first laparoscopic group, but without a significant difference among the three groups ($p = 0.09$). Our results show that the surgeon needed no apparent learning curve to reach their laparoscopic standards. However, further multicentric prospective studies are needed to confirm this conclusion.

Keywords: robotic; colorectal; colorectal cancer; laparoscopic; learning curve

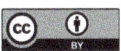

1. Introduction

Minimally invasive surgery represents nowadays the standard approach for the treatment of colorectal pathologies [1–3]. However, the complexity associated with laparoscopic colorectal surgery requires several skills to overcome the technical difficulties related to this type of procedure [4,5]. Thus, the safety and the feasibility of laparoscopic colorectal surgery are related to the surgeon's experience.

In this setting, several parameters have been investigated to define an adequate level of proficiency, but the number of cases needed to complete the learning curve is still not well defined [6–11], varying between 11 and 152 [6,9,11,12].

Recently, to overcome the technical challenges of laparoscopic surgery, a robotic approach has been introduced [13–15]. Its adoption to colorectal surgery has gained large consensus among the surgeons, because of its several facilities to overcome the difficulties of laparoscopic surgery.

In the setting of surgical expertise, most studies reported that robotic colorectal surgery has a shorter learning curve, reaching the plateau after 15–25 cases [12,16].

However, the results of the comparison between robotic and laparoscopic colorectal surgery during the learning curve are still under debate. This study reports the surgical outcomes obtained by the transition from laparoscopic to robotic approach in colorectal cancer surgery to establish in which type of approach the proficiency is easier to reach.

2. Materials and Methods

After the University Institutional Review Board of a tertiary referral colorectal center approval, a retrospective chart review of the minimally invasive colorectal resection for cancer performed by a single surgeon (M.M.) between 1 January 2014 and 31 March 2021 was conducted.

Patients who underwent colorectal resection for benign conditions and emergency cases were excluded.

Data about the first consecutive 15 laparoscopic (Group A) and the first 15 consecutive robotic cases (Group B) were extracted, adopting as a comparator of proficiency data about the last 15 laparoscopic colorectal cancer resections (Group C). Specifically, laparoscopic colorectal cancer surgery was introduced in our institution in 2014, while robotic-assisted surgery was adopted in 2018. Thus, the enrolment period ranged from 2014 (first 15 laparoscopic cases) to 2021 (last 15 laparoscopic cases) throughout 2018 (first 15 robotic cases).

2.1. Surgical Technique and Perioperative Management

When laparoscopy was introduced in the institution, the surgeon had no experience as the first surgeon in colorectal procedures, as well as for the robotic colorectal procedures when the robotic platform was introduced.

All the patients underwent preoperative antibiotics and heparin prophylaxis as described previously [17].

All the surgical interventions were performed by the same surgeon (M.M.), who had no experience as the first surgeon in laparoscopic colorectal procedures at the beginning of the enrolment period. Similarly, the surgeon had no experience in robotic colorectal procedures at the enrolment of the first 15 robotic cases, but with adequate expertise in laparoscopic colorectal surgery.

All the patients underwent surgical procedures were under general anesthesia. In right colectomy, after identifying the ileocolic pedicle, the peritoneum was dissected towards the transverse colon, and the Toldt's fascia was separated by the Gerota's plane, preserving the duodenum, the right gonadal vessels, and the right ureter. After the ligation of the ileocolic pedicles, the right colic artery (if present), and the right branch of the middle colic artery, the right hemicolectomy was performed with a linear stapler (or with a robotic stapler during the robotic procedure), and an intracorporeal side-to-side isoperistaltic anastomosis was performed. In the left colectomy, after a coloepiploic detachment, the splenic flexure was completely mobilized by creating a window under the Inferior Mesenteric Vein (IMV) to separate the mesocolon from the pancreatic tail. After identifying the Inferior Mesenteric Artery (IMA) origin, the Toldt's fascia was completely separated by the retroperitoneal plane, preserving the left ureter and the gonadal vessels. Then the IMV and IMA were ligated at their origin, a left hemicolectomy was performed, and an end-to-end Knight Griffen colorectal anastomosis was performed. In the case of splenic flexure resection, the transverse and descending colon were completely mobilized, the left branch of the middle colic artery and the left colic artery were ligated at their origin, and a splenic flexure resection was performed. In the case of transverse colon resection, both colic flexures were mobilized, and the wedge resection of the transverse colon and the mesentery between the two branches of the middle colic artery was performed. In the case of segmental colonic resection, an intracorporeal, isoperistaltic, side-to-side anastomosis was performed. In rectal anterior resection the procedure followed the surgical steps of the left hemicolectomy. In addition, a complete TME was performed, and in the case of middle- and low-rectal cancers, a protective loop ileostomy was performed after the Knight–Griffen colorectal anastomosis.

The postoperative period has been homogenized according to ERAS protocol [18].

2.2. Outcomes and Data Collection

Collected data of the three cohorts included gender, age, Body Mass Index (BMI), American Society of Anesthesiologists risk class (ASA), Charlson Comorbidity Index (CCI), tumor localization, and TNM stage, type of resection.

Intraoperative outcomes to predict the feasibility of the surgical approach were: Operative time, number of harvested nodes, and conversion rate.

Postoperative complications were recorded according to Clavien–Dindo (CD) classification [19], such as nausea and vomit, postoperative pain, ileus, surgical wound complications, abdominal or bowel bleeding, anastomotic leakage, need of Intensive Care Unit (ICU), and death.

Postoperative recovery outcomes were evaluated in terms of time to first flatus, time to first stools, and length of hospital stay.

The term anastomotic leakage included all conditions with clinical or radiologic anastomotic dehiscence, with or without needing surgical revision. Any bleeding has been considered if required blood transfusions. The term postoperative pain included the situations in which extra analgesia was needed for moderate or severe pain in the postoperative period. The term ileus included the situations in which the bowel movements were absent for over 72 postoperative hours. If the condition required prokinetics, it was inserted in the group of Clavien Dindo I complications group; on the contrary, the ileus requiring the insertion of the nasogastric tube was inserted in the Clavien Dindo II complications group. The term conversion included all situations in which a laparotomy was needed or in which, during the procedure, an extracorporeal anastomosis was preferred.

2.3. Statistical Analysis

Statistical analysis was performed by using SPSS version 26.0 (IBM, Armonk, NY, USA). Continuous data were expressed as mean ± SD; categorical variables were expressed as %. Continuous variables were compared among the groups by ANOVA test, and a Bonferroni post-hoc analysis was performed to investigate group differences on multiple dependent variables in the case of significance; categorical variables are compared by the $\chi 2$ test; when the minimum expected value was <5, the Fisher's exact test was adopted. A p value of <0.05 was defined as statistically significant.

A subgroup analysis of the intraoperative outcomes was performed according to the tumor localization and consequent surgical procedures to exclude any bias-related to any surgical challenge.

3. Results

Our analysis included 45 patients, 15 in each group. Demographic data are reported in Table 1.

No significant difference was found among the three groups in terms of gender ($p = 0.765$), age ($p = 0.814$), BMI ($p = 0.900$), ASA Score ($p = 0.557$), Charlson Score ($p = 0.978$), tumor localization ($p = 0.776$), TNM ($p = 0.946$, $p = 0.497$ and $p = 1.000$, respectively) and type of surgical resection ($p = 0.739$).

Intraoperative outcomes, postoperative complications, and recovery outcomes are shown in Table 2.

Operative time was significantly longer in the first 15 laparoscopic cases ($p = 0.001$), and the Bonferroni post-hoc test confirmed this significance between Group A and both Group B and Group C ($p = 0.003$ and $p = 0.008$, respectively), while no significance was found between Group B and Group C ($p = 0.998$).

Table 1. Demographic data of the included patients.

Patients' Characteristics	Group A (n = 15)	Group B (n = 15)	Group C (n = 15)	p Value
Gender				0.765
M	7 (46.7)	8 (53.3)	9 (6.2)	
F	8 (53.3)	7 (46.7)	6 (40.0)	
Age	72.07 ± 7.9	70.53 ± 13.51	69.53 ± 10.44	0.814
BMI	26.4 ± 4.2	25.8 ± 4.03	26.16 ± 2.04	0.900
ASA Score				0.557
I	0 (0)	0 (0)	1 (6.7)	
II	11 (73.3)	8 (53.3)	9 (60)	
III	4 (26.7)	6 (40.0)	5 (33.3)	
IV	0 (0)	1 (6.7)	0 (0)	
Charlson Score	6.07 ± 1.8	6.13 ± 2	6.2 ± 1.26	0.978
Tumour localization				0.776
Caecum	2 (13.3)	2 (13.3)	0 (0)	
Right Colon	2 (13.3)	3 (20.0)	4 (26.7)	
Hepatic flexure	1 (6.7)	0 (0)	1 (6.7)	
Transverse colon	0 (0)	0 (0)	1 (6.7)	
Splenic flexure	0 (0)	0 (0)	1 (6.7)	
Descending colon	4 (26.7)	3 (20)	2 (13.3)	
Sigma	1 (6.7)	0 (0)	1 (6.7)	
Rectum	5 (33.3)	7 (46.7)	5 (33.3)	
T Classification				0.946
1	1 (6.7)	2 (13.3)	1 (6.7)	
2	5 (33.3)	3 (20.0)	5 (33.3)	
3	6 (40.0)	8 (53.3)	7 (46.7)	
4	3 (20.0)	2 (13.3)	2 (13.3)	
N Classification				0.497
0	9 (60)	6 (40.0)	10 (66.7)	
1	6 (40.0)	8 (53.3)	4 (26.7)	
2	0 (0)	1 (6.7)	1 (6.7)	
M Classification				1.000
0	14 (93.3)	14 (93.3)	14 (93.3)	
1	1 (6.7)	1 (6.7)	1 (6.7)	
Type of resection				0.739
Right hemicolectomy	5 (33.3)	5 (33.3)	5 (33.3)	
Transverse resection	0 (0)	0 (0)	1 (6.7)	
Splenic flexure resection	0 (0)	0 (0)	1 (6.7)	
Left hemicolectomy	5 (33.3)	3 (20.0)	3 (20.0)	
Rectal anterior resection	5 (33.3)	6 (40.0)	5 (33.3)	
Abdomino-perineal resection	0 (0)	1 (6.7)	0 (0)	

Dichotomous variables are expressed by number and (percentage); continuous variables by mean ± standard deviation. M: male; F: female; BMI: Body Mass Index; ASA: American Society of Anesthesiologists.

Table 2. Intraoperative outcomes, postoperative complications and recovery outcomes.

Outcomes	Group A (n = 15)	Group B (n = 15)	Group C (n = 15)	p Value
Intraoperative outcomes				
Operative time (min)	233 ± 55.48	169.66 ± 46.27	177 ± 42	0.001
Harvested nodes	17.73 ± 4.62	23 ± 3	21.53 ± 4.59	0.003
Conversion	1 (6.7)	1 (6.7)	0 (0)	0.593
Postoperative complications				
Clavien Dindo				
I	7 (46.7)	2 (13.3)	3 (20.0)	0.09
Nausea	4 (26.7)	1 (6.7)	1 (6.7)	
Ileus	3 (20.0)	1 (6.7)	2 (13.3)	
II	4 (26.7)	1 (6.7)	1 (6.7)	0.18
Wound infection	1 (6.7)	1 (6.7)	0 (0)	
Intraluminal bleeding	2 (13.3)	0 (0)	1 (6.7)	
Extraluminal bleeding	1 (6.7)	0 (0)4	0 (0)	
III	1 (6.7)	1 (6.7)	0 (0)	0.59
Anastomotic leakage	1 (6.7)	1 (6.7)	0 (0)	
IV	0 (0)	0 (0)	0 (0)	1.000
V	0 (0)	0 (0)	0 (0)	1.000
Overall complications	12 (80)	4 (26.6)	4 (26.6)	0.003
Recovery outcomes				
Time to first flatus (hrs)	56.53 ± 23.08	51.66 ± 19	49.47 ± 27.15	0.704
Time to first stool (hrs)	79.6 ± 21.06	77.47 ± 25.31	76.6 ± 28.71	0.945
Length of hospital stay (days)	4.5 ± 0.7	3.75 ± 0.93	4.34 ± 1.1	0.072

Dichotomous variables are expressed by number and (percentage); continuous variables by mean ± standard deviation. Hrs: hours.

Similarly, a significantly lower number of harvested nodes was retrieved in the first 15 laparoscopic cases ($p = 0.003$). Bonferroni post-hoc test confirmed that the number of harvested nodes was significantly lower in Group A over both Group B and Group C ($p = 0.003$ and $p = 0.047$, respectively), while no significance was present between Group B and Group C ($p = 0.944$).

The number of conversions was similar among the three groups ($p = 0.593$).

Clavien Dindo I complications were seven in Group A, two in Group B, and three in Group C, showing no differences among the three groups, but a trend toward significance ($p = 0.09$). Ileus was included in the Clavien Dindo I complications because it did not require the nasogastric tube insertion. In a one-to-one comparison between Group A and Group B, the significance was present ($p = 0.04$).

Clavien Dindo II complications were 4 in Group A and 1 in Group B and C, respectively, with no significant differences among the three groups ($p = 0.18$).

Similarly, Clavien Dindo III complications were 1 in both Group A and Group B, and 0 in Group C, with no significant differences among the groups ($p = 0.59$).

No patients were affected by postoperative CD IV complications, and no death (CD V) occurred.

The comparisons between the overall complication rate showed a significantly lower number of complications in the first 15 robotic cases ($p = 0.003$).

About recovery outcomes, no differences among the three groups were found in terms of time to first flatus ($p = 0.704$) and time to first stools ($p = 0.945$). Interestingly, robotic approach was associated with lower length of hospital stay, with a trend toward the significance ($p = 0.072$).

Subgroup Analysis

The results of the subgroup analyses on right hemicolectomies, left hemicolectomies, and anterior rectal resections are shown in Tables 3–5, respectively.

In the case of right hemicolectomy, subgroup analyses confirmed the results obtained in the main analysis. In fact, no differences were found in terms of conversions ($p = 0.287$), Clavien Dindo II complications ($p = 0.09$), Clavien Dindo III complications ($p = 0.56$), time to first flatus ($p = 0.666$), time to first stool ($p = 0.391$) and length of hospital stay ($p = 0.530$) among the three groups. Similarly, according to the main analysis, in Group A a longer operative time ($p < 0.0001$), a lower number of harvested nodes ($p = 0.006$), and a higher number of minor complications (Clavien Dindo I, $p = 0.02$) were present.

In the case of left hemicolectomy, there was no differences in terms of conversions ($p = 0.517$), Clavien Dindo II and Clavien Dindo III complications ($p = 0.52$ and $p = 0.23$, respectively), time to first flatus and stool ($p = 0.369$ and 0.992, respectively), length of hospital stay ($p = 0.216$) among the three groups, while a longer operative time and a lower number of harvested nodes were present in Group A ($p < 0.0001$ and $p = 0.022$, respectively), confirming the results of the main analysis. Differently to the latter, no differences were found in terms of Clavien Dindo I complications ($p = 0.23$) among the three groups in the case of left hemicolectomy.

In the case of anterior rectal resection, our subgroup analysis confirmed the longer operative time in Group A ($p < 0.0001$) and the non-significance among the three groups in terms of Clavien Dindo II complications ($p = 0.41$), time to first flatus and stools ($p = 0.812$ and $p = 0.638$) and length of hospital stay ($p = 0.110$). Interestingly, no statistical difference was found in terms of number of harvested nodes ($p = 0.729$) and postoperative Clavien Dindo I complications ($p = 0.09$).

Table 3. Intraoperative outcomes, postoperative complications and recovery outcomes on right hemicolectomies.

Outcomes	Group A (n = 15)	Group B (n = 15)	Group C (n = 15)	p Value
Intraoperative outcomes				
Operative time (min)	167 ± 4.47	114 ± 6.51	129 ± 6.51	<0.0001
Harvested nodes	16 ± 4.06	24.8 ± 2.1	21.2 ± 3.96	0.006
Conversion	2 (40)	1 (20)	0 (0)	0.287
Postoperative complications				
Clavien Dindo				
I	4 (80)	1 (20)	1 (20)	0.02
Nausea	2 (40)	0 (0)	0 (0)	
Ileus	2 (40)	1 (20)	0 (0)	
II	3 (60)	0 (0)	1 (20)	0.09
Wound infection	1 (20)	0 (0)	0 (0)	
Intraluminal bleeding	1 (20)	0 (0)	1 (20)	
Extraluminal bleeding	1 (20)	0 (0)	0 (0)	
III	1 (20)	0 (0)	0 (0)	0.56
Anastomotic leakage	1 (20)	0 (0)	0 (0)	
IV	0 (0)	0 (0)	0 (0)	1.000
V	0 (0)	0 (0)	0 (0)	1.000
Recovery outcomes				
Time to first flatus (hrs)	68.8 ± 29.31	64.2 ± 27.32	54 ± 21	0.666
Time to first stool (hrs)	93.6 ± 21.46	93.2 ± 32.73	74.4 ± 15.64	0.391
Length of hospital stay (days)	4.8 ± 0.83	4.3 ± 1.37	4.1 ± 0.57	0.530

Dichotomous variables are expressed by number and (percentage); continuous variables by mean ± standard deviation. Hrs: hours.

Table 4. Intraoperative outcomes, postoperative complications and recovery outcomes on left hemicolectomies.

Outcomes	Group A (n = 15)	Group B (n = 15)	Group C (n = 15)	p Value
Intraoperative outcomes				
Operative time (min)	235 ± 10	160 ± 13.23	193.33 ± 20.20	<0.0001
Harvested nodes	16 ± 2.45	22.66 ± 1.15	19 ± 3.63	0.022
Conversion	1 (20)	0 (0)	0 (0)	0.517
Postoperative complications				
Clavien Dindo				
I	2 (40)	0 (0)	0 (0)	0.02
Nausea	1 (20)	0 (0)	0 (0)	
Ileus	1 (20)	0 (0)	0 (0)	
II	1 (20)	0 (0)	0 (0)	0.52
Wound infection	0 (0)	0 (0)	0 (0)	
Intraluminal bleeding	0 (0)	0 (0)	0 (0)	
Extraluminal bleeding	0 (0)	0 (0)	0 (0)	
III	1 (20)	0 (0)	0 (0)	0.23
Anastomotic leakage	0 (0)	1 (33.3)	0 (0)	
IV	0 (0)	0 (0)	0 (0)	1.000
V	0 (0)	0 (0)	0 (0)	1.000
Recovery outcomes				
Time to first flatus (hrs)	49 ± 27.05	46.66 ± 8.08	38 ± 6.9	0.369
Time to first stool (hrs)	73.6 ± 22.74	72 ± 24	74.33 ± 20.59	0.992
Length of hospital stay (days)	4.5 ± 0.73	3.5 ± 0.8	4.11 ± 0.76	0.216

Dichotomous variables are expressed by number and (percentage); continuous variables by mean ± standard deviation. Hrs: hours.

Table 5. Intraoperative outcomes, postoperative complications and recovery outcomes on rectal anterior resection.

Outcomes	Group A (n = 5)	Group B (n = 6)	Group C (n = 5)	p Value
Intraoperative outcomes				
Operative time (mins)	297 ± 9	214 ± 6	221 ± 10	<0.0001
Harvested nodes	21.2 ± 5.44	21.5 ± 3.62	23.6 ± 6.42	0.729
Conversion	0 (0)	0 (0)	0 (0)	1.000
Postoperative complications				
Clavien Dindo				
I	2 (40)	0 (0)	2 (40)	0.09
Nausea	1 (20)	0 (0)	0 (0)	
Ileus	1 (20)	0 (0)	2 (40)	
II	0 (0)	0 (0)	1 (20)	0.41
Wound infection	0 (0)	0 (0)	0 (0)	
Intraluminal bleeding	0 (0)	0 (0)	0 (0)	
Extraluminal bleeding	0 (0)	1 (16.66)	0 (0)	
III	0 (0)	0 (0)	0 (0)	1.000
IV	0 (0)	0 (0)	0 (0)	1.000
V	0 (0)	0 (0)	0 (0)	1.000
Recovery outcomes				
Time to first flatus (hrs)	51.8 ± 10.26	44.33 ± 12.16	52.8 ± 39.43	0.812
Time to first stool (hrs)	71.6 ± 14.31	67 ± 18.14	83.4 ± 45.24	0.638
Length of hospital stay (days)	4.23 ± 0.56	3.46 ± 0.5	4.9 ± 1.7	0.110

Dichotomous variables are expressed by number and (percentage); continuous variables by mean ± standard deviation. Hrs: hours.

4. Discussion

A minimally invasive approach is nowadays considered the treatment of choice of colorectal malignancies, being associated with low postoperative comorbidities and short length of hospital stay [20–23].

Nevertheless, it is still adopted less than expected, because of the complex surgical skills that this approach requires [4,5]. Thus, it should be considered safe only in expert hands.

In this setting, the correct proficiency in laparoscopic colorectal surgery could be considered as completed when the predefined variables reach a steady state, and the outcomes are comparable with those in the current literature [24,25].

Currently, several parameters have been proposed to determine the adequate number of procedures to achieve adequate expertise, but no consensus has been still reached among the author, varying the number of procedures between 11 and 152 [6,7,9,12,26].

In recent years, robotic surgery has been introduced to overcome some challenging skills of conventional laparoscopic surgery.

In fact, the intrinsic facilities of the robotic platform, i.e., the three dimensional view for better visualization of the operative field and the EndoWrist® for more accurate movements in narrow spaces, allow to be less invasive and to obtain lower conversions rate over laparoscopic surgery [27–30].

Because of these facilities, the learning curve in robotic colorectal seems to be easier to complete, needing 15–25 cases to reach the plateau [12,16].

Furthermore, the learning curve of robotic surgery seems to be shorter in experienced laparoscopists [31].

The latter could depend on the fact that minimally invasive procedures have been standardized, and the differences between laparoscopic and robotic surgery are only related to the adoption of different surgical instruments.

During the last years, the interest in the adequate learning curve between robotic and laparoscopic colorectal surgery has become fervent.

Recently, Park et al. [32] compared 89 robotic and 89 laparoscopic rectal resections for cancer, demonstrating that the learning curve for robotic low anterior rectal resection was the 44th case, while for the laparoscopic approach, the 41st case. The authors assessed that the learning curves were similar, with similar clinicopathologic outcomes in both procedures.

On the contrary, De Angelis et al. [33] compared results from 30 robotic right colectomies and 50 laparoscopic right colectomies performed by a surgical fellow novice in minimally invasive colorectal surgery. The authors obtained that 16 was the number of cases necessary to complete the learning curve in the robotic group, while 25 in the laparoscopic one, concluding that the robotic approach was associated with a faster learning curve than conventional laparoscopy.

Being the debate about the learning curve between robotic and laparoscopic colorectal surgery still open, we decided to perform a comparison between the first 15 robotic and first 15 laparoscopic colorectal resections of a single surgeon, adopting as a comparator the last 15 laparoscopic cases, thus after the completion of the learning curve.

Our results showed that the first 15 robotic cases are associated with better postoperative outcomes than the first 15 laparoscopic cases. First, the operative time was significantly lower in the robotic group ($p = 0.003$), with a similar rate of conversion ($p = 0.593$).

From an oncologic point of view, in all groups, an adequate number of harvested nodes was obtained (>12), but a significantly higher number in the robotic group (Group B) was obtained ($p = 0.003$). Then, considering the postoperative complications, in the first laparoscopic group (Group A), a higher number of minor complications occurred (7 vs. 2, $p = 0.04$).

However, the safety of both laparoscopic and robotic procedures was confirmed by the low rate of major complications (1 anastomotic leakage in each group and no death).

Finally, the number of overall complications was significantly lower in the robotic group ($p = 0.003$).

These results were confirmed in the subgroup analysis after dividing the patients in accordance with the different types of resection (right hemicolectomy, left hemicolectomy, rectal anterior resection).

In the case of rectal resection, our results differed from the results by Park et al. [32]. In fact, the subgroups analysis confirmed that the robotic approach was associated with better outcomes over laparoscopy.

In the study by Park et al., the operative time between the laparoscopic and robotic groups was similar (about 202 and 208 min, respectively), as well as the mean number of harvested nodes (about 17 and 16, respectively). In our subgroup's analysis in the laparoscopic groups, the operative time was significantly longer (267 vs. 184 min, $p < 0.0001$), while the mean number of harvested nodes was similar. On the contrary, in the study by Park et al., five conversions occurred in the laparoscopic group, while 0 in the robotic. In our subgroup analysis, no conversions occurred in both subgroups.

Finally, our subgroup analysis differed from the study by Park et al. for the number of major postoperative complications (Clavien Dindo IV and V). In fact, Park et al. registered 11 major complications in the laparoscopic group, and 3 in the robotic group, while we had no major complications.

In the case of subgroup analysis on right colectomies, our results confirmed the results obtained in the main analysis. Furthermore, we can state that the robotic approach could be considered feasible (only one conversion in the robotic group was needed) and safe in terms of postoperative complications. In fact, only one minor complication occurred (ileus, Clavien Dindo I), while no major complications and deaths were registered. On the contrary, in the first laparoscopic group, seven minor complications occurred (Clavien Dindo I complications and two Clavien Dindo II complications), and one major complication (one anastomotic leakage).

Our results are in line with the results obtained by De Angelis et al. [33], in which no conversions were needed in the robotic group, and four minor complications occurred (CD I–II complications).

Interestingly, comparing the robotic group with the last 15 laparoscopic cases, no differences were found in all included outcomes.

The possible reason for these similarities was that the surgeon was already an expert in laparoscopic colorectal procedures.

However, it is important to underline that surgical training with the DaVinci XI® simulator has been performed by the surgeon before starting to adopt the robotic platform in colorectal procedures.

Odermatt et al. [31] has investigated the proficiency in rectal robotic procedures in experienced laparoscopist. In fact, comparing two surgeons with different expertise in laparoscopic rectal surgery (206 vs. 88 cases), the authors demonstrated that surgeon A needed no apparent learning process to reach their laparoscopic standards.

According to the current literature, our results showed that the surgeon needed no apparent learning curve to reach their laparoscopic standards.

Thus, we can state that a robotic approach to colorectal surgery could be considered safe and feasible in the hands of an expert laparoscopist.

A major limitation of the study must be addressed. First, the results are related to a single surgeon's experience and derived from a retrospective study. Then, the cohorts are very small, making the comparison powerless. For this reason, larger comparative studies are needed to give definitive conclusions.

Thus, further multicentric prospective studies with the involvement of different surgeons and larger cohorts and are needed to confirm the absence of a learning curve in robotic colorectal procedures in experienced laparoscopists.

Author Contributions: M.M. (Michele Manigrasso): conception and design of the study; S.V., P.A., A.D., A.M., C.S., A.C., S.A., S.D., N.D., M.M. (Mario Musella), A.V.: acquisition, analysis and interpretation of the data; G.D.D.P. and M.M.: interpretation of the data and critical revisions; G.D.D.P. and M.M. (Marco Milone): critical revisions and final approval. All authors have read and agreed to the published version of the manuscript.

Funding: This research received no external funding.

Institutional Review Board Statement: Ethical review and approval were waived for this study, due to retrospective design of the study.

Informed Consent Statement: Informed consent was obtained from all subjects involved in the study.

Data Availability Statement: Data are available by request to the corresponding author.

Conflicts of Interest: The authors have no conflict of interest to declare.

References

1. Kang, S.B.; Park, J.W.; Jeong, S.Y.; Nam, B.H.; Choi, H.S.; Kim, D.W.; Lim, S.B.; Lee, T.G.; Kim, D.Y.; Kim, J.S.; et al. Open versus laparoscopic surgery for mid or low rectal cancer after neoadjuvant chemoradiotherapy (COREAN trial): Short-term outcomes of an open-label randomised controlled trial. *Lancet Oncol.* 2010. [CrossRef]
2. Milone, M.; Manigrasso, M.; Velotti, N.; Torino, S.; Vozza, A.; Sarnelli, G.; Aprea, G.; Maione, F.; Gennarelli, N.; Musella, M.; et al. Completeness of total mesorectum excision of laparoscopic versus robotic surgery: A review with a meta-analysis. *Int. J. Colorectal Dis.* 2019, *34*, 983–991. [CrossRef]
3. Guillou, P.J.; Quirke, P.; Thorpe, H.; Walker, J.; Jayne, D.G.; Smith, A.M.H.; Heath, R.M.; Brown, J.M. Short-term endpoints of conventional versus laparoscopic-assisted surgery in patients with colorectal cancer (MRC CLASICC trial): Multicentre, randomised controlled trial. *Lancet* 2005, *365*, 1718–1726. [CrossRef]
4. Smith, C.D.; Farrell, T.M.; McNatt, S.S.; Metreveli, R.E. Assessing laparoscopic manipulative skills. *Am. J. Surg.* 2001, *181*, 547–550. [CrossRef]
5. Scott, D.J.; Young, W.N.; Tesfay, S.T.; Frawley, W.H.; Rege, R.V.; Jones, D.B. Laparoscopic skills training. *Am. J. Surg.* 2001, *182*, 137–142. [CrossRef]
6. Gkionis, I.G.; Flamourakis, M.E.; Tsagkataki, E.S.; Kaloeidi, E.I.; Spiridakis, K.G.; Kostakis, G.E.; Alegkakis, A.K.; Christodoulakis, M.S. Multidimensional analysis of the learning curve for laparoscopic colorectal surgery in a regional hospital: The implementation of a standardized surgical procedure counterbalances the lack of experience. *BMC Surg.* 2020, *20*. [CrossRef]
7. Miskovic, D.; Ni, M.; Wyles, S.M.; Tekkis, P.; Hanna, G.B. Learning curve and case selection in laparoscopic colorectal surgery: Systematic review and international multicenter analysis of 4852 cases. *Dis. Colon Rectum* 2012, *55*, 1300–1310. [CrossRef]
8. Schlachta, C.M.; Mamazza, J.; Seshadri, P.A.; Cadeddu, M.; Gregoire, R.; Poulin, E.C. Defining a learning curve for laparoscopic colorectal resections. *Dis. Colon Rectum* 2001, *44*, 217–222. [CrossRef] [PubMed]
9. Tekkis, P.P.; Senagore, A.J.; Delaney, C.P.; Fazio, V.W. Evaluation of the learning curve in laparoscopic colorectal surgery: Comparison of right-sided and left-sided resections. *Ann. Surg.* 2005, *242*, 83–91. [CrossRef]
10. Choi, D.H.; Jeong, W.K.; Lim, S.W.; Chung, T.S.; Park, J.I.; Lim, S.B.; Choi, H.S.; Nam, B.H.; Chang, H.J.; Jeong, S.Y. Learning curves for laparoscopic sigmoidectomy used to manage curable sigmoid colon cancer: Single-institute, three-surgeon experience. *Surg. Endosc.* 2009, *23*, 622–628. [CrossRef]
11. Dinçler, S.; Koller, M.T.; Steurer, J.; Bachmann, L.M.; Christen, D.; Buchmann, P.; Tekkis, P.P.; Windsor, A.C.J. Multidimensional analysis of learning curves in laparoscopic sigmoid resection: Eight-year results. *Dis. Colon Rectum* 2003, *46*, 1371–1378. [CrossRef] [PubMed]
12. Bokhari, M.B.; Patel, C.B.; Ramos-Valadez, D.I.; Ragupathi, M.; Haas, E.M. Learning curve for robotic-assisted laparoscopic colorectal surgery. *Surg. Endosc.* 2011, *25*, 855–860. [CrossRef] [PubMed]
13. Weber, P.A.; Merola, S.; Wasielewski, A.; Ballantyne, G.H.; Delaney, C.P. Telerobotic-assisted laparoscopic right and sigmoid colectomies for benign disease. *Dis. Colon Rectum* 2002, *45*, 1689–1696. [CrossRef]
14. Ceccarelli, G.; Andolfi, E.; Biancafarina, A.; Rocca, A.; Amato, M.; Milone, M.; Scricciolo, M.; Frezza, B.; Miranda, E.; De Prizio, M.; et al. Robot-assisted surgery in elderly and very elderly population: Our experience in oncologic and general surgery with literature review. *Aging Clin. Exp. Res.* 2017. [CrossRef] [PubMed]
15. Troisi, R.I.; Pegoraro, F.; Giglio, M.C.; Rompianesi, G.; Berardi, G.; Tomassini, F.; De Simone, G.; Aprea, G.; Montalti, R.; De Palma, G.D. Robotic approach to the liver: Open surgery in a closed abdomen or laparoscopic surgery with technical constraints? *Surg. Oncol.* 2020, *33*, 239–248. [CrossRef]
16. Jiménez-Rodríguez, R.M.; Díaz-Pavón, J.M.; De La Portilla De Juan, F.; Prendes-Sillero, E.; Dussort, H.C.; Padillo, J. Learning curve for robotic-assisted laparoscopic rectal cancer surgery. *Int. J. Colorectal Dis.* 2013, *28*, 815–821. [CrossRef]
17. Di Minno, M.; Milone, M.; Mastronardi, P.; Ambrosino, P.; Minno, A.; Parolari, A.; Tremoli, E.; Prisco, D. Perioperative Handling of Antiplatelet Drugs. A Critical Appraisal. *Curr. Drug Targets* 2013, *14*, 880–888. [CrossRef]

18. Gustafsson, U.O.; Scott, M.J.; Hubner, M.; Nygren, J.; Demartines, N.; Francis, N.; Rockall, T.A.; Young-Fadok, T.M.; Hill, A.G.; Soop, M.; et al. Guidelines for Perioperative Care in Elective Colorectal Surgery: Enhanced Recovery After Surgery (ERAS®) Society Recommendations: 2018. *World J. Surg.* **2019**, *43*, 659–695. [CrossRef]
19. Clavien, P.A.; Barkun, J.; De Oliveira, M.L.; Vauthey, J.N.; Dindo, D.; Schulick, R.D.; De Santibañes, E.; Pekolj, J.; Slankamenac, K.; Bassi, C.; et al. The clavien-dindo classification of surgical complications: Five-year experience. *Ann. Surg.* **2009**, *250*, 187–196. [CrossRef]
20. Chern, Y.J.; Hung, H.Y.; You, J.F.; Hsu, Y.J.; Chiang, J.M.; Hsieh, P.S.; Tsai, W.S. Advantage of laparoscopy surgery for elderly colorectal cancer patients without compromising oncologic outcome. *BMC Surg.* **2020**, *20*. [CrossRef]
21. Miyo, M.; Kato, T.; Takahashi, Y.; Miyake, M.; Toshiyama, R.; Hamakawa, T.; Sakai, K.; Nishikawa, K.; Miyamoto, A.; Hirao, M. Short-term and long-term outcomes of laparoscopic colectomy with multivisceral resection for surgical T4b colon cancer: Comparison with open colectomy. *Ann. Gastroenterol. Surg.* **2020**, *4*, 676–683. [CrossRef] [PubMed]
22. Garbarino, G.M.; Canali, G.; Tarantino, G.; Costa, G.; Ferri, M.; Balducci, G.; Pilozzi, E.; Berardi, G.; Mercantini, P. Laparoscopic versus open rectal resection: A 1:2 propensity score–matched analysis of oncological adequateness, short- and long-term outcomes. *Int. J. Colorectal Dis.* **2021**, *36*, 801–810. [CrossRef]
23. Milone, M.; Manigrasso, M.; Burati, M.; Velotti, N.; Milone, F.; De Palma, G.D. Surgical resection for rectal cancer. Is laparoscopic surgery as successful as open approach? A systematic review with meta-analysis. *PLoS ONE* **2018**, *13*, e0204887. [CrossRef]
24. Pitiakoudis, M.; Michailidis, L.; Zezos, P.; Kouklakis, G.; Simopoulos, C. Quality training in laparoscopic colorectal surgery: Does it improve clinical outcome? *Tech. Coloproctol.* **2011**, *15* (Suppl. 1), S17–S20. [CrossRef]
25. Cuschieri, A. Nature of human error: Implications for surgical practice. *Ann. Surg.* **2006**, *244*, 642–648. [CrossRef]
26. Simons, A.J.; Anthone, G.J.; Ortega, A.E.; Franklin, M.; Fleshman, J.; Geis, W.P.; Beart, R.W. Laparoscopic-assisted colectomy learning curve. *Dis. Colon Rectum* **1995**, *38*, 600–603. [CrossRef]
27. Jayne, D.; Pigazzi, A.; Marshall, H.; Croft, J.; Corrigan, N.; Copeland, J.; Quirke, P.; West, N.; Rautio, T.; Thomassen, N.; et al. Effect of robotic-assisted vs conventional laparoscopic surgery on risk of conversion to open laparotomy among patients undergoing resection for rectal cancer:the ROLARR randomized clinical trial. *JAMA J. Am. Med. Assoc.* **2017**, *318*, 1569–1580. [CrossRef] [PubMed]
28. Bhama, A.R.; Obias, V.; Welch, K.B.; Vandewarker, J.F.; Cleary, R.K. A comparison of laparoscopic and robotic colorectal surgery outcomes using the American College of Surgeons National Surgical Quality Improvement Program (ACS NSQIP) database. *Surg. Endosc.* **2016**, *30*, 1576–1584. [CrossRef] [PubMed]
29. Köckerling, F. Robotic vs. Standard Laparoscopic Technique—What is Better? *Front. Surg.* **2014**, *1*, 15. [CrossRef]
30. Zelhart, M.; Kaiser, A.M. Robotic versus laparoscopic versus open colorectal surgery: Towards defining criteria to the right choice. *Surg. Endosc.* **2018**, *32*, 24–38. [CrossRef]
31. Odermatt, M.; Ahmed, J.; Panteleimonitis, S.; Khan, J.; Parvaiz, A. Prior experience in laparoscopic rectal surgery can minimise the learning curve for robotic rectal resections: A cumulative sum analysis. *Surg. Endosc.* **2017**, *31*, 4067–4076. [CrossRef]
32. Park, E.J.; Kim, C.W.; Cho, M.S.; Kim, D.W.; Min, B.S.; Baik, S.H.; Lee, K.Y.; Kim, N.K. Is the learning curve of robotic low anterior resection shorter than laparoscopic low anterior resection for rectal cancer?: A comparative analysis of clinicopathologic outcomes between robotic and laparoscopic surgeries. *Medicine* **2014**, *93*. [CrossRef] [PubMed]
33. De'Angelis, N.; Lizzi, V.; Azoulay, D.; Brunetti, F. Robotic Versus Laparoscopic Right Colectomy for Colon Cancer: Analysis of the Initial Simultaneous Learning Curve of a Surgical Fellow. *J. Laparoendosc. Adv. Surg. Tech.* **2016**, *26*, 882–892. [CrossRef] [PubMed]

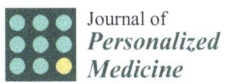

Review

Robotic Transanal Total Mesorectal Excision (RTaTME): State of the Art

Fabio Rondelli [1], Alessandro Sanguinetti [1], Andrea Polistena [2], Stefano Avenia [1], Claudio Marcacci [1], Graziano Ceccarelli [3], Walter Bugiantella [3] and Michele De Rosa [3],*

1. Department of General Surgery and Surgical Specialties, University of Perugia, "S. Maria" Hospital, 05100 Terni, Italy; rondellif@hotmail.com (F.R.); sanguinettiale@gmail.com (A.S.); stefano_avenia@libero.it (S.A.); claudio.marcacci@libero.it (C.M.)
2. Department of General and Laparoscopic Surgery–University Hospital, University of Rome, "Umberto I", 00161 Rome, Italy; apolis74@yahoo.it
3. Department of General and Robotic Surgery, "San Giovanni Battista" Hospital, USL Umbria 2, 06034 Foligno, Italy; graziano.ceccarelli@uslumbria2.it (G.C.); walter.bugiantella@uslumbria2.it (W.B.)
* Correspondence: michele.derosa@nhs.net

Abstract: Total mesorectal excision (TME) is the gold standard technique for the surgical management of rectal cancer. The transanal approach to the mesorectum was introduced to overcome the technical difficulties related to the distal rectal dissection. Since its inception, interest in transanal mesorectal excision has grown exponentially and it appears that the benefits are maximal in patients with mid-low rectal cancer where anatomical and pathological features represent the greatest challenges. Current evidence demonstrates that this approach is safe and feasible, with oncological and functional outcome comparable to conventional approaches, but with specific complications related to the technique. Robotics might potentially simplify the technical steps of distal rectal dissection, with a shorter learning curve compared to the laparoscopic transanal approach, but with higher costs. The objective of this review is to critically analyze the available literature concerning robotic transanal TME in order to define its role in the management of rectal cancer and to depict future perspectives in this field of research.

Keywords: rectal cancer; total mesorectal excision (TME); transanal total mesorectal excision (TaTME); robotic; robotic transanal total mesorectal excision (RTaTme); transanal surgery

1. Introduction

Total mesorectal excision (TME) is the standard procedure in the surgical treatment of rectal cancer [1]. In the last two decades this technique has revolutionized the results of rectal cancer surgery, demonstrating how surgical quality has a direct impact on local control and survival [2,3], the circumferential radial margin (CRM) and the integrity of mesorectal envelope being independent predictors of local recurrence [4–6]. Similarly, functional results can be considered a direct expression of the quality of surgery and are not always satisfying with conventional surgical techniques for rectal cancer treatment [7,8].

From the first report by Sylla et al. [9], transanal TME (TaTME) aroused great enthusiasm in the colorectal community, showing technical advantages compared to conventional open and laparoscopic approaches, preferentially in clinical scenarios considered "difficult" [10,11].

Indeed, even in the hands of expert surgeons, the rectal resection for distal cancers can be extremely difficult, and this is truer in patients with anterior-located lesions, narrow pelvis, obese, with bulky tumours, or treated with neo-adjuvant chemoradiotherapy, where a challenging distal rectal dissection may increase the risk of incomplete mesorectal excision [12,13].

Exposure of the operative field, rectal dissection, and distal cross-stapling of the rectum can be extremely challenging in these conditions, the latter increasing the risk of anastomotic leakage [14].

TaTME was conceived and developed with the aim of overcoming these limitations, mainly in middle-low tumours. The concept relies on a "bottom-up" (caudal to cephalad) or retrograde dissection technique, in which starting the rectal dissection from the perineum may be advantageous for the surgeon.

A magnified vision in line with pelvic structures, distal control of tumour margin, and improved identification and preservation of nervous structures make dissection from below safe and effective. Moreover, abdominal and pelvic structures and viscera are avoided, as they no longer need to be retracted cephalad for rectal mobilization and exposure.

Several case series have been published in the last eight years, suggesting that taTME is feasible and safe concerning short-term outcomes and quality of the resected specimen, with promising CRM involvement ranging from 0–6% [15].

However, despite this proven safety and feasibility, early reports have shown that TaTME is a challenging technique with a steep learning curve [16,17]. The occurrence of urethral injury, a serious complication directly related to the transanal phase of the operation, [10] and recent evidence of the higher involvement of the distal resection margin (DRM) when compared with a robotic low anterior resection [18] underline how relevant are a deep knowledge of pelvic anatomy and the acquisition of advanced surgical skills.

In this light, the introduction of robotic technology with a stable 3D vision may offer the possibility of performing very complex tasks with ambidextrous movements, decreasing tremor and improved dexterity, thus allowing a better dissection, especially in confined surgical fields [19].

All these advantages would potentially help overcome the steep learning curve related to the complexity of TaTME, making robotic assistance a gold standard for this approach.

2. Device and Technique

2.1. Robotic Platform

Directly derived from military projects aiming to develop a technology to be used in situations where the expert surgeon is away from the patient, the concept of robotic surgery has become a reality and achieved great success in clinical practice over three decades of scientific and technological progress.

In 1985, the PUMA 560 robotic system was introduced into an operating theatre to orient a needle for a neurosurgical biopsy under computer tomography, providing more accurate and steady guidance compared to a human hand [20]. A transurethral resection of the prostate (TURP) was subsequently performed by Davies et al. using the same technology [21].

Shortly afterwards, the PROBOT was developed by Imperial College, London, and designed specifically to undertake a TURP, while parallel developments led to the introduction of the ROBODOC system (Integrated Surgical Systems, Sacramento, CA, USA), designed to improve the precision of total hip arthroplasties [22]. Currently, ROBODOC is marketed by Curexo Technology Corporation and is the only FDA-approved robot for orthopedic surgery.

At the end of the 20th century, abdominal surgery was revolutionized by the introduction of laparoscopy. In 1994, the Automated Endoscopic System for Optimal Positioning 1000 (AESOP 1000; Computer Motion, Santa Barbara, CA, USA) became the first laparoscopic camera holder to be approved by the FDA and commercialized. It consisted of a table-mounted voice-controlled laparoscopic camera system that adjusted its position following surgeon's orders, allowing greater image stability and sometimes avoiding the need for an assistant [20].

In 1998, with the introduction of Zeus (Computer Motion, Santa Barbara, CA, USA), the concept of tele-robotics or telepresence was finally applied, with the surgeon sat at a console distant from the robot operating on the patient. With three arms, each independently attached to the surgical table, i.e., one AESOP arm and two surgical arms with four degrees of freedom, a console with a Storz 3D imaging system (Karl Storz Endoscopy, Santa Barbara, CA, USA) and two handles to manipulate the two surgical arms of the telerobot, the Zeus robotic system made a highly relevant mark in the development of cardiac surgery and allowed, in 2001, a transatlantic cholecystectomy with the surgeon operating in New York while the patient was situated physically in Strasbourg, France.

Around the time that ZEUS was being developed, the da Vinci® robot (Intuitive Surgical, Sunnyvale, CA, USA) was introduced. Its console is composed of a computer, a 3D imaging system, and two "masters" that manipulate the arms of the robot and are filtered by the computer to suppress manual tremor. The first da Vinci® robot had three arms, one for the camera and two for surgical instruments, but the latest model has one extra arm for the surgical instruments. Differently to ZEUS, the da Vinci® robot is attached to operative trocars rather than to the surgical table. Hallmark features of this platform are the binocular endoscopic vision which creates a truly 3D experience and specifically designed instruments endowed with Endowrist® technology which, by imitating the human wrist, allow for seven degrees of freedom, 180° of articulation and 540° of rotation [23].

After preliminary experiences such as the undertaking of a cholecystectomy by Himpens in Belgium [24], and a mitral valve replacement by Carpentier et al. [25], in 2000 the da Vinci® obtained FDA approval for general laparoscopic procedures and became the first operative surgical robot in the US.

In 2003 Computer Motion was merged with Intuitive Surgical, the ZEUS and da Vinci® systems were effectively unified and, as a result, further innovations and improvements were focused on the da Vinci® platform, which has subsequently dominated the world of robotic surgery for almost a decade.

From 2014 a more advanced and versatile version of da Vinci®, the Xi platform, has become available, offering the opportunity to perform multi-quadrant single-docking procedures with consequently decreased operative time. Augmented-reality software allows the assessment of intestinal perfusion or real-time three-dimensional (3D) anatomical simulation of abdominal structures [26,27].

Future Direction: New Robotic Platforms

Since its inception in colorectal surgery, the da Vinci® Surgical System has passed through the evolution of different platforms, and published reports on robotic transanal surgery have shown the feasibility of this approach with currently available systems, but not without remarkable limitations.

The game-changing SP (single-port) da Vinci® Robotic platform has been recently introduced and approved by the FDA for urological procedures, anticipating what is expected to happen soon in colorectal surgery, where pre-clinical or preliminary pilot studies have already demonstrated its feasibility and how promising it might be, mainly in transanal and endoscopic procedures.

Despite the limited clinical use of robotic surgery, driven by economic costs and limited access, the technological advancement in this field of research is under continuous progression.

This list of available surgical robots is non-exhaustive, and many of these projects are confidential at present, with each day bringing newly developed technology.

The Senhance Surgical Robotic System (TransEnterix, Morrisville, NC, USA) obtained clearance by the FDA in October 2017 for gynecological and colorectal procedures [28]. The system includes a "cockpit" that serves as a remote-control station unit, up to four manipulator arms, with their own individual carts, and a HD-3D-technology camera, as well as a haptic feedback system.

The most exciting areas of innovation are single-port and natural orifice surgery, where new robotic platforms with flexible arms and camera are under development.

The Flex® Robotic System and Flex® Colorectal (CR) Drive (MedRobotics, Corp. Raynham, MA, USA), after pilot experiences in oral surgery, proved their feasibility in a cadaveric model and in miscellaneous surgical procedures, gaining FDA approval [29].

Being a semi-robotic platform with no robotic effectors, it does not fully express the potential of current technology, but its special design for transanal endoluminal applications makes it also suitable for more complex tasks such TaTME, as already tested in a preclinical setting.

Other single incision platforms such the Single Port Orifice Robotic Technology–SPORT (Titan Medical Company, Toronto, ON, Canada) or the multi-trocar platforms such as Versius (Cambridge Medical Robotics, Cambridge, UK), Revo-I (model MSR-5000; Meerecompany Inc., Seongnam, Republic of Korea), MiroSurge (Medtronic, Minneapolis, MN, USA), and Medicaroid (Kobe, Japan) are expected to bring further advancement in this field.

Verb Surgical, born in 2015 thanks to the collaboration between Google and Johnson & Johnson, introduced artificial intelligence to robotic systems with the aim of starting a new era of robotic-guided, rather than robot-assisted, surgery. The long-term plan would be to develop a surgery technology fully performed by robots, but this page is yet to be written [30].

2.2. Transanal Device

In 1983 TEM (Transanal Endoscopic Microsurgery) was conceived by Professor Gerard Buess who, in cooperation with Richard Wolf, created and developed the platform for endoscopic rectal surgery, with the aim of treating benign lesions of the high and middle rectum not reachable by a conventional transanal approach [31].

Based on this model, Karl Storz developed the TEO (Transanal Endoscopic Operations-Storz, Tuttlingen, Germany), a rigid operative rectoscope which is compatible with many standard laparoscopic instruments and units, and with no need for a dedicated platform.

An evolution and simplification of TEM was introduced in 2009 by Atallah et al. who, by adapting a device already conceived for single-port surgery, created TAMIS (Trans-Anal Minimally Invasive Surgery), a hybrid platform midway between TEM and single-port laparoscopy, using a multiport device placed in the anal canal as an access system, with conventional scope and laparoscopic instruments [32].

To date, two transanal platforms, GelPoint Path (Applied Medical, Rancho Santa Margarita, CA, USA) and SILS Port (Covidien, Mansfield, MA, USA) have gained FDA approval for TAMIS. Clinical studies published so far have demonstrated that both platforms, rigid and non-disposable, e.g, TEM/TEO, and flexible and disposable, e.g., TAMIS, could be equally used for this technique, but TAMIS is the preferred option for surgeons dedicated to transanal surgery because, compared to TEM, it offers a better angle of vision, a soft and less traumatic platform, an economic advantage and an easier set-up [33,34].

A self-designed custom-made transanal access platform, the PAT (Developia-IDIVAL, Santander, Spain), closed with an 80-mm GelPOINT gel cap (Applied Medical, Rancho Santa Margarita, CA, USA) for trocar placement, has been described by Gomez Ruiz et al. [35].

2.3. Surgical Technique

Despite the attempt at standardization, with the development of experience and the dissemination of this approach many different technical modifications have been introduced, although the pivotal principle of this procedure remains the same: to provide a complete mobilization of the rectum up to the pelvic floor, regardless of the platform and the device used.

After induction of general anesthesia, patient is catheterized and put in lithotomy position. The procedure is carried out either with two different surgical teams working simultaneously or with a two-step approach, using the same surgical team for both operative phases.

The majority of the experiences reported so far refer to a hybrid procedure that incorporates an abdominal phase to achieve proximal colonic mobilization, inferior mesenteric vessel division and partial rectal dissection, and the transanal part of the operation where the rectal dissection is completed "bottom-up", joining the surgical plane previously developed.

Abdominal phase: this part of the operation has been described with different variations, either performed simultaneously in a two team approach, or in a sequential model, being the first or the last step in the operation, according to the surgeon's preference. Similarly, laparoscopic multiport/single-port or robotic-assisted procedures have been described.

Regardless of the approach, operative steps are performed according to the standardized technique of rectal anterior resection with identification and ligation of the inferior mesenteric vessels, full mobilization of the splenic flexure and circumferential incision of the peritoneal reflection to start the rectal dissection posteriorly along the sacral plane, developing it laterally, paying attention not to damage the hypogastric nerves and ureters. Anteriorly, the peritoneal reflection should only be incised, without performing any further dissection manoeuver.

Transanal phase: after pneumoperitoneum release, the transanal phase of the operation can begin using the TAMIS approach with a disposable single-site device, or the reusable platform with rigid rectoscope TEM/TEO. The adoption of a self-designed transanal access port proctoscope PAT (Developia-IDIVAL, Santander, Spain), closed with an 80-mm GelPOINT gel cap (Applied Medical, Rancho Santa Margarita, CA, USA) for trocar placement, has been reported [35].

The placement of a self-fixing anal retractor (Lone Star Medical Products Inc., Houston, TX, USA) may be useful to better expose the anal canal and, once the tumor distance from the anal verge is verified, the procedure can start immediately with an intersphincteric resection or with straight positioning of the anal access system and the creation of a pressure of 8 to 10 mmHg to the pneumopelvis.

In patients with tumors located ≤3 cm from the anal verge, a partial intersphincteric resection can be performed, by circumferential dissection of the mucosa and internal sphincter muscle at least 1 cm below the distal margin of the tumor, developing the plane cranially for 1–2 cm. A purse-string suture is then placed to seal the rectum below the tumor and the transanal access platform is inserted. The robotic trocars are then directly introduced through the GelPOINT Path or, using a trocar in trocar technique, inserted in the gelPOINT path trocars. The da Vinci® system patient cart is positioned near the lower left side of the patient. A 30-degree-angle videoscope, hot shears with monopolar diathermy on the right and a fenestrated grasper (or Maryland grasper) with bipolar cautery on the left are commonly used. An accessory 12-mm trocar is operated by a patient-side assistant, who assists in tissue countertraction or manipulates suction and irrigation modules. If available, an AirSEAL System (Conmed, Utica, NY, USA) and 5-mm or 8-mm valveless trocar can be used for the assistant to stabilize the pneumopelvis. In patients with tumors higher than 3 cm from the anal verge, where an adequate distal resection margin can be obtained without intersphinteric resection, the transanal device is set up directly and the rectum insufflated with CO_2, establishing the pneumo-rectum.

The rectal mucosa is marked circumferentially with a monopolar hook and a full thickness rectotomy is begun, usually posteriorly, where the plane between presacral fascia and mesorectum is more easily identified, but slightly laterally where the anococcygeal ligament is less easily entered.

The rectal division is performed by opening the different layers of the rectal wall joining the mesorectal plane, which is insufflated to ease the pelvic dissection and RtaTME.

The posterior plane is developed first in the pre-sacral avascular space, along the mesorectal fascia which is kept intact. The anterior plane is approached afterwards, keeping the dissection in front of or behind the Denonvillier's fascia according to the rectal cancer position in male patients, and dissecting the rectum from the posterior vagina in females. The lateral dissection comes last in order to minimize injuries to the neurovascular structures. Once TME is completed and the peritoneal cavity is accessed, the specimen can be extracted transanally or transabdominally through a suprapubic Pfannenstiel incision using an Alexis wound retractor (Applied Medical Inc., Rancho Santa Margarita, CA, USA). If the transanal route is chosen, the colo-rectal segment is carefully exteriorized and divided, after having checked for the presence of an adequate blood supply.

Different anastomotic techniques have been described according to the surgeon's experience and the choice should be tailored depending on case specifics and the height of the tumor.

In the case of lower cancers with a short rectal stump, a conventional hand-sewn coloanal anastomosis (lateroterminal when feasible) is performed, while if the rectal stump is long enough to allow a pursestring closure around the anvil of a stapler, a mechanical end-to-end anastomosis should be optioned.

Defunctioning loop ileostomy should be considered to protect low anastomosis, and pelvic drain can be left intra-abdominally.

3. Outcomes

Recent reports show similar clinical and oncological results in comparing robotic and laparoscopic trans-abdominal surgical procedures so, at present, no significant benefit of robotic over laparoscopic surgery seems to be detectable, except perhaps in conversion rates [36].

The application of robotics to TaTME appears to be the next logical step in the evolution of minimal access surgery, allowing the technical benefits of an advanced surgical platform, whilst adhering to the principles of NOTES. Despite the literature on RtaTME being in its infancy, this exciting new trend is rising and the results coming from available preclinical or pilot reports are promising in terms of mesorectal integrity, resection margins, number of intraoperatively harvested lymph nodes and conversion rate.

After a preliminary experimental approach in a cadaveric model [37], the first in-human application of robotic technology to TaTME, termed robotic-assisted transanal surgery for TME (RATS-TME), was reported in 2013 [38].

Therefore, after demonstrating the feasibility, Atallah et al. published a case series with the first three human cases performed at a single institution. In all cases, tumors were located in the distal 5 cm of the rectum, no involvement of the distal and circumferential resection margins was detected and no major morbidity or mortality on short-term follow-up were reported [39].

Parallel experience led to the publication of a case of RTaTME performed on a 48-year-old female with a rectal cancer 8 cm from the anal verge, who underwent a sequential laparoscopic and RTaTME using the da Vinci® Si System with the GelPoint Path. The specimen was transanally extracted and an end-to-end stapled anastomosis was fashioned using a circular stapler. The total operative time was 250 min, with an estimated blood loss of 50 mL. No complication was recorded and the postoperative stay was 3 days. The histological report showed a complete mesorectal excision with free distal and circumferential margins [40].

In the single-center preliminary experience of Atallah, from a dataset of 18 robotic miscellaneous transanal procedures, four cases (three male) of distal rectal cancer were treated via a sequential hybrid abdominal laparoscopic and RTaTME (one more patient was added to the previously reported case series.) [39]. The mean operative time was 376 min with an estimated mean blood loss of 200 mL. There was no intra-operative morbidity and the mean postoperative length of stay was 4.3 days. Mesorectal quality was graded as complete or near complete and an R0 resection was performed in all four cases. Concerning morbidity, one wound hematoma, one subsegmental pulmonary embolism (asymptomatic) and recurrent deep vein thrombosis, and a high ileostomy output were recorded. No local or distant recurrences were found in any of the patients after an average 8-month follow-up [41].

Huscher et al. published the results of seven patients (four women) with rectal cancer who underwent a sequential hybrid laparoscopic transabdominal and RTaTME, showing how the combination of robotics and transanal access is feasible and could improve results in rectal cancer surgery. The mean operative time was 165.7 min and no anastomotic leakage was recorded. One patient presented post-operative gastrointestinal bleeding, presumably from the anastomosis, requiring transfusion. The mean hospital stay was 4.8 days. Pathology assessment revealed a complete or near-complete mesorectum and an R0 resection in all cases [42].

Gomez Ruiz et al. performed a pilot study of robotic-assisted laparoscopic transanal proctectomy with TME, enrolling five patients. Mean operative time was 398 ± 88 min with no intraoperative complications. Mean length of hospital stay was 6 ± 1 days. A Clavien II, grade B anastomotic leakage developed in one patient postoperatively. In all cases, specimens showed complete mesorectal excision with negative proximal, distal and circumferential margins. All patients were disease-free at their initial 3-month follow-up [35].

Kuo et al. reported a series of 15 patients (8 males) who underwent a combined sequential single-site plus one port (R-SSPO) robotic transabdominal operation followed by RTaTME performed by a single surgeon adopting the da Vinci® Si surgical system with the da Vinci® Single-Site platform.

Median operative time was 473 min and the estimated blood loss was 33 mL. Conversion to conventional laparoscopy was required in two patients, one due to bleeding during the transanal phase and another due to a left ureteric transection. Reported complications included an intestinal obstruction requiring surgical adhesiolysis and a superficial wound infection. The mean length of hospital stay was 12.2 days. All specimens were reported as complete mesorectum with clear circumferential and distal resection margins [43].

Monsellato et al. reported three consecutive cases (two male) of RTaTME: in two cases a sequential approach with a transanal phase and a subsequent robotic transabdominal operation was performed, and in the third case a simultaneous laparoscopic transabdominal and robotic perineal approach was employed. With a mean operative time of 530 min, no intra-operative or post-operative complications and excellent (Quirke 3 grade) TME quality in all cases, the authors demonstrated that this approach is feasible, safe and with good early post-operative outcomes [44].

In the single-centre experience reported by Hu et al. a total of twenty patients (12 male) underwent RtaTME via a simultaneous two-team approach, with the "abdominal team" working via a laparoscopic single-port technique at ileostomy site, while the "transanal team" operated via the DaVinci Xi system with a GelPoint Path. The mean estimated intraoperative blood loss was 88 mL and circular stapling was used to restore continuity in 80% of study patients. The overall postoperative complication rate was 35%, including one pelvic abscess, and the mean distal margin length was 3.1 ± 1.3 cm. They reported that all patients had complete or near complete mesorectal resections and three patients had CRM involved by cancer cells (≤1 mm) [45].

Ye et al. reported 13 cases of RTaTME in patients with rectal cancer demonstrating the feasibility of this innovative approach. The median docking time was 18 min, median transanal phase time was 95 min, and median total operation time was 240 min. Median estimated blood loss was 60 mL, the median number of lymph nodes retrieved was 15 and median length of postoperative hospital stay was 7 days, without mortality recorded. Three postoperative complications including one anastomotic leak and one prolonged ileus were reported, with no requirement for further intervention. Patients were followed up for a median of 15 months, and no local tumor recurrences, metastasis or deaths were reported [46].

The results of these experiences are summarized in Table 1.

Table 1. Summary of published experience of RTaTME performed with da Vinci® Robotic platform.

	Atallah (2013)	Atallah (2014)	Verheijen (2014)	Huscher (2015)	Gomez-Ruiz (2015)	Kuo (2016)	Monsellato (2019)	Hu (2020)	Ye (2020)
Number of patients	1	3	1	7	5	15	3	20	13
Abdominal approach	Laparoscopic	Laparoscopic	Laparoscopic	Laparoscopic	Robotic	Single port robotic + assistant port	Robotic 2, laparoscopic 1	Laparoscopic	Robotic 9, Laparoscopic 4
Transanal platform	GelPoint Path (daVinci® Si)	GelPoint Path (daVinci® Si)	GelPoint Path (daVinci® Si)	GelPoint Path (daVinci® Si)	PAT * + GelPoint Path (daVinci® Si)	GelPoint Path (daVinci® Si)	GelPoint Path (daVinci® Si)	GelPoint Path (daVinci® Xi)	GelPoint Path (daVinci® Si)
Two-team approach	No	No	No	No	No	No	1/3	20/20	4/13
BL (mL)	140	200	50	n/a	90 (25–120)	33 (30–50)	n/a	82 (30–500)	60 (50–100)
LOS (days)	No	4.3	3		6 (5–7)	12.2 (10–14)	10 (7–15)	8.8 (6–24)	7 (6–10)
Conversion	No	No	No	No	No	2/15	No	No	No
Hand-sewn anastomosis	0/1	2/3	0/1	0/7	2/5	15/15	3/3	2/20	8/13
Defunctioning stoma	Terminal ileostomy	Yes	Yes	Yes	Yes	5/15	Yes	14/18	Yes
Operative time (min)	381	376	205	165.7 (85–220)	398 (270–450)	473 (335–569)	550 (440–600)	172.3 (135–215)	240 (195–270)
Complications	No	1 Pulmonary embolism 1 Peristomal dermatitis/ dehydration	No	1 anastomotic bleeding	1 anastomotic leak	1 mechanical bowel obstruction, 1 wound infection	1 acute renal failure	7/20 (no anastomotic leaks reported)	1 post-op ileus 1 duodenal hemorrage 1 anastomotic leakage
TME quality C/NC/I	0/1/0	1/2/0	1/0/0	6/1/0	5/0/0	15/0/0	3/0/0	18/2/0	8/5/0
CRM involvement	No	No	No	No	No	No	No	3/20	No
Distal margin involvement	No	No	No	No	No	No	No	No	No

BL: Blood loss; LOS: Length of hospital stay, C: Complete; NC: Near complete; I: Incomplete; * PAT ('Puerto Acceso Transanal'—Developia-HUMV, Santander, Spain).

Emerging Robotic Systems

Despite the well described benefits, the presence of external arm clashes and internal conflicts make the multi-arm robot inappropriate for single port surgery.

The introduction of the robotic platform based on single-port access and the implementation of smaller, more flexible robotic systems designed for true natural orifice procedures, may represent the start of a new era for robot-assisted transanal surgery (Table 2).

In a correspondence article, Samalavicius et al. reported on a 57-year-old patient with an ulcerated rectal tumour 5 cm from the anal verge who underwent robotic-assisted TaTME using a Senhance Transenterix robotic system. After failure of long-course chemoradiotherapy and a watch-and-wait strategy, the patient underwent an uneventful procedure, demonstrating that RTaTME using the Senhance robotic system is a good and feasible option for low-lying rectal cancer [47].

Atallah et al. demonstrated in a cadaveric model the preclinical feasibility of the Versius surgical modular robotic system for taTME. Using this modular robotic system, one surgeon performed the abdominal portion of the operation, including colonic mobilization and vascular pedicle ligation, while simultaneously a second surgeon performed the transanal portion of the operation to the point of rendezvous at the peritoneal refection, where the operation was completed cooperatively. The operation was successfully completed in 195 min demonstrating the theoretical advantage of reducing surgical time and thereby reducing overall operative costs [48].

Table 2. Summary of published experience of RTaTME performed with emerging robotic platforms.

	Samalavicius (2020)	Atallah (2019)	Carmicheal (2019)	Ribeiro (2021)	Kneist (2020)
Number of cases	1 patient	1 fresh human cadaver	6 fresh human cadavers	2 fresh cadavers	1 fresh human cadaver
Robotic platform	Senhance Transenterix	Versius	Flex® System	daVinci® SP	daVinci® SP
Abdominal approach	Robotic	Robotic with Versius	n/a	n/a	Robotic with daVinci® SP
Transanal platform	n/a	GelPoint Path	n/a	GelPoint Path	GelPoint Path
Two-team approach	n/a	Yes	n/a	n/a	No
Hand-sewn anastomosis	Yes	n/a	n/a	n/a	n/a
Operative time (min)	n/a	195	n/a	n/a	232
Complications	No	n/a	n/a	n/a	n/a
TME quality	n/a	Near complete	Complete 4 Incomplete 2	Complete 3	Good
CRM involvement	No	n/a	n/a	n/a	n/a
Distal margin involvement	No	n/a	n/a	n/a	n/a

In 2017 the United States Food and Drug Administration approved the Flex® Robotic System and Flex® Colorectal (CR) Drive (MedRobotics, Corp. Raynham, MA, USA), a semi-robotic apparatus for colorectal surgery specifically indicated for transanal endoluminal applications, as well as for more radical resection. Atallah et al. used the flexible robotic system to perform taTME, showing its feasibility and potentiality to perform operative tasks not otherwise possible with conventional methods [49].

Similarly, taTME was performed by two surgeons in six fresh human cadaveric specimens using the same platform, with or without transabdominal laparoscopic assistance, simulating both mid- and low-rectal resections [50].

In a cadaveric study, the da Vinci® SP Surgical System was shown to be a realistic platform for the future of endoluminal surgery [51] and in 2020 the first clinical experience performing a single-port left colectomy using the SP robot (SPr SILS left colectomy) was described [52]. In a subsequent feasibility study, Dr. Marks expanded the use of the SP robot performing TaTME, including transanal splenic flexure release and high ligation of the IMA, but the results of these experiences have not yet been published.

Recently Ribero et al. published a preclinical study to establish the technical feasibility of RtaTME using the da Vinci® SP, simulating two clinical scenarios of rectal cancer at different heights from the anal verge (at 1 cm and at >4 cm respectively), in two fresh cadavers. The GelPOINT Path was used as transanal access platform through which the 2.5 cm single port robotic trocar and a 10 mm sleeve were inserted. A complete taTME was performed with an intact mesorectal fascia in both cases. Operation times were 124 and 106 min with about 15 min of non-console time for robot positioning and docking [53].

In a preclinical study in a male human cadaver the da Vinci® SP Surgical System was employed to realize the transanal and abdominal parts of the taTME procedure, in a sequential fashion with a one-team approach. This experience demonstrated the technical feasibility of a dual field procedure, with operative time of 189 min for the perineal phase and 43 min for the abdominal procedure, and good quality of resected specimen [54].

With these advances, the SP robot demonstrates significant surgical milestones in the field of transanal and other natural orifice surgery.

4. Benefits and Limitations

4.1. Technical Advantages

Compared to conventional laparoscopy, current robotic platforms provide a stable camera with a magnified 3DHD vision delivering an immersive surgical experience, with true depth perception which allows the clear identification of tissue planes and anatomical structures.

Modelled after the human wrist, the EndoWrist® instruments offer a greater range of motion than the human hand, providing maximum responsiveness and allowing rapid and precise suturing, dissection and tissue manipulation [20].

These technical advantages, more relevant in such a restricted surgical field, are expected to allow a fine TME with preservation of the integrity of the fascia and consequent optimal oncological results. On the other hand, the better identification and preservation of autonomic nerves should result in improved functional outcomes, with reduced sexual dysfunction, anterior resection syndrome or urinary retention.

Finally, but no less important, robotics offers optimal ergonomics for operating surgeons, with reduced musculoskeletal discomfort, and this could reflect a better quality of surgery, especially for such challenging technical operations.

4.2. Technical Limitations

The loss of force feedback, coupled with the inherent ability of robotic surgical systems to apply strong compressive and shear forces, have led to an increased risk of excessive tissue trauma, representing the major technical limitation of the available robotic platforms [55,56].

With the aims of imitating natural touch and improving the effectiveness of haptic feedback in tissue grasping and manipulation, in a benchmark study by Abiri et al. a multi-modal pneumatic feedback system, designed to allow for tactile, kinesthetic and vibrotactile feedback, was mounted on a da Vinci® Surgical System, demonstrating the possibility of achieving average grip forces closer to those normally possible with the human hand [57].

With the advancement of technology, it appears mandatory that haptic feedback modalities are developed, becoming a standard feature of commercially available surgical robots.

As a consequence, new-generation robotic platforms such as the Senhance Surgical Robotic System and the REVO-I Robot Platform incorporate haptic feedback systems [58].

Moreover and more importantly, da Vinci® robotic arms are large and intrusive, making it very challenging to work in the setting of single-port or transanal surgery, because of external clashes and collisions. At this stage, current experiences of robotic-assisted transanal surgery have demonstrated the feasibility of the approach, but have highlighted the limitations of the available robotic systems, relying on the potential benefits of emerging flexible or miniaturized systems.

4.3. Costs

Despite the efforts aimed at containing increasing expenditure, overall worldwide health care spending remains on an unsustainable course. As a consequence, in consideration of limited health resources, a relevant focus has been placed on the assessment of the economic impact of robotics, given that the attributed increase in costs, associated with equivocal evidence of improved clinical outcomes, is the most significant barrier preventing the diffusion of this technology.

It is the case that da Vinci®'s supremacy in the market of robotic surgery, in the absence of real competition, whilst producing a potential stagnation in the advancement of technology, has mostly led to a growth in costs. On the other hand, the accurate assessment of the financial impact of robotic surgery is a challenging operation, as total costs include direct, indirect and intangible costs.

Direct costs can be fixed costs (to buy and maintain the robotic system), and variable costs (consumable instruments), but to better understand whether robotic surgery is beneficial compared to other available techniques, it is mandatory to also capture indirect costs (loss of productivity, trips to hospital) and out-of-pocket costs borne by patients after discharge.

No economic data are available concerning RTaTME but almost all studies on robotic TME showed higher costs compared with laparoscopic TME, with similar overall clinical outcomes. After a learning curve for robotic TME, the operative costs could be reduced, but the total costs including fixed costs would still be higher because of the expensive purchasing charge for the robotic system (average cost of a robotic platform is $1–$2.3 million) [59].

The ROLARR trial showed that health-care costs in the robotic-assisted laparoscopic group (£11,853 or $13,668) were higher than in the conventional laparoscopic group (£10,874 or $12,556), because of a longer mean use of the operating theatre and the mean cost of instruments [60].

Baek et al. in a cost analysis from a single institute in South Korea reported that operative charges were significantly higher in the robotic surgery group (8849 vs. 2289 USD, $p \leq 0.001$), while the charge for anesthesia, laboratory, radiology, nursing care and medical therapy was not different between two groups [61].

On the other hand, Kim et al., in a propensity score-matching analysis of cost-effectiveness of robotic versus laparoscopic surgery, showed similar short-term clinical outcomes, but higher costs in all categories of charges for the robotic group (total hospital charges, patients' payment, operative charges, anesthetic charges, and postoperative management charges) [62].

Ramji et al., comparing the clinical and economic outcomes between open, laparoscopic and robotic approaches to rectal cancer surgery, did not find any difference for total and operative costs between the open and laparoscopic method, whereas the median costs of each robotic operation increased approximately by 6000 CAD [63].

In the experience of Ielpo et al. comparing clinical outcomes and costs of robotic versus laparoscopic surgery for rectal cancer, the mean overall costs were similar in both groups (7279.31 vs. 6879.80, EUR, $p = 0.44$), but fixed costs for robotic surgery were not included, thus minimizing the real financial impact of robotic devices on health spending [64].

Morelli et al. demonstrated that total costs (12,283.5 vs. 7619.8 EUR, $p < 0.001$), and variable costs (10,614.6 vs. 7585.4 EUR, $p < 0.001$) were higher in the robotic TME group compared with the laparoscopic TME group, as well as within the robotic group itself in the first phase of the learning curve, reflecting how the advancement of robotic experience produced a reduction of operative time and consequently of overall costs. Excluding fixed costs, the variable operative costs were similar between the robotic group, for the achievement of proficiency, and the laparoscopic TME group ($p = 0.084$) [65].

This demonstrates how relevant is robotic expertise to the potential reduction of indirect costs, alongside institutional case volume, standardization of procedures and efficiency of surgical teams.

Despite that analysis of indirect costs is not available in the literature, it is conceivable that the described potential advantages of robotic surgery in terms of reduction of conversion rate and hospital stay may translate into lower expenditure.

A recent retrospective, propensity score-weighed analysis using insurance claims from the MarketScan database showed that the robotic approach was associated with lower out-of-pocket costs for five types of common oncological procedures compared to open surgery [66].

The analysis of indirect costs and the evaluation of quality of life measures, including sexual, urinary and bowel functions, require further research to accurately compare the outcomes of the different surgical alternatives.

So far, results from the available literature suggest that robotic-assisted surgery for rectal cancer is unlikely to be cost-saving, mainly considering the cost of purchase and maintenance of the system.

In the near future, positive competition among companies will foster the introduction of new robotic systems and the expected gradual decrease of the platform price will make it cost-effective, with the same clinical outcomes as alternative operation techniques.

5. Learning Curve of RTaTME

For such a challenging surgical procedure, one of the main areas of research is to identify the phases of the learning curve and to establish appropriate training, in order to guarantee patients' safety and to provide inexpert surgeons with adequate proctorship.

Despite the fact that robotic surgery is generally more intuitive and easier to learn than laparoscopic surgery, a learning curve is unavoidable and special training programs for the development of new surgical skills appear mandatory. FDA enforced companies responsible for robotic systems to develop dedicated, structured educational programs for surgeons and an official certification based on a formal curriculum for skills and procedures has been recommended also by The European Association of Endoscopic Surgeons (EAES).

Supporters of the TaTME technique have highlighted the potential benefits, mainly in selected high-risk patients, without ignoring that the new bottom-up approach is associated with a significant learning curve which, from the evaluation of major post-operative complications, is estimated at 40–50 cases [67].

On the other hand, robotic transabdominal TME should include at least 20–23 cases to gain proficiency, which is in any case faster than for laparoscopy [68,69].

Being still in its infancy, no formal assessment of the learning curve for RTaTME is reported in the literature, but it is intuitive that the steep learning curve of so complex a technique would probably be favoured by robotic technology.

"Operative time", "bleeding" or "conversion" have been evaluated as markers of expertise in most of the publications [69–71], but the most critical variable to be assessed in rectal cancer surgery is the difference between learning and competent surgeons in terms of the quality of the resected specimen [72].

If robotics does not modify the operative steps and the intrinsic complexity of this procedure, it may ease or simplify its technical aspects, making minimally invasive surgery feasible by less experienced surgeons in more patients, thus shortening the time needed for the achievement of proficiency.

On the other hand, limitations imposed by the currently available robotic platforms may at this stage counterbalance the advantages, making the learning curve steeper than expected.

6. Conclusions

Robotic-assisted surgery was introduced at the beginning of the new millennium, showing obvious advantages over laparoscopy in terms of visualization, manipulation and ergonomics.

With proper training, TaTME can be considered a real game-changer in the surgical management of rectal cancer. The accuracy of transanal dissection may be improved by the use of robotic assistance, which expresses its potentialities even better in confined spaces such as the pelvic outlet.

To date only a few experiences have demonstrated the feasibility and safety of this approach, with oncological results expected to be not inferior compared to conventional TaTME.

Increased costs, poor availability and dedicated training are still relevant barriers which prevent the wide adoption of this system, also because, at this stage, no important benefits have been demonstrated yet for robotics compared with the other available surgical alternatives.

In the near future, emerging robotic platforms will lead to major competition and consequent reduction of costs, while the development of miniaturization of the surgical instrumentation will start a new era for endoluminal surgery.

These advancements, associated with technical refinements and standardized training programmes, may allow robotic surgery to become the gold standard for TaTME.

Author Contributions: M.D.R. and F.R. were responsible for the conceptualization, literature review, and writing—original draft preparation, review and editing. G.C. and A.S. were responsible for the project supervision, writing—review and editing. A.P., S.A., C.M. and W.B. contributed to the writing—review and editing. All authors have read and agreed to the published version of the manuscript.

Funding: This research received no external funding.

Institutional Review Board Statement: Not applicable.

Informed Consent Statement: Not applicable.

Conflicts of Interest: The authors declare no conflict of interest.

References

1. Heald, R.J.; Husband, E.M.; Ryall, R.D. The mesorectum in rectal cancer surgery: The clue to pelvic recurrence? *Br. J. Surg.* **1982**, *69*, 613–616. [CrossRef] [PubMed]
2. Heald, R.J.; Ryall, R.D. Recurrence and survival after total mesorectal excision for rectal cancer. *Lancet* **1986**, *327*, 1479–1482. [CrossRef]
3. Bernardshaw, S.V.; Øvrebø, K.; Eide, G.E.; Skarstein, A.; Røkke, O. Treatment of rectal cancer: Reduction of local recurrence after the introduction of TME-experience from one University Hospital. *Dig. Surg.* **2006**, *23*, 51–59. [CrossRef] [PubMed]
4. Quirke, P.; Steele, R.; Monson, J.; Grieve, R.; Khanna, S.; Couture, J.; O'Callaghan, C.; Myint, A.S.; Bessell, E.; Thompson, L.C.; et al. Effect of the plane of surgery achieved on local recurrence in patients with operable rectal cancer: A prospective study using data from the MRC CR07 and NCIC-CTG CO16 randomised clinical trial. *Lancet* **2009**, *373*, 821–828. [CrossRef]
5. Maslekar, S.; Sharma, A.; Macdonald, A.; Gunn, J.; Monson, J.R.; Hartley, J.E. Mesorectal grades predict recurrences after curative resection for rectal cancer. *Dis. Colon Rectum* **2007**, *50*, 168–175. [CrossRef]
6. Baik, S.H.; Kim, N.K.; Lee, K.Y.; Sohn, S.K.; Cho, C.H.; Kim, M.J.; Kim, H.; Shinn, R.K. Factors influencing pathologic results after total mesorectal excision for rectal cancer: Analysis of consecutive 100 cases. *Ann. Surg. Oncol.* **2008**, *15*, 721–728. [CrossRef] [PubMed]
7. Dulskas, A.; Miliauskas, P.; Tikuisis, R.; Escalante, R.; Samalavicius, N.E. The functional results of radical rectal cancer surgery: Review of the literature. *Acta Chir. Belg.* **2016**, *116*, 1–10. [CrossRef]
8. Nocera, F.; Angehrn, F.; von Flüe, M.; Steinemann, D.C. Optimising functional outcomes in rectal cancer surgery. *Langenbeck's Arch. Surg.* **2021**, *406*, 233–250. [CrossRef]
9. Sylla, P.; Rattner, D.W.; Delgado, S.; Lacy, A.M. NOTES transanal rectal cancer resection using transanal endoscopic microsurgery and laparoscopic assistance. *Surg. Endosc.* **2010**, *24*, 1205–1210. [CrossRef]
10. Rouanet, P.; Mourregot, A.; Azar, C.C.; Carrere, S.; Gutowski, M.; Quenet, F.; Saint-Aubert, B.; Colombo, P.E. Transanal endoscopic proctectomy: An innovative procedure for difficult resection of rectal tumorsin men with narrow pelvis. *Dis. Colon Rectum* **2013**, *56*, 408–415. [CrossRef]
11. De Rosa, M.; Rondelli, F.; Boni, M.; Ermili, F.; Bugiantella, W.; Mariani, L.; Ceccarelli, G.; Giuliani, A. Transanal total mesorectal excision (TaTME): Single-centre early experience in a selected population. *Updates Surg.* **2019**, *71*, 157–163. [CrossRef] [PubMed]
12. García-Granero, E.; Faiz, O.; Flor-Lorente, B.; García-Botello, S.; Esclápez, P.; Cervantes, A. Prognostic implications of circumferential location of distal rectal cancer. *Colorectal Dis.* **2011**, *13*, 650–657. [CrossRef]
13. You, J.F.; Tang, R.; Changchien, C.R.; Chen, J.S.; You, Y.T.; Chiang, J.M.; Yeh, C.Y.; Hsieh, P.S.; Tsai, W.S.; Fan, C.W.; et al. Effect of body mass index on the outcome of patients with rectal cancer receiving curative anterior resection: Disparity between the upper and lower rectum. *Ann. Surg.* **2009**, *249*, 783–787. [CrossRef] [PubMed]
14. Ito, M.; Sugito, M.; Kobayashi, A.; Nishizawa, Y.; Tsunoda, Y.; Saito, N. Relationship between multiple numbers of stapler firings during rectal division and anastomotic leakage after laparoscopic rectal resection. *Int. J. Color Dis.* **2008**, *23*, 703–707. [CrossRef]
15. De Rosa, M.; Wynn, G.; Rondelli, F.; Ceccarelli, G. Transanal total mesorectal excision for rectal cancer: State of the art. *Mini Invasive Surg.* **2020**, *4*, 34. [CrossRef]
16. Persiani, R.; Agnes, A.; Belia, F.; D'Ugo, D.; Biondi, A. The learning curve of TaTME for mid-low rectal cancer: A comprehensive analysis from a five-year institutional experience. *Surg. Endosc.* **2020**. [CrossRef]

17. Koedam, T.W.A.; Veltcamp Helbach, M.; van de Ven, P.M.; Kruyt, P.M.; van Heek, N.T.; Bonjer, H.J.; Tuynman, J.B.; Sietses, C. Transanal total mesorectal excision for rectal cancer: Evaluation of the learning curve. *Tech. Coloproctol.* **2018**, *22*, 279–287. [CrossRef]
18. Lee, L.; de Lacy, B.; Gomez Ruiz, M.; Liberman, A.S.; Albert, M.R.; Monson, J.R.T.; Lacy, A.; Kim, S.H.; Atallah, S.B. A multicenter matched comparison of transanal and robotic total mesorectal excision for mid and low-rectal adenocarcinoma. *Ann. Surg.* **2019**, *270*, 1110–1116. [CrossRef] [PubMed]
19. Wexner, S.D. Robotic transanal minimally invasive surgery. *Colorectal Dis.* **2020**, *22*, 1217–1218. [CrossRef]
20. Leal Ghezzi, T.; Campos Corleta, O. 30 Years of Robotic Surgery. *World. J. Surg.* **2016**, *40*, 2550–2557. [CrossRef]
21. Davies, B.L.; Hibberd, R.D.; Ng, W.S.; Timoney, A.G.; Wickham, J.E. The development of a surgeon robot for prostatectomies. *Proc. Inst. Mech. Eng. H* **1991**, *205*, 35–38. [CrossRef] [PubMed]
22. Stefano, G.B. Robotic Surgery: Fast Forward to Telemedicine. *Med. Sci. Monit.* **2017**, *17*, 1856. [CrossRef]
23. Pugin, F.; Bucher, P.; Morel, P. History of robotic surgery: From AESOP® and ZEUS® to da Vinci®. *J. Visc. Surg.* **2011**, *148* (Suppl. S6), e3–e8. [CrossRef] [PubMed]
24. Himpens, J.; Leman, G.; Cadiere, G.B. Telesurgical laparoscopic cholecystectomy. *Surg. Endosc.* **1998**, *12*, 1091. [CrossRef] [PubMed]
25. Carpentier, A.; Loulmet, D.; Aupècle, B.; Kieffer, J.P.; Tournay, D.; Guibourt, P.; Fiemeyer, A.; Méléard, D.; Richomme, P.; Cardon, C. Chirurgie à coeur ouvert assistée par ordinateur. Premier cas opéré avec succès. *C. R. de l'Academie des Sci. Ser. III Sci. de la Vie* **1998**, *321*, 437–442. [CrossRef]
26. Atallah, S.; Parra-Davila, E.; Melani, A.; Romagnolo, L.G.; Larach, S.W.; Marescaux, J. Robotic-assisted stereotactic real-time navigation: Initial clinical experience and feasibility for rectal cancer surgery. *Tech. Coloproctol.* **2019**, *23*, 53–63. [CrossRef]
27. Porpiglia, F.; Checcucci, E.; Amparore, D.; Autorino, R.; Piana, A.; Bellin, A.; Piazzolla, P.; Massa, F.; Bollito, E.; Gned, D.; et al. Augmented-reality robot-assisted radical prostatectomy using hyper-accuracy three-dimensional reconstruction (HA3D) technology: A radiological and pathological study. *BJU Int.* **2019**, *123*, 834–845. [CrossRef]
28. U. S. Food and Drug FDA Clears New Robotically-Assisted Surgical Device for Adult Patients. 2017. Available online: http://news.doximity.com/entries/9699292?authenticated=false (accessed on 26 April 2021).
29. Taylor, N.P. FDA Clears Medrobotics' Robotic Surgical Platform for Expanded Use. 2018. Available online: https://www.fiercebiotech.com/medtech/fda-clears-medrobotics-robotic-surgical-platform-for-expanded-use (accessed on 26 April 2021).
30. Peters, B.S.; Armijo, P.R.; Krause, C.; Choudhury, S.A.; Oleynikov, D. Review of emerging surgical robotic technology. *Surg. Endosc.* **2018**, *32*, 1636–1655. [CrossRef]
31. Buess, G.; Mentges, B.; Manncke, K.; Starlinger, M.; Becker, H.D. Technique and results of transanal endoscopic microsurgery in early rectal cancer. *Am. J. Surg.* **1992**, *163*, 63–69. [CrossRef]
32. Atallah, S.; Albert, M.; Larach, S. Transanal minimally invasive surgery: A giant leap forward. *Surg. Endosc.* **2010**, *24*, 2200–2205. [CrossRef] [PubMed]
33. Fernández-Hevia, M.; Delgado, S.; Castells, A.; Tasende, M.; Momblan, D.; Díaz del Gobbo, G.; DeLacy, B.; Balust, J.; Lacy, A.M. Transanal total mesorectal excision in rectal cancer: Short-term outcomes in comparison with laparoscopic surgery. *Ann. Surg.* **2015**, *261*, 221–227. [CrossRef] [PubMed]
34. McLemore, E.C.; Coker, A.; Jacobsen, G.; Talamini, M.A.; Horgan, S. eTAMIS: Endoscopic visualization for transanal minimally invasive surgery. *Surg. Endosc.* **2013**, *27*, 1842–1845. [CrossRef]
35. Gomez Ruiz, M.; Parra, I.M.; Palazuelos, C.M.; Martin, J.A.; Fernandez, C.C.; Diego, J.C.; Gomez Fleitas, M. Robotic-assisted laparoscopic transanal total mesorectal excision for rectal cancer: A prospective pilot study. *Dis. Colon Rectum* **2015**, *58*, 145–153. [CrossRef] [PubMed]
36. Park, E.J.; Cho, M.S.; Baek, S.J.; Hur, H.; Min, B.S.; Baik, S.H.; Lee, K.Y.; Kim, N.K. Long-term oncologic outcomes of robotic low anterior resection for rectal cancer: A comparative study with laparoscopic surgery. *Ann. Surg.* **2015**, *261*, 129–137. [CrossRef] [PubMed]
37. Atallah, S.B.; Albert, M.R.; deBeche-Adams, T.H.; Larach, S.W. Robotic transanal minimally invasive surgery in a cadaveric model. *Tech. Coloproctol.* **2011**, *15*, 461–464. [CrossRef] [PubMed]
38. Atallah, S.; Nassif, G.; Polavarapu, H.; deBeche-Adams, T.; Ouyang, J.; Albert, M.; Larach, S. Robotic-assisted transanal surgery for total mesorectal excision (RATS-TME): A description of a novel surgical approach with video demonstration. *Tech. Coloproctol.* **2013**, *17*, 441–447. [CrossRef]
39. Atallah, S.; Martin-Perez, B.; Pinan, J.; Quinteros, F.; Schoonyoung, H.; Albert, M.; Larach, S. Robotic transanal total mesorectal excision: A pilot study. *Tech. Coloproctol.* **2014**, *18*, 1047–1053. [CrossRef]
40. Verheijen, P.M.; Consten, E.C.; Broeders, I.A. Robotic transanal total mesorectal excision for rectal cancer: Experience with a first case. *Int. J. Med. Robot.* **2014**, *10*, 423–426. [CrossRef]
41. Atallah, S.; Martin-Perez, B.; Parra-Davila, E.; deBeche-Adams, T.; Nassif, G.; Albert, M.; Larach, S. Robotic transanal surgery for local excision of rectal neoplasia, transanal total mesorectal excision, and repair of complex fistulae: Clinical experience with the first 18 cases at a single institution. *Tech. Coloproctol.* **2015**, *19*, 401–410. [CrossRef]
42. Huscher, C.G.S.; Bretagnol, F.; Ponzano, C. Robotic-assisted Transanal Total Mesorectal Excision: The Key against the Achilles' Heel of Rectal Cancer? *Ann. Surg.* **2015**, *261*, e120–e121. [CrossRef]

43. Kuo, L.J.; Ngu, J.C.; Tong, Y.S.; Chen, C.C. Combined robotic transanal total mesorectal excision (R-taTME) and single-site plus one-port (R-SSPO) technique for ultra-low rectal surgery-initial experience with a new operation approach. *Int. J. Colorectal Dis.* **2017**, *32*, 249–254. [CrossRef]
44. Monsellato, I.; Morello, A.; Prati, M.; Argenio, G.; Piscioneri, D.; Lenti, L.M.; Priora, F. Robotic transanal total mesorectal excision: A new perspective for low rectal cancer treatment. A case series. *Int. J. Surg. Case Rep.* **2019**, *61*, 86–90. [CrossRef] [PubMed]
45. Hu, J.M.; Chu, C.H.; Jiang, J.K.; Lai, Y.L.; Huang, I.P.; Cheng, A.Y.; Yang, S.H.; Chen, C.C. Robotic transanal total mesorectal excision assisted by laparoscopic transabdominal approach: A preliminary twenty-case series report. *Asian J. Surg.* **2020**, *43*, 330–338. [CrossRef] [PubMed]
46. Ye, J.; Shen, H.; Li, F.; Tian, Y.; Gao, Y.; Zhao, S.; Liu, B.; Tong, W. Robotic-assisted transanal total mesorectal excision for rectal cancer: Technique and results from a single institution. *Tech. Coloproctol.* **2020**, *25*, 693–700. [CrossRef]
47. Samalavicius, N.E.; Janusonis, V.; Smolskas, E.; Dulskas, A. Transanal and robotic total mesorectal excision (robotic-assisted TaTME) using the Senhance® robotic system—A video vignette. *Colorectal Dis.* **2020**, *22*, 114–115. [CrossRef] [PubMed]
48. Atallah, S.; Parra-Davila, E.; Melani, A.G.F. Assessment of the Versius surgical robotic system for dual-field synchronous transanal total mesorectal excision (taTME) in a preclinical model: Will tomorrow's surgical robots promise newfound options? *Tech. Coloproctol.* **2019**, *23*, 471–477. [CrossRef] [PubMed]
49. Atallah, S. Assessment of a flexible robotic system for endoluminal applications and transanal total mesorectal excision (taTME): Could this be the solution we have been searching for? *Tech. Coloproctol.* **2017**, *21*, 809–814. [CrossRef]
50. Carmichael, H.; D'Andrea, A.P.; Skancke, M.; Obias, V.; Sylla, P. Feasibility of transanal total mesorectal excision (taTME) using the Medrobotics Flex® System. *Surg. Endosc.* **2020**, *34*, 485–491. [CrossRef]
51. Marks, J.; Ng, S.; Mak, T. Robotic transanal surgery (RTAS) with utilization of a next-generation single-port system: A cadaveric feasibility study. *Tech. Coloproctol.* **2017**, *21*, 541–545. [CrossRef]
52. Marks, J.H.; Salem, J.F.; Anderson, B.K.; Josse, J.M.; Schoonyoung, H.P. Single-port left colectomy: First clinical experience using the SP robot (rSILS). *Tech. Coloproctol.* **2020**, *24*, 57–63. [CrossRef]
53. Ribero, D.; Baldassarri, D.; Spinoglio, G. Robotic taTME using the da Vinci SP: Technical notes in a cadaveric model. *Updates Surg.* **2021**. [CrossRef] [PubMed]
54. Kneist, W.; Stein, H.; Rheinwald, M. Da Vinci Single-Port robot-assisted transanal mesorectal excision: A promising preclinical experience. *Surg. Endosc.* **2020**, *34*, 3232–3235. [CrossRef]
55. Van Der Meijden, O.A.J.; Schijven, M.P. The value of haptic feedback in conventional and robot-assisted minimal invasive surgery and virtual reality training: A current review. *Surg. Endosc. Other Interv. Tech.* **2009**, *23*, 1180–1190. [CrossRef] [PubMed]
56. Enayati, N.; De Momi, E.; Ferrigno, G. Haptics in robot-assisted surgery: Challenges and benefts. *IEEE Rev. Biomed. Eng.* **2016**, *9*, 49–65. [CrossRef] [PubMed]
57. Abiri, A.; Pensa, J.; Tao, A.; Ma, J.; Juo, Y.Y.; Askari, S.J.; Bisley, J.; Rosen, J.; Dutson, E.P.; Grundfest, W.S. Multi-Modal haptic feedback for grip force reduction in robotic surgery. *Sci. Rep.* **2019**, *9*, 5016. [CrossRef]
58. Rao, P.P. Robotic surgery: New robots and finally some real competition! *World J. Urol.* **2018**, *36*, 537–541. [CrossRef] [PubMed]
59. Prewitt, R.; Bochkarev, V.; McBride, C.L.; Kinney, S.; Oleynikov, D. The patterns and costs of the Da Vinci robotic surgery system in a large academic institution. *J. Robot. Surg.* **2008**, *2*, 17–20. [CrossRef]
60. Jayne, D.; Pigazzi, A.; Marshall, H.; Croft, J.; Corrigan, N.; Copeland, J.; Quirke, P.; West, N.; Rautio, T.; Thomassen, N.; et al. Effect of Robotic-Assisted vs Conventional Laparoscopic Surgery on Risk of Conversion to Open Laparotomy among Patients Undergoing Resection for Rectal Cancer: The ROLARR Randomized Clinical Trial. *JAMA* **2017**, *24*, 1569–1580. [CrossRef]
61. Baek, S.J.; Kim, S.H.; Cho, J.S.; Shin, J.W.; Kim, J. Robotic versus conventional laparoscopic surgery for rectal cancer: A cost analysis from a single institute in Korea. *World J. Surg.* **2012**, *36*, 2722–2729. [CrossRef]
62. Kim, C.W.; Baik, S.H.; Roh, Y.H.; Kang, J.; Hur, H.; Min, B.S.; Lee, K.Y.; Kim, N.K. Cost-effectiveness of robotic surgery for rectal cancer focusing on short-term outcomes: A propensity score-matching analysis. *Medicine* **2015**, *94*, e823. [CrossRef] [PubMed]
63. Ramji, K.M.; Cleghorn, M.C.; Josse, J.M.; MacNeill, A.; O'Brien, C.; Urbach, D.; Quereshy, F.A. Comparison of clinical and economic outcomes between robotic, laparoscopic, and open rectal cancer surgery: Early experience at a tertiary care center. *Surg. Endosc.* **2016**, *30*, 1337–1343. [CrossRef] [PubMed]
64. Ielpo, B.; Duran, H.; Diaz, E.; Fabra, I.; Caruso, R.; Malavé, L.; Ferri, V.; Nuñez, J.; Ruiz-Ocaña, A.; Jorge, E.; et al. Robotic versus laparoscopic surgery for rectal cancer: A comparative study of clinical outcomes and costs. *Int. J. Colorectal Dis.* **2017**, *32*, 1423–1429. [CrossRef] [PubMed]
65. Morelli, L.; Guadagni, S.; Lorenzoni, V.; Di Franco, G.; Cobuccio, L.; Palmeri, M.; Caprili, G.; D'Isidoro, C.; Moglia, A.; Ferrari, V.; et al. Robot-assisted versus laparoscopic rectal resection for cancer in a single surgeon's experience: A cost analysis covering the initial 50 robotic cases with the da Vinci Si. *Int. J. Colorectal Dis.* **2016**, *3*, 1639–1648. [CrossRef] [PubMed]
66. Nabi, J.; Friedlander, D.F.; Chen, X.; Cole, A.P.; Hu, J.C.; Kibel, A.S.; Dasgupta, P.; Trinh, Q.D. Assessment of out-of-Pocket Costs for Robotic Cancer Surgery in US Adults. *JAMA Netw. Open.* **2020**, *3*, e1919185. [CrossRef]
67. D'Andrea, A.P.; McLemore, E.C.; Bonaccorso, A.; Cuevas, J.M.; Basam, M.; Tsay, A.T.; Bhasin, D.; Attaluri, V.; Sylla, P. Transanal total mesorectal excision (taTME) for rectal cancer: Beyond the learning curve. *Surg. Endosc.* **2020**, *34*, 4101–4109. [CrossRef]
68. Jimenez-Rodriguez, R.M.; Diaz-Pavon, J.M.; de la Portilla de Juan, F.; Prendes-Sillero, E.; Dussort, H.C.; Padillo, J. Learning curve for robotic-assisted laparoscopic rectal cancer surgery. *Int. J. Colorectal Dis.* **2013**, *28*, 815–821. [CrossRef]

69. Yamaguchi, T.; Kinugasa, Y.; Shiomi, A.; Sato, S.; Yamakawa, Y.; Kagawa, H.; Tomioka, H.; Mori, K. Learning curve for robotic-assisted surgery for rectal cancer: Use of the cumulative sum method. *Surg. Endosc.* **2015**, *29*, 1679–1685. [CrossRef]
70. Sng, K.K.; Hara, M.; Shin, J.W.; Yoo, B.E.; Yang, K.S.; Kim, S.H. The multiphasic learning curve for robot-assisted rectal surgery. *Surg. Endosc.* **2013**, *27*, 3297–3307. [CrossRef] [PubMed]
71. Mohd Azman, Z.A.; Kim, S.H. A review on robotic surgery in rectal cancer. *Transl. Gastroenterol. Hepatol.* **2016**, *1*, 5. [CrossRef]
72. Gachabayov, M.; Kim, S.H.; Jimenez-Rodriguez, R.; Kuo, L.J.; Cianchi, F.; Tulina, I.; Tsarkov, P.; Bergamaschi, R. Impact of robotic learning curve on histopathology in rectal cancer: A pooled analysis. *Surg. Oncol.* **2020**, *34*, 121–125. [CrossRef]

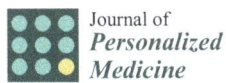

Review

Robotic versus Laparoscopic Surgery for Spleen-Preserving Distal Pancreatectomies: Systematic Review and Meta-Analysis

Gianluca Rompianesi , Roberto Montalti * , Luisa Ambrosio and Roberto Ivan Troisi

Division of Hepato-Bilio-Pancreatic, Minimally Invasive and Robotic Surgery, Department of Clinical Medicine and Surgery, Federico II University Hospital, Via S.Pansini 5, 80131 Naples, Italy; gianluca.rompianesi@unina.it (G.R.); luisa.ambrosio@unina.it (L.A.); roberto.troisi@unina.it (R.I.T.)
* Correspondence: roberto.montalti@unina.it; Tel.: +39-081-7462732

Abstract: Background: When oncologically feasible, avoiding unnecessary splenectomies prevents patients who are undergoing distal pancreatectomy (DP) from facing significant thromboembolic and infective risks. Methods: A systematic search of MEDLINE, Embase, and Web Of Science identified 11 studies reporting outcomes of 323 patients undergoing intended spleen-preserving minimally invasive robotic DP (SP-RADP) and 362 laparoscopic DP (SP-LADP) in order to compare the spleen preservation rates of the two techniques. The risk of bias was evaluated according to the Newcastle–Ottawa Scale. Results: SP-RADP showed superior results over the laparoscopic approach, with an inferior spleen preservation failure risk difference (RD) of 0.24 (95% CI 0.15, 0.33), reduced open conversion rate (RD of −0.05 (95% CI −0.09, −0.01)), reduced blood loss (mean difference of −138 mL (95% CI −205, −71)), and mean difference in hospital length of stay of −1.5 days (95% CI −2.8, −0.2), with similar operative time, clinically relevant postoperative pancreatic fistula (ISGPS grade B/C), and Clavien–Dindo grade ≥3 postoperative complications. Conclusion: Both SP-RADP and SP-LADP proved to be safe and effective procedures, with minimal perioperative mortality and low postoperative morbidity. The robotic approach proved to be superior to the laparoscopic approach in terms of spleen preservation rate, intraoperative blood loss, and hospital length of stay.

Keywords: robotic distal pancreatectomy; laparoscopic distal pancreatectomy; spleen-preserving distal pancreatectomy; minimally-invasive distal pancreatectomy; systematic review; meta-analysis

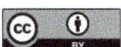

1. Introduction

The decision on preserving the spleen when performing a distal pancreatectomy (DP) is usually based on the balance between achieving an adequate oncological clearance and avoiding complications related to asplenia. Spleen-preserving DP has therefore been mainly reserved for surgeries performed for benign indications or to excise lesions with a low malignant potential. With the advent of minimally invasive surgery, in the early 1990s, surgeons around the world started to explore the potential of the laparoscopic approach in pancreatic surgery [1,2] and, almost a decade later, of the robotic-assisted technique [3]. Minimally invasive pancreatic surgery has been progressively gaining widespread popularity, and advancements in surgical skills have removed most of the technical restrictions, allowing the safe and effective execution of complex procedures, including laparoscopic spleen-preserving distal pancreatectomy (SP-LADP) [4] and robot-assisted spleen-preserving distal pancreatectomy (SP-RADP) [5].

This systematic review and meta-analysis aims to summarize all of the available evidence regarding spleen-preserving DP and compare results and outcomes of minimally invasive SP-RADP and SP-LADP techniques.

2. Materials and Methods

This systematic review and meta-analysis was conducted in accordance with the preferred reporting items for systematic reviews and meta-analyses (PRISMA 2020 Statement [6]) and was registered on PROSPERO (CRD42021239032).

2.1. Search Strategy

MEDLINE, Embase, and Web Of Science electronic databases were searched using the following terms: "pancrea*" AND "robot*" AND "laparoscop*" AND "sple*". The last search was run on 1 February 2021 with no language or publication status restrictions. Additional potentially relevant studies were identified from the reference lists of selected studies.

2.2. Study Selection

For inclusion, studies had to (1) include patients undergoing DP for any disease; (2) include procedures performed robotically and laparoscopically; and (3) report data on patients undergoing DP with the intent of preserving the spleen. Case reports, reviews, and communications, as well as non-human studies, were excluded. Two reviewers (G.R. and L.A.) independently screened the results of the electronic search at title and abstract levels. The full texts of the selected references were also retrieved for further analysis and data extraction. When duplicate reports from the same study were identified, only the most recent publication was included.

2.3. Data Extraction and Quality Assessment

Two reviewers (G.R. and L.A.) extracted data from each selected study regarding the first author; publication year; country of origin; study design; number of patients undergoing SP-RADP and SP-LADP; patients characteristics (age, sex, body mass index (BMI)); underlying disease requiring DP; American Society of Anesthesiologists (ASA) score; tumor size; conversion rate; blood loss; pancreatic stump closure technique; splenic vessel preservation and technique (Warshaw vs. Kimura); blood transfusion requirement; length of surgery; data on postoperative morbidity, including prevalence and grading of the clinical severity of postoperative pancreatic fistula (POPF) according to the ISGPS definition [7]; complications and grading according to the Clavien–Dindo classification [8]; re-operation rate; length of stay (LOS); mortality; and length of follow-up. The quality and risk of bias of each included study was evaluated independently by two reviewers (G.R. and L.A.) according to the Newcastle–Ottawa Scale for evaluating the quality of non-randomized studies in meta-analyses [9]. The level of evidence was rated according to the Grading of Recommendations, Assessment, Development and Evaluations (GRADE) system [10]. Any disagreement was resolved through discussion in order to reach consensus across the study team.

2.4. Statistical Analysis and Data Synthesis

The primary outcome was the spleen preservation failure rate. Secondary outcomes included intraoperative blood loss, operative time, prevalence of clinically relevant POPF (grade B/C), prevalence of postoperative complications (Clavien–Dindo [8] grades ≥ 3), hospital LOS, and mortality. For the analysis, values expressed as median (range) were converted to average $\pm$ standard deviation using Wan's method [11]. To pool proportions, we used random-effects or fixed-effect modelling according to the DerSimonian and Laird method [12,13] to take into account heterogeneity. The presence of heterogeneity among the studies was assessed using Cochran's Q test and quantified with the I^2 inconsistency index, with 25, 50, and 75% considered as thresholds for low, moderate, and high statistical heterogeneity, respectively. Heterogeneity was evaluated by sensitivity analysis [14]. Statistical analyses were performed using Review Manager version 5.3.

3. Results

3.1. Studies Selection

Eleven studies met the inclusion criteria and were included in the systematic review and meta-analysis [15–25] (Figure 1).

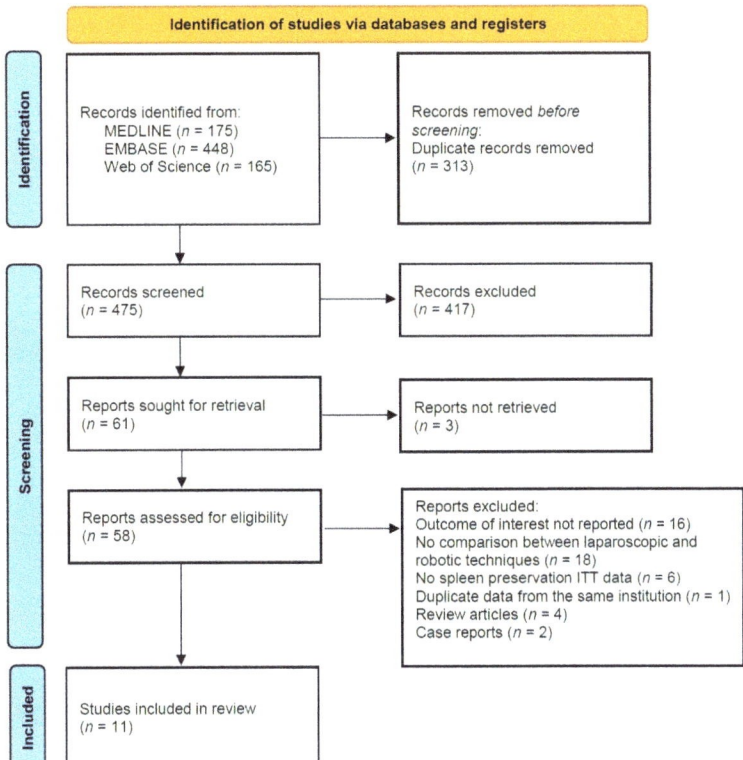

Figure 1. PRISMA flow diagram. ITT: intention-to-treat.

3.2. Studies Characteristics

The characteristics of the selected studies are reported in Table 1. A total of 323 patients undergoing SP-RADP and 362 patients undergoing SP-LADP were included in this meta-analysis. Eight included series (72.7%) were retrospective cohort studies [16–18,21–25], two were matched cohort studies (18.2%) [15,19], and one was a case-control study (9.1%) [20]. The reported median follow-up was 27 months (range 6.5–47) for SP-RADP and 33.5 months (range 32–75.5) for SP-LADP. The most frequent indications for surgery were neuroendocrine tumors (NET) in 61 SP-RADP and 52 SP-LADP, mucinous cystic neoplasms in 37 SP-RADP and 28 SP-LADP, intraductal papillary mucinous neoplasms (IPMN) in 15 SP-RADP and 28 SP-LADP, and pseudopapillary tumors in 18 SP-RADP and 17 SP-LADP.

Table 1. Summary of the selected studies with patients' characteristics and quality assessment according to the Newcastle–Ottawa scale (NOS). NA: not available.

Author and Year	Study Type	N Rob/Lap	Age, Years Rob–Lap	Sex (F) Rob/Lap	Lesion Size, mm Rob–Lap	BMI Rob–Lap	ASA Rob–Lap	NOS Assessment Selection	Comparability	Outcome
Chen et al., 2015	Matched cohort	47/33	55.6 ± 14.3–55.8 ± 16.2	31/21	31.25 ± 3.4–29 ± 3.4	24.4 ± 2.9–24.8 ± 2.7	2.5 ± 0.7–1.91 ± 0.3	3*	2*	3*
Eckhardt et al., 2016	Cohort	12/29	50.5 ± 14.4–55 ± 16.8	8/17	22 ± 10.4–38 ± 3	24.00 ± 3.4–27.3 ± 4.3	NA	3*	1*	3*
Hong et al., 2020	Cohort	31/57	NA	NA	36.5 ± 17.4–29.8 ± 19.5	NA	NA	3*	1*	3*
Kang et al., 2011	Cohort	20/25	44.5 ± 15.9–56.5 ± 13.9	12/14	35 ± 13–30 ± 14	24.2 ± 2.9–23.4 ± 2.6	NA	3*	1*	3*
Liu et al., 2017	Matched cohort	76/77	NA	NA	NA	NA	NA	3*	2*	3*
Morelli et al., 2016	Case-control	15/15	58.2 ± 13.7–49.3 ± 17.1	9/13	29.9 ± 16.5–26.9 ± 13.5	26.4 ± 3.1–26.1 ± 1.9	2.40 ± 0.5–2.30 ± 0.5	2*	2*	3*
Nell et al., 2016	Cohort	5/9	NA	NA	NA	NA	NA	3*	1*	3*
Najafi et al., 2020	Cohort	24/32	NA	NA	NA	NA	NA	3*	1*	3*
Souche et al. 2018	Cohort	13/13	NA	NA	NA	NA	NA	3*	1*	3*
Yang et al., 2020	Cohort	37/41	42.9 ± 14–51.3 ± 14.6	23/27	27 ± 12–42 ± 33	23.5 ± 3.2–24.1 ± 3.4	1.41 ± 0.6–1.58 ± 0.8	3*	1*	3*
Zhang et al., 2017	Cohort	43/31	47.9 ± 10.5–48.7 ± 12.3	23/19	17.5 ± 2.7–16.5 ± 2.4	23.3 ± 2.7–23.9 ± 3.2	1.26 ± 0.4–1.39 ± 0.5	3*	1*	3*

3.3. Quality Assessment and Publication Bias

The results of the quality assessment of the 11 included studies according to the guidelines of the Newcastle–Ottawa Scale are reported in Table 1.

3.4. Spleen Preservation Rate

All selected studies reported the number of procedures intended to be spleen preserving and the spleen preservation failure rate for both the robotic and laparoscopic techniques. The risk difference (RD) of spleen preservation failures was 0.24 (95% CI 0.15, 0.33), favoring the robotic approach and with moderate heterogeneity (I^2 = 63%) (Figure 2). Heterogeneity was evaluated by sensitivity analysis, and the results are summarized in Table 2.

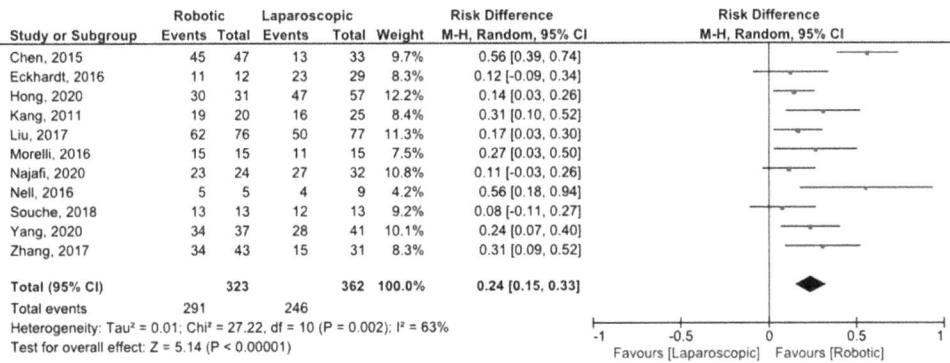

Figure 2. Spleen preservation rate forest plot.

Table 2. Sensitivity analysis by sequential omission of each individual study. Meta-analysis estimates, given the named study is omitted. CI: confidence interval.

Study Omitted	Risk Difference [95% CI] (<1 Favors Robotic)	Test of Heterogeneity Chi^2	p	Quantification of Heterogeneity
Chen et al., 2015	0.19 [0.13, 0.25]	10.51	0.31	df = 9; I^2 = 14%
Eckhardt et al., 2016	0.25 [0.15, 0.35]	26.40	0.002	df = 9; I^2 = 66%
Hong et al., 2020	0.25 [0.15, 0.36]	24.73	0.003	df = 9; I^2 = 64%
Kang et al., 2011	0.23 [0.14, 0.33]	26.49	0.002	df = 9; I^2 = 66%
Liu et al., 2017	0.25 [0.15, 0.36]	27.61	0.001	df = 9; I^2 = 67%
Morelli et al., 2016	0.24 [0.14, 0.34]	27.11	0.001	df = 9; I^2 = 67%
Najafi et al., 2020	0.25 [0.16, 0.35]	24.78	0.003	df = 9; I^2 = 64%
Nell et al., 2016	0.23 [0.13, 0.32]	24.15	0.004	df = 9; I^2 = 63%
Souche et al., 2018	0.26 [0.16, 0.25]	24.49	0.004	df = 9; I^2 = 63%
Yang et al., 2020	0.24 [0.14, 0.34]	27.30	0.001	df = 9; I^2 = 67%
Zhang et al., 2017	0.23 [0.14, 0.33]	26.34	0.002	df = 9; I^2 = 66%

3.5. Patient Characteristics and Operative Details

Only four series [16,21,25,26] reported the average ASA score (median value of 1.9, range 1.3–2.5 for SP-RADP; 1.7, range 1.4–2.3 for SP-LADP), while preoperative BMI was described in six series [16,17,19,21,25,26] (median value of 24.1, range 23.3–26.4 for SP-RADP; 24.4, range 23.4–27.3 for SP-LADP). Of the groups reporting the incidence of previous abdominal surgery [16,17,21], 5 out of 15 patients in both groups had had previous surgery in one study [20], with no patients undergoing previous surgery in the other two reports. All other patients' characteristics are summarized in Table 1.

Eight of the included studies [15,16,18,20,21,23–25] reported the conversion rate, with an RD of −0.05 (95% CI −0.09, −0.01) and moderate heterogeneity ($I^2 = 26\%$) of being converted to "open" technique favoring the robotic approach. Unfortunately, no study described the reason for conversion. The intraoperative blood loss (Figure 3), as reported in seven series [16,17,19,21,22,25,26], was significantly lower for the robotic group, with a mean difference of −138 mL (95% CI −205, −71) and high heterogeneity ($I^2 = 97\%$). There was no statistical difference in the operative time between the two groups (Figure 3), reported by nine series [15–18,20,21,23–25], with a mean difference of 6.1 min (95% CI −40, 52) and high heterogeneity ($I^2 = 97\%$). Four studies [17,23–25] reported the distal pancreatic stump closure technique, which was with an endo-GIA stapler in all cases in both groups. Eight studies [15,16,18,20,21,23–25] reported data on spleen preservation techniques, including a total of 211 robotic and 219 laparoscopic procedures. The Kimura technique [26] was adopted in 159 out of the 196 patients (81.1%) undergoing SP-RADP (the remaining 18.9% of patients had the pancreatic resection performed according to the technique described by Warshaw [27]) and in 84 out of the 154 SP-LADP (54.5%), with the Warshaw technique being adopted for the remaining 45.5%.

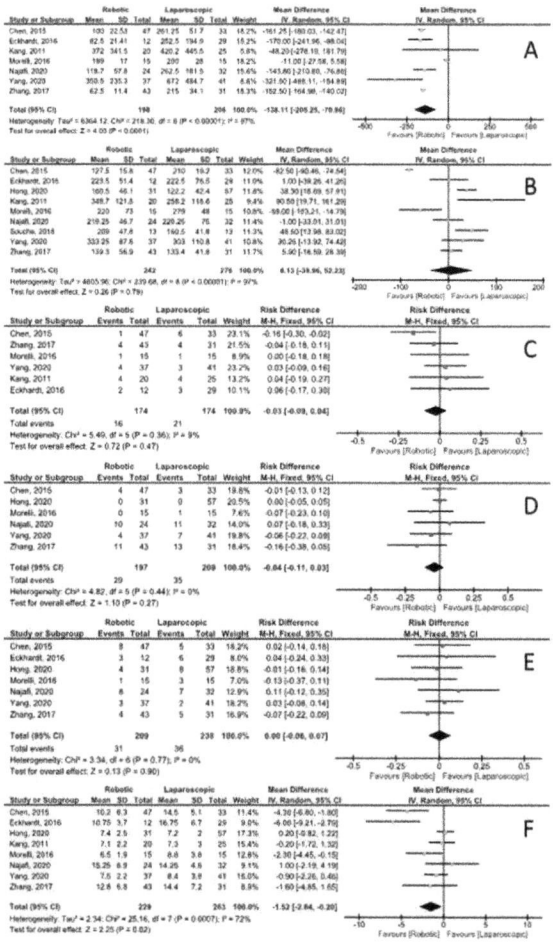

Figure 3. Secondary outcomes forest plots: (**A**) intraoperative blood loss (mL); (**B**) operative time (min); (**C**) perioperative blood transfusions; (**D**) Clavien–Dindo grade ≥3 complications; (**E**) postoperative pancreatic fistula grade B/C; (**F**) hospital length of stay (days).

3.6. Postoperative Morbidity and Outcomes

Eight series [15–18,20,21,24,25] reported the perioperative mortality, with no cases of 30-day deaths. Seven studies [15–17,20,21,24,27] described the prevalence of POPF. The RD of clinically relevant POPF (ISGPS grade B/C) was 0.00 (95% CI −0.06, 0.07) with no heterogeneity ($I^2 = 0\%$). The RD of Clavien–Dindo grade ≥3 postoperative complications, as reported in six series [16,18,21,22,25,26], was −0.04 (95% CI −0.11, 0.03) with no heterogeneity ($I^2 = 0\%$). The mean hospital LOS difference was −1.5 days (95% CI −2.8, −0.2) in favor of SP-RADP and with high heterogeneity ($I^2 = 0\%$). Data on overall postoperative complications, Clavien–Dindo grade 1–2 postoperative complications, biochemical leaks, and postoperative bleeding episodes are reported in Table 3.

Table 3. Risk differences between robotic and laparoscopic spleen-preserving distal pancreatectomies. CI: confidence interval; POPF: postoperative pancreatic fistula.

Outcome	Studies	Risk Difference [95% CI] (<1 Favors Robotic)	Test of Heterogeneity Chi²	p	Quantification of Heterogeneity
Spleen preserving failure	16–26	−0.25 [−0.30, −0.19]	27.22	0.002	df = 10; $I^2 = 63\%$
Open conversions	16, 17, 19, 21, 22, 24–26	−0.05 [−0.09, −0.01]	9.41	0.22	df = 7; $I^2 = 26\%$
Overall complications	16–19, 21, 25, 26	−0.06 [−0.14, 0.02]	2.15	0.91	df = 6; $I^2 = 0\%$
Complications—Clavien–Dindo grade 1–2	16, 18, 21	−0.02 [−0.15, 0.11]	1.00	0.61	df = 2; $I^2 = 0\%$
Complications—Clavien–Dindo grade ≥3	16, 18, 21, 22, 25, 26	−0.04 [−0.11, 0.03]	4.82	0.44	df = 5; $I^2 = 0\%$
POPF grade B/C	16–18, 21, 22, 25, 26	0.00 [−0.06, 0.07]	3.34	0.77	df = 6; $I^2 = 0\%$
Biochemical leaks	16–18, 21, 26	−0.04 [−0.14, 0.05]	1.01	0.91	df = 4; $I^2 = 0\%$
Intra-/post-operative blood transfusions	16, 17, 19, 21, 25, 26	−0.03 [−0.09, 0.04]	5.49	0.36	df = 5; $I^2 = 9\%$
Reoperation rate	16, 17, 21, 22, 26	0.01 [−0.05, 0.07]	3.86	0.42	df = 4; $I^2 = 0\%$
Hospital length of stay	16–19, 21, 22, 25, 26	−1.52 [−2.84, −0.20]	25.16	<0.001	df = 7; $I^2 = 72\%$

3.7. Quality of Evidence

The level of evidence was rated according to GRADE and is summarized in Table 4.

Table 4. Robotic versus laparoscopic surgery for spleen-preserving distal pancreatectomies. * The risk in the intervention group (and its 95% confidence interval) is based on the assumed risk in the comparison group and the relative effect of the intervention (and its 95% CI). CI: Confidence interval; RR: Risk ratio; MD: Mean difference.

Outcomes	N of Participants (Studies) Follow up	Certainty of the Evidence (GRADE)	Relative Effect (95% CI)	Anticipated Absolute Effects	
				Risk with Laparoscopic Approach	Risk Difference with Robotic Approach
Spleen preservation rate	685 (11 observational studies)	⊕⊕○○ LOW	RR 1.31 (1.16 to 1.48)	680 per 1000	211 more per 1000 (109 more to 326 more)
Blood Loss	404 (7 observational studies)	⊕⊕○○ LOW	-	Mean blood loss was 233.3 mL	MD 138.11 lower (205.25 lower to 70.96 lower)
Operative time	518 (9 observational studies)	⊕⊕○○ LOW	-	Mean operative time was 206.1 min	MD 6.13 higher (39.96 lower to 52.23 higher)
Pancreatic fistula grade B–C	447 (7 observational studies)	⊕⊕○○ LOW	RR 1.03 (0.66 to 1.60)	151 per 1000	5 more per 1000 (51 fewer to 91 more)
Complications Clavien–Dindo 3–4	406 (6 observational studies)	⊕⊕○○ LOW	RR 0.79 (0.52 to 1.20)	167 per 1000	35 fewer per 1000 (80 fewer to 33 more)
Hospital length of stay	492 (8 observational studies)	⊕⊕○○ LOW	-	Mean hospital stay was 9.8 days	MD 1.52 lower (2.84 lower to 0.2 lower)
Perioperative bleeding	143 (3 observational studies)	⊕⊕○○ LOW	RR 0.93 (0.24 to 3.63)	55 per 1000	4 fewer per 1000 (42 fewer to 144 more)

4. Discussion

To the best of our knowledge, this systematic review and meta-analysis is the first report summarizing all the available evidence on patients undergoing spleen-preserving distal pancreatectomy with robotic and laparoscopic techniques. All published studies comparing these two minimally invasive surgical approaches were screened in order to analyze the intention-to-treat population of patients undergoing DP where the spleen was intended to be preserved and to evaluate whether the surgical technique would have an impact on the spleen preservation success rate.

The spleen holds the largest lymphoid tissue mass in the body, producing early immunoglobulins M and containing macrophages that act as barriers against encapsulated pathogens. Avoiding unnecessary splenectomies prevents those patients undergoing DP from facing significant thromboembolic [28] and infective risks [29]. The most serious post-splenectomy complication is overwhelming post-splenectomy infection (OPSI), which can start with flu-like symptoms but can rapidly progress to septic shock, coma, and disseminated intravascular coagulation [30]. OPSI can represent a major medical emergency, with a mortality rate that can be up to 50–70% [31,32], a yearly incidence of 0.23%, and a lifetime risk of approximately 5%. The risk is greater within the first two years postoperatively but can vary depending on patient risk factors, such as age, immunological status, and indication for splenectomy [33,34]. In order to protect splenectomized individuals from such complications, prophylactic pneumococcal, Haemophilus influenzae type b, meningococcal, and annual influenza vaccinations are usually performed. Despite these risks, splenectomy is routinely performed alongside DP for pancreatic adenocarcinoma in order to achieve an adequate oncological clearance, given the high risk of lymph node involvement [35]. Spleen preservation should be considered in all patients undergoing DP for benign indications or pre-malignant/low-grade tumors, as it has been shown to be a safe procedure that can reduce perioperative morbidity and enable better long-term outcomes [36–39]. The spleen can be preserved despite the excision of the splenic vessels, as firstly described by Warshaw in 1988 [27], or with splenic vessel preservation, as demonstrated by Kimura et al. almost a decade later [26]. Both approaches have been shown to have comparable short- and long-term results in a recent international multicentric retrospective study [40] and carry fewer complications when performed with a minimally invasive technique. After early experiences of laparoscopic DP [1,2], the minimally invasive approach to pancreatic surgery has progressively gained popularity, with safety and efficacy profiles comparable to open surgery, together with reduced blood loss and a faster recovery time [41–45]. According to the most recent evidence-based guidelines, minimally invasive DP should be considered over open DP for all patients with benign and low-grade malignant tumors [46]. The robotic technique, with its superior accuracy, 3D vision, greater range of motion and precision [47], and excellent safety and efficacy profile in complex oncological surgery [48,49], has been utilized by several surgeons when performing pancreatic procedures [5,50,51].

This meta-analysis showed that the robotic approach is more effective than laparoscopy in allowing spleen preservation during DP, with an RD of spleen preservation failures of 0.24 (95% CI 0.15, 0.33), with reduced intraoperative blood loss (mean difference of -138 mL (95% CI -205, -71)) and similar operative time (mean difference of 6.1 min (95% CI -40, 52)). Patients undergoing SP-RADP were also less likely to experience intraoperative conversion to the "open" technique, with 3/201 open conversions (1.5%) in the robotic group and 15/219 (6.8%) in the laparoscopic group, with an RD of -0.05 (95% CI -0.09, -0.01) [15,16,18,20,21,23–25]. It was not possible to identify the proportion of patients where splenic vessel excision (Warshaw technique) was planned preoperatively, but a higher proportion of splenic vessel preservation was observed in patients undergoing SP-RADP (159/196 patients (81.1%)) versus SP-LADP (84/154 (54.5%)). With the exception of cases of tumor proximity or vascular involvement of the splenic vessels, when splenectomy or the Warshaw technique are usually the preferred choices, the Kimura technique is generally the preferred approach. The higher proportion of successful splenic vessel preservations in the robotic group, coupled with the superior spleen preservation rate, could reflect the more precise vascular dissection of the small tributaries of the splenic artery and vein that can be performed robotically. No differences in overall, clinically significant complications (Clavien–Dindo grade ≥ 3) and POPF were observed between the two groups, but patients undergoing SP-RADP had a significantly shorter hospital LOS, with a mean difference of -1.5 days (95% CI -2.8, -0.2).

Due to the lack of long-term follow-up data, the postoperative morbidity results of the present meta-analysis could underestimate the possible beneficial effects of the robotic approach in terms of expected lower incidence of complications related to the occurrence of splenic infarctions and asplenia-related infections due to the significantly higher proportion of successful splenic and splenic vessel preservation in patients undergoing SP-RADP. Prevalence of overall complications, of Clavien–Dindo grade ≥ 3 complications, and of clinically relevant POPF were similar to those reported in the literature following minimally invasive DP and open DP [40], with overall complications reported in 31.5% and 45.4%, Clavien–Dindo grade ≥ 3 complications in 14.7% and 16.7%, and clinically relevant POPF in 14.8% and 15.1% of patients undergoing SP-RADP and SP-LADP, respectively.

Unfortunately, there was no randomized controlled trial directly comparing SP-RADP and SP-LADP that could be included in the present analysis. We performed a sensitivity analysis in order to further investigate the moderate heterogeneity ($I^2 = 63\%$) of the main outcome.

In conclusion, both SP-RADP and SP-LADP proved to be safe and effective procedures, with minimal perioperative mortality and low postoperative morbidity. The robotic approach proved to be superior to the laparoscopic approach in terms of spleen preservation rate, intraoperative blood loss, and hospital length of stay. Future prospective and randomized studies with a longer follow-up could better evaluate the possible differences between these two techniques in terms of mid- to long-term complications and outcomes.

Author Contributions: Conceptualization, R.M. and G.R.; methodology, G.R.; software, R.M.; validation, R.I.T.; formal analysis, L.A.; resources, L.A.; writing—original draft preparation, G.R.; writing—review and editing, R.M. and R.I.T. All authors have read and agreed to the published version of the manuscript.

Funding: This research received no external funding.

Data Availability Statement: The data used for this manuscript are available upon request of the reviewers.

Conflicts of Interest: The authors declare no conflict of interest.

Abbreviations

ASA:	American Society of Anesthesiologists
BMI:	body mass index
CI:	confidence interval
DP:	distal pancreatectomy
IPMN:	intraductal papillary mucinous neoplasm
LOS:	length of stay
NET:	neuroendocrine tumors
OPSI:	overwhelming post-splenectomy infection
POPF:	postoperative pancreatic fistula
RD:	risk difference
SP-LADP:	spleen-preserving laparoscopic-assisted distal pancreatectomy
SP-RADP:	spleen-preserving robot-assisted distal pancreatectomy

References

1. Gagner, M.; Pomp, A.; Herrera, M.F. Early experience with laparoscopic resections of islet cell tumors. *Surgery* **1996**, *120*, 1051–1054. [CrossRef]
2. Cuschieri, A. Laparoscopic surgery of the pancreas. *J. R. Coll. Surg. Edinb.* **1994**, *39*, 178–184. [PubMed]

3. Melvin, W.S.; Needleman, B.; Krause, K.R.; Ellison, E.C. Robotic Resection of Pancreatic Neuroendocrine Tumor. *J. Laparoendosc. Adv. Surg. Tech.* **2003**, *13*, 33–36. [CrossRef]
4. Masson, B.; Fernández-Cruz, L.; Sa-Cunha, A.; Adam, J.-P.; Jacquin, A.; Laurent, C.; Collet, D. Laparoscopic Spleen-Preserving Distal Pancreatectomy: Splenic vessel preservation compared with the Warshaw technique. *JAMA Surg.* **2013**, *148*, 246–252. [CrossRef]
5. Esposito, A.; Casetti, L.; De Pastena, M.; Ramera, M.; Montagnini, G.; Landoni, L.; Bassi, C.; Salvia, R. Robotic spleen-preserving distal pancreatectomy: The Verona experience. *Updat. Surg.* **2020**, *73*, 923–928. [CrossRef]
6. Page, M.J.; McKenzie, J.E.; Bossuyt, P.M.; Boutron, I.; Hoffmann, T.C.; Mulrow, C.D.; Shamseer, L.; Tetzlaff, J.M.; Akl, E.A.; Brennan, S.E.; et al. The PRISMA 2020 statement: An updated guideline for reporting systematic reviews. *BMJ* **2021**, *372*, n71. [CrossRef] [PubMed]
7. Bassi, C.; Marchegiani, G.; Dervenis, C.; Sarr, M.; Abu Hilal, M.; Adham, M.; Allen, P.; Andersson, R.; Asbun, H.J.; Besselink, M.G.; et al. International Study Group on Pancreatic Surgery (ISGPS). The 2016 update of the International Study Group (ISGPS) definition and grading of postoperative pancreatic fistula: 11 Years After. *Surgery* **2017**, *161*, 584–591. [CrossRef]
8. Dindo, D.; Demartines, N.; Clavien, P.-A. Classification of Surgical Complications: A new proposal with evaluation in a cohort of 6336 patients and results of a survey. *Ann. Surg.* **2004**, *240*, 205–213. [CrossRef]
9. Wells, G.; Shea, B.; O'Connell, D.; Peterson, J.; Welch, V.; Losos, M.; Tugwell, P. The Newcastle-Ottawa Scale (NOS) for Assessing the Quality of Nonrandomised Studies in Meta-Analyses. Available online: http://www.ohri.ca/programs/clinical_epidemiology/oxford.asp (accessed on 1 June 2021).
10. Hultcrantz, M.; Rind, D.; Akl, E.A.; Treweek, S.; Mustafa, R.A.; Iorio, A.; Alper, B.S.; Meerpohl, J.; Murad, M.H.; Ansari, M.T.; et al. The GRADE Working Group clarifies the construct of certainty of evidence. *J. Clin. Epidemiol.* **2017**, *87*, 4–13. [CrossRef] [PubMed]
11. Wan, X.; Wang, W.; Liu, J.; Tong, T. Estimating the sample mean and standard deviation from the sample size, median, range and/or interquartile range. *BMC Med Res. Methodol.* **2014**, *14*, 1–13. [CrossRef]
12. Higgins, J.P.T.; Thompson, S.G. Quantifying heterogeneity in a meta-analysis. *Stat. Med.* **2002**, *21*, 1539–1558. [CrossRef] [PubMed]
13. DerSimonian, R.; Laird, N. Meta-analysis in clinical trials. *Control. Clin. Trials* **1986**, *7*, 177–188. [CrossRef]
14. Higgins, J.P.T.; Thompson, S.G.; Deeks, J.J.; Altman, D.G. Measuring inconsistency in meta-analyses. *BMJ* **2003**, *327*, 557–560. [CrossRef]
15. Chen, S.; Zhan, Q.; Chen, J.-Z.; Jin, J.-B.; Deng, X.-X.; Chen, H.; Shen, B.-Y.; Peng, C.-H.; Li, H.-W. Robotic approach improves spleen-preserving rate and shortens postoperative hospital stay of laparoscopic distal pancreatectomy: A matched cohort study. *Surg. Endosc.* **2015**, *29*, 3507–3518. [CrossRef] [PubMed]
16. Eckhardt, S.; Schicker, C.; Maurer, E.; Fendrich, V.; Bartsch, D.K. Robotic-Assisted Approach Improves Vessel Preservation in Spleen-Preserving Distal Pancreatectomy. *Dig. Surg.* **2016**, *33*, 406–413. [CrossRef] [PubMed]
17. Hong, S.; Song, K.B.; Madkhali, A.A.; Hwang, K.; Yoo, D.; Lee, J.W.; Youn, W.Y.; Alshammary, S.; Park, Y.; Lee, W.; et al. Robotic versus laparoscopic distal pancreatectomy for left-sided pancreatic tumors: A single surgeon's experience of 228 consecutive cases. *Surg. Endosc.* **2020**, *34*, 2465–2473. [CrossRef] [PubMed]
18. Kang, C.M.; Kim, D.H.; Lee, W.J.; Chi, H.S. Conventional laparoscopic and robot-assisted spleen-preserving pancreatectomy: Does da Vinci have clinical advantages? *Surg. Endosc.* **2011**, *25*, 2004–2009. [CrossRef] [PubMed]
19. Liu, R.; Liu, Q.; Zhao, Z.-M.; Tan, X.-L.; Gao, Y.-X.; Zhao, G.-D. Robotic versus laparoscopic distal pancreatectomy: A propensity score-matched study. *J. Surg. Oncol.* **2017**, *116*, 461–469. [CrossRef]
20. Morelli, L.; Guadagni, S.; Palmeri, M.; Di Franco, G.; Caprili, G.; D'Isidoro, C.; Bastiani, L.; Di Candio, G.; Pietrabissa, A.; Mosca, F. A Case-Control Comparison of Surgical and Functional Outcomes of Robotic-Assisted Spleen-Preserving Left Side Pancreatectomy versus Pure Laparoscopy. *J. Pancreas* **2016**, *17*, 30–35.
21. Najafi, N.; Mintziras, I.; Wiese, D.; Albers, M.B.; Maurer, E.; Bartsch, D.K. A retrospective comparison of robotic versus laparoscopic distal pancreatic resection and enucleation for potentially benign pancreatic neoplasms. *Surg. Today* **2020**, *50*, 872–880. [CrossRef] [PubMed]
22. Nell, S.; Brunaud, L.; Ayav, A.; Bonsing, B.A.; Koerkamp, B.G.; van Dijkum, E.J.N.; Kazemier, G.; de Kleine, R.H.; Hagendoorn, J.; Molenaar, I.Q.; et al. Robot-assisted spleen preserving pancreatic surgery in MEN1 patients. *J. Surg. Oncol.* **2016**, *114*, 456–461. [CrossRef] [PubMed]
23. Souche, R.; Herrero, A.; Bourel, G.; Chauvat, J.; Pirlet, I.; Guillon, F.; Nocca, D.; Borie, F.; Mercier, G.; Fabre, J.-M. Robotic versus laparoscopic distal pancreatectomy: A French prospective single-center experience and cost-effectiveness analysis. *Surg. Endosc.* **2018**, *32*, 3562–3569. [CrossRef] [PubMed]
24. Yang, S.J.; Hwang, H.K.; Kang, C.M.; Lee, W.J. Revisiting the potential advantage of robotic surgical system in spleen-preserving distal pancreatectomy over conventional laparoscopic approach. *Ann. Transl. Med.* **2020**, *8*, 188. [CrossRef]
25. Zhang, J.; Jin, J.; Chen, S.; Gu, J.; Zhu, Y.; Qin, K.; Zhan, Q.; Cheng, D.; Chen, H.; Deng, X.; et al. Minimally invasive distal pancreatectomy for PNETs: Laparoscopic or robotic approach? *Oncotarget* **2017**, *8*, 33872–33883. [CrossRef] [PubMed]
26. Kimura, W.; Inoue, T.; Futakawa, N.; Shinkai, H.; Han, I.; Muto, T. Spleen-preserving distal pancreatectomy with conservation of the splenic artery and vein. *Surgery* **1996**, *120*, 885–890. [CrossRef]
27. Warshaw, A.L. Conservation of the Spleen With Distal Pancreatectomy. *Arch. Surg.* **1988**, *123*, 550–553. [CrossRef]

28. Rottenstreich, A.; Kleinstern, G.; Spectre, G.; Da'As, N.; Ziv, E.; Kalish, Y. Thromboembolic Events Following Splenectomy: Risk Factors, Prevention, Management and Outcomes. *World J. Surg.* **2018**, *42*, 675–681. [CrossRef] [PubMed]
29. Hansen, K.; Singer, D.B. Asplenic-hyposplenic Overwhelming Sepsis: Postsplenectomy Sepsis Revisited. *Pediatr. Dev. Pathol.* **2001**, *4*, 105–121. [CrossRef]
30. Tahir, F.; Ahmed, J.; Malik, F. Post-splenectomy Sepsis: A Review of the Literature. *Cureus* **2020**, *12*, e6898. [CrossRef]
31. Sinwar, P.D. Overwhelming post splenectomy infection syndrome—Review study. *Int. J. Surg.* **2014**, *12*, 1314–1316. [CrossRef] [PubMed]
32. Sarangi, J.; Coleby, M.; Trivella, M.; Reilly, S. Prevention of post splenectomy sepsis: A population based approach. *J. Public Health* **1997**, *19*, 208–212. [CrossRef]
33. Davidson, R.; Wall, R. Prevention and management of infections in patients without a spleen. *Clin. Microbiol. Infect.* **2001**, *7*, 657–660. [CrossRef]
34. Edgren, G.; Almqvist, R.; Hartman, M.; Utter, G.H. Splenectomy and the Risk of Sepsis: A population-based cohort study. *Ann. Surg.* **2014**, *260*, 1081–1087. [CrossRef] [PubMed]
35. Jain, G.; Chakravartty, S.; Patel, A.G. Spleen-preserving distal pancreatectomy with and without splenic vessel ligation: A systematic review. *HPB* **2013**, *15*, 403–410. [CrossRef] [PubMed]
36. Shoup, M.; Brennan, M.; McWhite, K.; Leung, D.H.Y.; Klimstra, D.; Conlon, K.C. The Value of Splenic Preservation with Distal Pancreatectomy. *Arch. Surg.* **2002**, *137*, 164–168. [CrossRef] [PubMed]
37. Lillemoe, K.D.; Kaushal, S.; Cameron, J.L.; Sohn, T.A.; Pitt, H.A.; Yeo, C.J. Distal Pancreatectomy: Indications and Outcomes in 235 Patients. *Ann. Surg.* **1999**, *229*, 693–698; discussion 698–700. [CrossRef] [PubMed]
38. Carrère, N.; Abid, S.; Julio, C.H.; Bloom, E.; Pradère, B. Spleen-preserving Distal Pancreatectomy with Excision of Splenic Artery and Vein: A Case-matched Comparison with Conventional Distal Pancreatectomy with Splenectomy. *World J. Surg.* **2007**, *31*, 375–382. [CrossRef]
39. Jusoh, A.C.; Ammori, B.J. Laparoscopic versus open distal pancreatectomy: A systematic review of comparative studies. *Surg. Endosc.* **2012**, *26*, 904–913. [CrossRef]
40. Paiella, S.; De Pastena, M.; Korrel, M.; Pan, T.L.; Butturini, G.; Nessi, C.; De Robertis, R.; Landoni, L.; Casetti, L.; Giardino, A.; et al. Long term outcome after minimally invasive and open Warshaw and Kimura techniques for spleen-preserving distal pancreatectomy: International multicenter retrospective study. *Eur. J. Surg. Oncol.* **2019**, *45*, 1668–1673. [CrossRef]
41. Iacobone, M.; Citton, M.; Nitti, N. Laparoscopic distal pancreatectomy: Up-to-date and literature review. *World J. Gastroenterol.* **2012**, *18*, 5329–5337. [CrossRef]
42. Merchant, N.B.; Parikh, A.A.; Kooby, D.A. Should All Distal Pancreatectomies Be Performed Laparoscopically? *Adv. Surg.* **2009**, *43*, 283–300. [CrossRef]
43. Butturini, G.; Damoli, I.; Crepaz, L.; Malleo, G.; Marchegiani, G.; Daskalaki, D.; Esposito, A.; Cingarlini, S.; Salvia, R.; Bassi, C. A prospective non-randomised single-center study comparing laparoscopic and robotic distal pancreatectomy. *Surg. Endosc.* **2015**, *29*, 3163–3170. [CrossRef] [PubMed]
44. Cao, H.S.T.; Lopez, N.; Chang, D.C.; Lowy, A.M.; Bouvet, M.; Baumgartner, J.M.; Talamini, M.A.; Sicklick, J.K. Improved Perioperative Outcomes with Minimally Invasive Distal Pancreatectomy: Results from a population-based analysis. *JAMA Surg.* **2014**, *149*, 237–243. [CrossRef]
45. De Rooij, T.; Van Hilst, J.; Van Santvoort, H.; Boerma, D.; Boezem, P.V.D.; Daams, F.; Van Dam, R.; DeJong, C.; Van Duyn, E.; Dijkgraaf, M.; et al. Minimally Invasive Versus Open Distal Pancreatectomy (LEOPARD): A Multicenter Patient-blinded Randomized Controlled Trial. *Ann. Surg.* **2019**, *269*, 2–9. [CrossRef] [PubMed]
46. Asbun, H.J.; Moekotte, A.L.; Vissers, F.L.; Kunzler, F.; Cipriani, F.; Alseidi, A.; D'Angelica, M.I.; Balduzzi, A.; Bassi, C.; Björnsson, B.; et al. The Miami International Evidence-based Guidelines on Minimally Invasive Pancreas Resection. *Ann. Surg.* **2020**, *271*, 1–14. [CrossRef] [PubMed]
47. Troisi, R.I.; Pegoraro, F.; Giglio, M.C.; Rompianesi, G.; Berardi, G.; Tomassini, F.; De Simone, G.; Aprea, G.; Montalti, R.; De Palma, G.D. Robotic approach to the liver: Open surgery in a closed abdomen or laparoscopic surgery with technical constraints? *Surg. Oncol.* **2020**, *33*, 239–248. [CrossRef]
48. Hu, Y.; Strong, V.E. Robotic Surgery and Oncologic Outcomes. *JAMA Oncol.* **2020**, *6*, 1537–1539. [CrossRef] [PubMed]
49. Ceccarelli, G.; Andolfi, E.; Biancafarina, A.; Rocca, A.; Amato, M.; Milone, M.; Scricciolo, M.; Frezza, B.; Miranda, E.; De Prizio, M.; et al. Robot-assisted surgery in elderly and very elderly population: Our experience in oncologic and general surgery with literature review. *Aging Clin. Exp. Res.* **2017**, *29*, 55–63. [CrossRef] [PubMed]
50. Daouadi, M.; Zureikat, A.; Zenati, M.S.; Choudry, H.; Tsung, A.; Bartlett, D.L.; Hughes, S.J.; Lee, K.K.; Moser, A.J.; Zeh, H.J. Robot-Assisted Minimally Invasive Distal Pancreatectomy Is Superior to the Laparoscopic Technique. *Ann. Surg.* **2013**, *257*, 128–132. [CrossRef]
51. Huang, B.; Feng, L.; Zhao, J. Systematic review and meta-analysis of robotic versus laparoscopic distal pancreatectomy for benign and malignant pancreatic lesions. *Surg. Endosc.* **2016**, *30*, 4078–4085. [CrossRef]

Review

Updates on Robotic CME for Right Colon Cancer: A Qualitative Systematic Review

Wanda Petz *, Simona Borin and Uberto Fumagalli Romario

Division of Digestive Surgery, IEO European Institute of Oncology IRCCS, 20141 Milano, Italy; simona.borin@ieo.it (S.B.); uberto.fumagalliromario@ieo.it (U.F.R.)
* Correspondence: wanda.petz@ieo.it

Abstract: Background. Complete mesocolic excision (CME) is a surgical technique introduced with the aim of ameliorating the oncologic results of colectomy. Various experiences have demonstrated favorable oncologic results of CME in comparison with standard colectomy, in which the principles of CME are not respected. The majority of the literature refers to open or laparoscopic CME. This review analyses current evidence regarding robotic CME for right colectomy. Methods. An extensive Medline (Pub Med) search for relevant case series, restricted to papers published in English, was performed, censoring video vignettes and case reports. Results. Fourteen studies (ten retrospective, four comparative series of robotic versus laparoscopic CME) were included, with patient numbers ranging from 20 to 202. Four different approaches to CME are described, which also depend on the robotic platform utilized. Intraoperative and early clinical results were good, with a low conversion and anastomotic leak rate and a majority of Clavien–Dindo complications being Grades I and II. Oncologic adequacy of the surgical specimens was found to be good, although a homogeneous histopathologic evaluation was not provided. Conclusions. Further large studies are warranted to define long-term oncologic results of robotic right colectomy with CME and its eventual benefits in comparison to laparoscopy.

Keywords: complete mesocolic excision; robotic surgery; right colectomy

1. Background

Complete mesocolic excision (CME) with central vessel ligation (CVL) is a surgical technique first described by West [1] in 2008 and Hohenberger [2] in 2009.

By analogy with the concept of total mesorectal excision (TME) for rectal cancer, and with the aim of improving the radicality of surgery and, therefore, of ameliorating the oncologic results of colectomy for cancer, it involves the complete removal of an intact mesocolic envelope surrounding the colon.

In addition, the technique implies ligature of the supplying vessels at their origin from mesenteric artery and vein, and an extended lymphadenectomy, superimposable to the D3 dissection described by Japanese authors [3].

The surgical community has shown a growing interest in this more radical approach to colon cancer, suggesting that it could play a role in ameliorating the oncologic results of right colectomy [4–14]; however, large randomized clinical trials providing a high level of evidence are lacking.

Therefore, the guidelines of the major international scientific societies still do not mention the need to perform a CME when approaching a colonic cancer [15,16], while the same guidelines make TME for rectal cancer mandatory [17,18].

Regarding the surgical approach to CME, the techniques most used are the open and the laparoscopic techniques, although the latter has been recognized as being technically more challenging, especially with regard to vascular dissection [19].

In this paper, we shall focus on the robotic approach to CME for surgery of right colon cancer, analyzing current evidence and providing a summary of its eventual benefits.

2. Methods

The Preferred Reporting Outcomes for Systematic Reviews and Meta-Analyses (PRISMA) guidelines were followed [20] and an extensive Medline (Pub Med) search for relevant case series was performed. The search strategy included "complete mesocolic excision" AND "robotic" AND "right colon" OR "right colectomy" OR "right hemicolectomy".

Inclusion criteria were English language and detailed description of the surgical technique, including all the particular technical aspects of CME with CVL. Exclusion criteria were case reports, video vignettes and case series in which the CME technique was employed for colonic resections different from right or extended right colectomy; if a single centre published more than a paper, only the one including the greater number of patients was included.

The quality of each included study was assessed using the Newcastle–Ottawa Scale (NOS) [21] and the risk of bias was considered high if NOS total score was <7 or low if NOS total score was 7 or more.

A single reviewer (WP) screened each record retrieved and collected data from each report. Outcomes for which data were sought were: number of patients included in the study, type of robotic platform utilized, details of surgical technique (patient and trocar position, sequence of surgical steps, technique of anastomosis), conversion rate, operative time, intra and postoperative complications, number of retrieved lymph nodes, overall and disease-free survival.

Continuous data are presented as median and range, while categorical data are presented as percentages.

3. Results

After duplicate censoring, fourteen studies were included in this review [22–35], and the publication dates ranged from 2013 to 2021.

There are ten retrospective non comparative case series [22,23,27–31,33–35] and four comparative studies (three retrospective and one prospective) of robotic versus laparoscopic CME for right colectomy [24–26,32]; the patient number ranges from 20 to 202.

Characteristics and principal results of the included studies are reported in Table 1.

According to the NOS score obtained, the risk of bias was high in 4 studies and low in the remaining 10 (Table 2).

Table 1. Characteristics and principal results of the included studies.

Author	Year	Type of Study (Retrosp./Prosp.)	Type of Study (Comp./Non Comp.)	Pat. N	Conversion Rate	Mortality	Leaks	OS	DFS
Trastulli [22]	2013	retrospective	non comparative	20	0	0	0	nd	nd
Petz [23]	2017	retrospective	non comparative	20	0	0	0	nd	nd
Spinoglio [24]	2018	retrospective	comparative	202	0	1%	1%	77% (5 years)	85% (5 years)
Ngu [25]	2018	retrospective	comparative	23	0	nd	nd	nd	nd
Yozgatli [26]	2019	prospective	comparative	96	0	nd	0	nd	nd
Yang [27]	2019	retrospective	non comparative	66	1.5%	0	0	nd	nd
Shulte am Esch [28]	2019	retrospective	non comparative	31	0	0	0	nd	nd
Bae [29]	2019	retrospective	non comparative	43	0	0	2.3%	93.6% (55 months)	81.1% (55 months)
Ramachandra [30]	2020	retrospective	non comparative	52	3.84%	0	1.92%	nd	nd
Petz [31]	2020	retrospective	non comparative	50	0	0	2%	nd	nd
Ceccarelli [32]	2020	retrospective	comparative	55	0	0	0	nd	nd
Larach [33]	2021	retrospective	non comparative	20	0	0	0	nd	nd
Siddiqui [34]	2021	retrospective	non comparative	77	0	0	0	94% (3 years)	94% (3 years)
Bianchi [35]	2021	retrospective	non comparative	161	3.7%	0	0.6%	nd	nd

Pat. n: patients number; retrosp.: retrospective; prosp.: prospective; comp.: comprative; non comp.: non comparativend: not defined; OS: overall survival; DFS: disease-free survival.

Table 2. Risk of bias.

Author	Type of Study	NOS	Overall Risk of Biases
Trastulli [22]	non comparative	7 (S4, C1, O2)	low
Petz [23]	non comparative	7 (S4, C1, O2)	low
Spinoglio [24]	comparative	6 (S2, C1, E3)	high
Ngu [25]	comparative	6 (S2, C1, E3)	high
Yozgatli [26]	comparative	6 (S2, C1, E3)	high
Yang [27]	non comparative	7 (S4, C1, O2)	low
Shulte am Esch [28]	non comparative	7 (S4, C1, O2)	low
Bae [29]	non comparative	8 (S4, C1, O3)	low
Ramachandra [30]	non comparative	7 (S4, C1, O2)	low
Petz [31]	non comparative	7 (S4, C1, O2)	low
Ceccarelli [32]	comparative	6 (S2, C1, E3)	high
Larach [33]	non comparative	7 (S4, C1, O2)	low
Siddiqui [34]	non comparative	8 (S4, C1, O3)	low
Bianchi [35]	non comparative	7 (S4, C1, O2)	low

NOS: Newcastle–Ottawa Scale; S: selection; C: comparison; O: outcomes; E: exposure.

4. Technical Considerations

The da Vinci Xi robotic platform has been utilized in nine of the fourteen studies [23,25,28,30,31,33,35], the Si platform in two [22,24], the X platform in one [35] and both the Si and the Xi in the remaining two [29,32].

Four different approaches to colonic dissection, CME and lymphadenectomy are reported, the difference essentially residing in the sequence of surgical steps and the direction of detachment of the mesocolon from the retroperitoneum: a "medial-to-lateral" approach [22,24,30,32], a "bottom-to-up" approach [23,25,28,29,31,35], a "top-to-down" approach [26] and a "superior mesenteric vein first" approach [27,33,34].

Patient position on the operative table is similar for the "medial-to-lateral", the "bottom-to-up" and the "superior mesenteric vein first" approaches: the patient is supine and the operative table is in a slight Trendelenburg position and rotated to the left, in order to expose the surgical field by moving the small bowel in the left abdominal quadrants.

In the "top-to-down" approach, conversely, the patient is in a 30° reverse Trendelenburg position in the first phase of surgery, to facilitate entrance in the lesser sac through the gastrocolic ligament; a different docking is performed in the second part of the procedure.

In the "medial-to lateral" approach, when using the da Vinci Si® platform, trocars are positioned in the left abdomen with the camera in the left flank (Figure 1a,b); while using the da Vinci Xi® system, all the trocars are along the same line with an oblique costofemoral layout (Figure 2).

With the third robotic arm suspending cranially the transverse mesocolon, the procedure starts with opening of the peritoneum just below the prominence of ileocolic vessels and along the left side of superior mesenteric vein (SMV); the ileocolic artery and vein are then easily identified, dissected and ligated. Subsequently, vascular dissection proceeds cranially with ligature of right colic vessels, middle colic vein and right branch of middle colic artery.

CME is performed once vascular dissection is completed, by sharp separation of posterior mesocolic fascia from retroperitoneum.

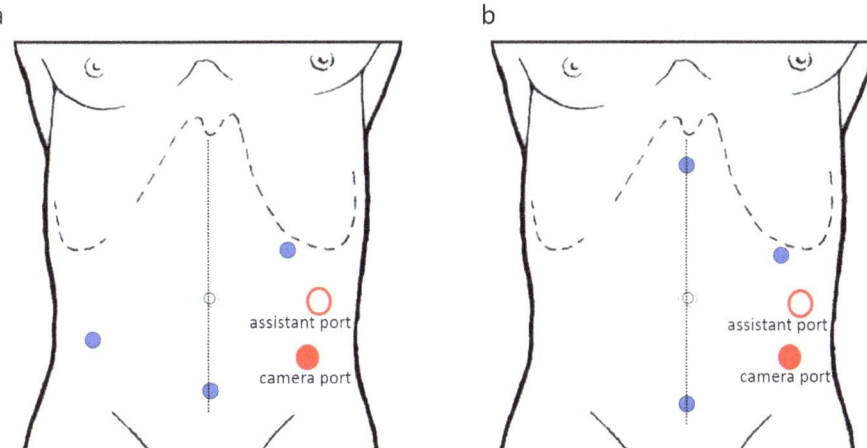

Figure 1. (a,b): trocars position for "medial-to-lateral" approach with the da Vinci Si® system.

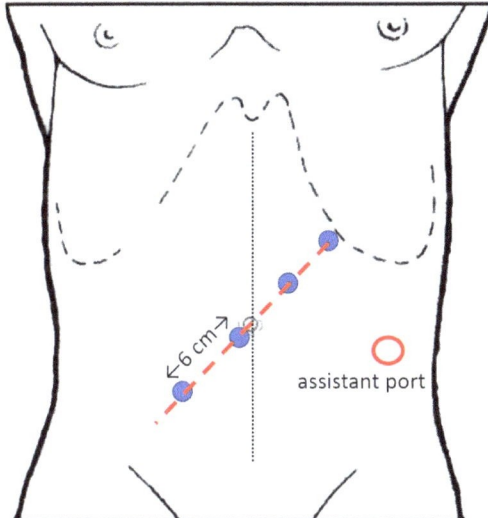

Figure 2. Trocars position for "medial-to-lateral", "SMV first" and "top-to-down" approach with the da Vinci Xi® system.

This is similar to the "superior mesenteric vein first" approach described by Yang [27] and adopted by other authors [33,34]; the vascular dissection is performed first, exposing the anterior aspect of the SMV by removing the lymphatic tissue covering it, and sequentially ligating the right colic and right branches of middle colic vessels; afterwards the CME is performed by sharp dissection of the ascending and transverse mesocolon from retroperitoneum, exposing the duodenum and the head of the pancreas, and proceeding from medial to lateral until the right colo-parietal area.

The "bottom-to-up" approach has been introduced with the da Vinci Xi® platform, which allows the thinner robotic arms to be positioned on the same suprapubic line (Figure 3): with this different vision, frontal to the axis of superior mesenteric vessels, the dissection starts with the incision of the root of mesentery and proceeds cranially developing the retro-mesocolic plane, separating ascending and right mesocolon from the retroperitoneum and joining the ventral aspect of the duodenum and the pancreatic head. Once the is CME completed, vascular dissection is performed, exposing the ventral aspect of SMV and ligating the ileocolic, right colic and right branches of the middle colic vessels.

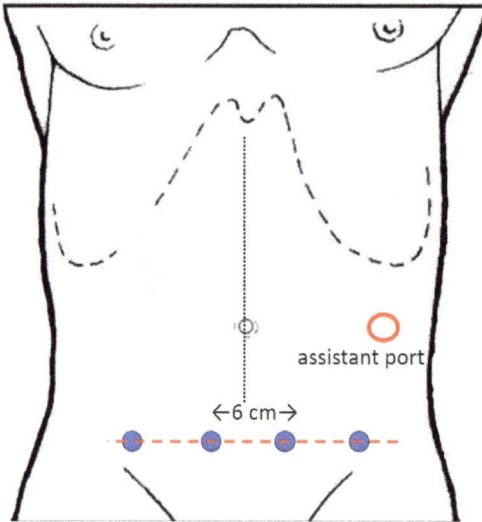

Figure 3. Trocars position for "bottom-to-up" approach with the da Vinci Xi® system.

The "top-to-down" technique has been proposed [26] for the surgical approach to cancer of the distal ascending colon, hepatic flexure or proximal transverse colon: with an oblique offset costofemoral trocars layout (Figure 2), the procedure starts with opening of the gastrocolic ligament and the identification and section of gastroepiploic vessels; the gastro-epiploic vein is then used as a guide to identify and dissect the gastro-colic trunk and, subsequently, the SMV, with removal of the lymphatic and fatty tissue of its anterior aspect. The second phase of the surgical procedure entails a robot redocking with a change of patient position to a 30° Trendelenburg; with the same trocars layout, the vascular dissection is performed and then the CME is realized with a medial-to-lateral direction.

The ileo-colic anastomosis was performed intracorporeally in ten out of the fourteen studies [22–25,29,31–35] and extracorporeally in two [28,30]; both the techniques have been utilized in two studies [26,27], in which, however, the number of patients receiving intracorporeal or extracorporeal anastomosis is not specified.

5. Clinical Outcomes

5.1. Operative Results

Conversion rate was reported in all the studies and ranged from 0 to 3.8%; among the four comparative series of robotic versus laparoscopic CME, only Spinoglio [24] reported a significantly higher conversion rate in the laparoscopic than in the robotic group (7% vs. 0).

The mean reported operative time was 236 min; in all the four comparative studies, operative time in the robotic group was significantly higher than in the laparoscopic group.

Intraoperative complications were only reported by Yozgatli [26], who described two cases of minor vascular injuries that were repaired robotically and did not require conversion to open surgery. In the comparative series from Spinoglio [24], a patient in the laparoscopic group had an intraoperative lesion of SMV.

5.2. Early Clinical Results

Postoperative complications were detailed in all the studies, with a mean incidence of 22% and no significant differences found in the four comparative studies of robotic versus laparoscopic CME.

The majority of complications were Clavien–Dindo Grade I–II, while median incidence of Clavien–Dindo Grade III–IV complications was 2.8% (range 0–11.5%).

Anastomotic leak rate was very low (0–2%) with the majority of the studies (ten out of fourteen) [22,23,26–28,32–34] reporting no leaks in the study population.

Early postoperative mortality was declared in only one study [24] and related to a sudden cardiac death.

6. Oncologic Outcomes

Adequacy of resection was mainly evaluated by reporting the median number of harvested lymph nodes, which totalled 32 (range 19–41) considering all the studies; in the comparative series published by Ngu [25] and Yozgatli [26], significantly more lymph nodes were retrieved in the robotic group in comparison with the laparoscopic group (41 vs. 31 and 41 vs. 33, respectively), while differences were not significant in the remaining two comparative series.

The length of the specimen was only reported in four studies [22–24,31] and its median value was 38.5 cm.

The integrity of the mesocolon was reported in only one study [22].

Only three studies reported on long-term oncologic outcomes: Spinoglio [24], with a median follow up of 60 months, described a 5-year overall survival (OS) rate of 77% vs. 73%, a 5-year cancer specific survival (CSS) of 90% vs. 85% and a 5-year disease-free survival (DFS) of 85% vs. 83%, respectively, in the robotic versus the laparoscopic group; in the specific subgroup of stage III patients, 5-year DFS was 81% versus 68%. Although more noticeable, this, as the other oncologic outcomes, did not differ significantly among the two groups.

In the study from Bae [29], median follow up was 55 months, and OS and DFS were 93% and 81%, respectively.

Siddiqui [34] reported an OS and a DFS of 94%. However, follow up was shorter (3 years).

A summary of clinical and oncologic outcomes of the four different surgical approaches described ("medial to lateral", "bottom-up", "top-to-down" and "SMV first") is depicted in Table 3.

Table 3. Clinical and oncologic outcomes of robotic CME for right colectomy.

	Surgical Approach				
	Medial-to-Lateral	Bottom-Up	Top-to-Down	SMV First	p
Pat. n.	329	328	96	163	
Op. time (median, min)	248	238	286	180	0.07 *
Conversions (median)	0.9%	0.6%	0	0.6%	0.88 °
Postop. compl (median, Dindo III–IV)	3.8%	5.1%	3%	1.8%	0.18 °
Harvested LN (median)	24	34	41	33	0.15 *

*: one way ANOVA test; °: Chi-square test; Pat.: patients; SMV: superior mesenteric vein; Op.: operative; min: minutes; Postop.: postoperative; compl.: complications; LN: lymph nodes.

7. Discussion

This review underlines the feasibility and safety of the robotic approach to CME with CVL for right colon cancer; in all the reported studies, operative, clinical and oncologic outcomes were good, with a very low rate of conversions to open surgery, a low rate of postoperative serious complications and anastomotic leaks, and satisfactory oncologic results.

Although laparoscopic surgery is considered the gold standard treatment for colon cancer owing to its better short-term outcomes in comparison to open surgery [36–38], laparoscopic right colectomy with CME is generally adopted by expert surgeons in high volume Centers [39–41].

One of the major concerns regarding the adoption of minimally invasive CME is its intrinsic technical challenge [42]. This is particularly the case when approaching right colectomy. In fact, the extensive dissection of the superior mesenteric vein and artery, to perform an extended lymphadenectomy, and the posterior approach to the transverse mesocolon to expose the second duodenum and the head of pancreas are undoubtedly more complex than the corresponding procedure for left colectomy. In the left colectomy, the dissection plane from the left Toldt's and Gerota's fascia is easier to approach, and only two major vessels (the inferior mesenteric artery and vein) have to be isolated and sectioned.

Vascular anatomy of the right colon is more complex [43]; right colonic vessels are not always constant, as the course of ICA after its emergence from SMA (anterior or posterior to SMV). Furthermore, the dissection of Henle's trunk and the preservation of its pancreatic and gastroepiploic afferents presents an added difficulty.

Surgeons performing a robotic approach to the vascular dissection of a right colectomy with CME are of the opinion that the robotic assistance can play a role in decreasing its technical difficulties; this concept has been widely reported by all the authors of the papers included in this review.

Similarly, some authors have raised concerns of a major risk of vascular injury when CME started to become surgically widespread [44]. This concern was confirmed by preliminary results of an ongoing randomized, controlled, phase 3 superiority trial on laparoscopic right colectomy with CME versus D2 lymphadenectomy [45]. However, it has not been confirmed in our present review of robotic series, as only one author described two cases of minor vascular injury, both of which were successfully repaired and did not require conversion to open surgery. Robotics would, therefore, seem to promise great potential in assuring the feasibility of complex and precise surgical maneuvers.

The operative feasibility of robotic CME is confirmed by the very low incidence of conversions to open surgery (0% in eleven out of the fourteen included studies); in the largest comparative series [24], a significant lower conversion rate in the robotic group is reported.

This is in accordance with evidence from the peer-reviewed published medical literature regarding robotic versus laparoscopic colorectal surgery, where the low conversion rate is accepted as one of the predominant advantages of robotics [46,47]

Finally, the dexterity of the robotic platform with the seven degrees of freedom of surgical instruments has been evoked as decisive in increasing the use of intracorporeal anastomosis (ICA) in comparison to laparoscopic surgery [48–51]; in all but two studies included in this review [28,30], an ICA was performed and the specimen was extracted through a Pfannenstiel incision. Although level 1 evidence from the literature concerning the advantages of ICA over extracorporeal anastomosis (ECA) after right colectomy is still lacking, [52,53] a recent systematic review and meta-analysis including more than 4400 patients [54] demonstrated that patients receiving an ICA had a significantly lower incidence of conversion to open surgery, total complications, anastomotic leakage, surgical site infection and incisional hernia compared to the ECA group.

If the surgical principles of CME are respected, patients' oncologic outcomes are likely to improve, as has been shown in previous series, although these are mainly retrospective and non-randomized [4–14].

Therefore, assessment of the adequacy of the surgical resection is mandatory when considering CME surgery; this has been evaluated by number of harvested lymph nodes, length of surgical specimen, distance of tumor from the vessels ligation site, integrity of the mesocolon and plane of surgery achieved. However, all these parameters are not always detailed in the studies reporting on CME, which makes it difficult to obtain definitive and homogeneous results.

Recently, Benz [55] proposed a new classification of surgical specimens of right colectomy with CME, with the aim of standardizing the histopathological evaluation. It takes into account two main parameters: the integrity of the mesocolon and the completeness of tissue removal. The focus, therefore, is on one of the key factors of CME, that is the clearance of the part of the mesocolon covering the anterior surface of SMV between the stumps of ileo-colic and middle colic vessels.

In new trials on CME for right colon cancer, a homogeneous adoption of this new classification is suggested, to standardize and, therefore, compare results.

Among the studies included in this review, only Trastulli [22] mentioned that the quality of mesocolic excision was assessed referring to the West classification of plane of resection, while in all the other studies the only evaluated histopathologic parameters were number of harvested lymph nodes and [22–24,31] the length of specimen.

It can, therefore, only be affirmed that the number of lymph nodes number was oncologically appropriate, and that in two of the comparative series, more lymph nodes were retrieved in the robotic group than in the laparoscopic group. However, in the majority of the reported series, principles of CME were declared by authors when describing the surgical technique but could not be verified on surgical specimens.

Regarding oncologic results, understood in terms of OS and DFS, these were very good but only reported in three papers.

The results of the four different approaches to robotic CME described in this review are shown in Table 2. Excluding the "top-to-down" approach reported only in one series [26], clinical and oncologic outcomes of the "medial-to-lateral", "bottom-to-up" and "SMV-first" approach do not show statistically significant differences.

Nevertheless, the number of harvested lymph nodes is greater in the "bottom-to up" and in the "SMV first" approaches in comparison with the "medial-to-lateral".

One of the advantages of the "bottom-to-up" approach is the frontal vision of superior mesenteric vascular axis, that can make extensive vascular dissection and D3 lymphadenectomy easier to perform in comparison with the "medial-to-lateral" approach.

Even the "SMV-first" approach is focused on the extensive vascular dissection prior to any other surgical manoeuvre; these technical details, if confirmed by larger scale randomized trials, could in part explain the greater lymph-nodes yield with these two approaches.

In conclusion, this review asserts the feasibility of the robotic approach to CME and CVL for right colectomy; this allows for a low conversion rate, the successful management of any intraoperative complications that might arise, and good clinical outcomes.

Oncologic results should be evaluated, in future trials, by a rigorous assessment of the surgical specimen [55] and by long-term survival rates.

Author Contributions: Conceptualization, W.P.; methodology, W.P.; software, W.P., S.B.; validation, W.P.; formal analysis, W.P.; investigation, W.P.; resources, W.P.; data curation, W.P.; writing—original draft prepewration, W.P.; writing—review and editing, W.P., U.F.R.; visualization, W.P., S.B., U.F.R.; supervision, W.P., U.F.R.; project administration, W.P., U.F.R. All authors have read and agreed to the published version of the manuscript.

Funding: This work was partially realized with the Italian Ministry of Health with Ricerca Corrente and 5×1000 funds.

Institutional Review Board Statement: Ethical review and approval were waived for this study, due to the fact that it represents a review of already published articles and no added data on patients were included.

Informed Consent Statement: Patient consent was waived as patient data were already published in the articles analyzed.

Data Availability Statement: All data were retrieved by PubMed search.

Conflicts of Interest: The authors declare no conflict of interests.

References

1. West, N.P.; Morris, E.J.; Rotimi, O.; Cairns, A.; Finan, P.J.; Quirke, P. Pathology grading of colon cancer surgical resection and its association with survival: A retrospective observational study. *Lancet Oncol.* **2008**, *9*, 857–865. [CrossRef]
2. Hohenberger, W.; Weber, K.; Matzel, K.; Papadopoulos, T.; Merkel, S. Standardized surgery for colonic cancer: Complete mesocolic excision and central ligation—Technical notes and outcome. *Colorectal Dis.* **2009**, *11*, 354–364. [CrossRef] [PubMed]
3. Japanese Society for Cancer of the Colon and Rectum. *Japanese Classification of Colorectal Carcinoma*, 2nd ed.; Kanehara & Co., Ltd.: Tokyo, Japan, 2009.
4. Bokey, E.L.; Chapuis, P.H.; Dent, O.F.; Mander, B.J.; Bissett, I.; Newland, R.C. Surgical Technique and Survival in Patients Having a Curative Resection for Colon Cancer. *Dis. Colon Rectum* **2003**, *46*, 860–866. [CrossRef] [PubMed]
5. Ovrebo, K.; Rokke, O. Extended lymph node dissection in colorectal cancer surgery. Reliability and reproducibility in assessments of operative reports. *Int. J. Colorectal Dis.* **2010**, *25*, 213–222. [CrossRef] [PubMed]
6. West, N.P.; Hohenberger, W.; Weber, K.; Perrakis, A.; Finan, P.J.; Quirke, P. Complete Mesocolic Excision with Central Vascular Ligation Produces an Oncologically Superior Specimen Compared with Standard Surgery for Carcinoma of the Colon. *J. Clin. Oncol.* **2010**, *28*, 272–278. [CrossRef]
7. Storli, K.E.; Søndenaa, K.; Furnes, B.; Nesvik, I.; Gudlaugsson, E.; Bukholm, I.; Eide, G.E. Short term results of complete (D3) vs. standard (D2) mesenteric excision in colon cancer shows improved outcome of complete mesenteric excision in patients with TNM stages I–II. *Tech. Coloproctol.* **2013**, *18*, 557–564. [CrossRef]
8. Søndenaa, K.; Quirke, P.; Hohenberger, W.; Sugihara, K.; Kobayashi, H.; Kessler, H.; Brown, G.; Tudyka, V.; D'Hoore, A.; Kennedy, R.H.; et al. The rationale behind complete mesocolic excision (CME) and a central vascular ligation for colon cancer in open and laparoscopic surgery. *Int. J. Colorectal Dis.* **2014**, *29*, 419–428. [CrossRef]
9. Bertelsen, C.A.; Neuenschwander, A.U.; Jansen, J.E.; Wilhelmsen, M.; Kirkegaard-Klitbo, A.; Tenma, J.R.; Bols, B.; Ingeholm, P.; Rasmussen, L.A.; Jepsen, L.V.; et al. Disease-free survival after complete mesocolic excision compared with conventional colon cancer surgery: A retrospective, population-based study. *Lancet Oncol.* **2015**, *16*, 161–168. [CrossRef]
10. Liang, J.-T.; Lai, H.-S.; Huang, J.; Sun, C.-T. Long-term oncologic results of laparoscopic D3 lymphadenectomy with complete mesocolic excision for right-sided colon cancer with clinically positive lymph nodes. *Surg. Endosc.* **2015**, *29*, 2394–2401. [CrossRef]
11. Spinoglio, G.; Marano, A.; Bianchi, P.P.; Priora, F.; Lenti, L.M.; Ravazzoni, F.; Formisano, G. Robotic Right Colectomy with Modified Complete Mesocolic Excision: Long-Term Oncologic Outcomes. *Ann. Surg. Oncol.* **2016**, *23*, 684–691. [CrossRef]
12. Bernhoff, R.; Martling, A.; Sjövall, A.; Granath, F.; Hohenberger, W.; Holm, T. Improved survival after an educational project on colon cancer management in the county of Stockholm—A population based cohort study. *Eur. J. Surg. Oncol. (EJSO)* **2015**, *41*, 1479–1484. [CrossRef] [PubMed]
13. Paquette, I.M.; Madoff, R.D.; Sigurdson, E.R.; Chang, G.J. Impact of Proximal Vascular Ligation on Survival of Patients with Colon Cancer. *Ann. Surg. Oncol.* **2016**, *25*, 38–45. [CrossRef] [PubMed]
14. Ow, Z.G.W.; Sim, W.; Nistala, K.R.Y.; Ng, C.H.; Koh, F.H.-X.; Wong, N.W.; Foo, F.J.; Tan, K.-K.; Chong, C.S. Comparing complete mesocolic excision versus conventional colectomy for colon cancer: A systematic review and meta-analysis. *Eur. J. Surg. Oncol. (EJSO)* **2021**, *47*, 732–737. [CrossRef] [PubMed]
15. Argilés, G.; Tabernero, J.; Labianca, R.; Hochhauser, D.; Salazar, R.; Iveson, T.; Laurent-Puig, P.; Quirke, P.; Yoshino, T.; Taieb, J.; et al. Localised colon cancer: ESMO Clinical Practice Guidelines for diagnosis, treatment and follow-up. *Ann. Oncol.* **2020**, *31*, 1291–1305. [CrossRef]
16. NCCN Clinical Practice Guidelines in Oncology (NCCN Guidelines®). Colon Cancer. Version 2.2021—21 January. Available online: https://www.nccn.org/professionals/physician_gls/pdf/colon.pdf (accessed on 15 April 2021).
17. Glynne-Jones, R.; Wyrwicz, L.; Tiret, E.; Brown, G.; Rödel, C.; Cervantes, A.; Arnold, D. Rectal cancer: ESMO Clinical Practice Guidelines for diagnosis, treatment and follow-up. *Ann. Oncol.* **2017**, *28*, iv22–iv40. [CrossRef]
18. NCCN Clinical Practice Guidelines in Oncology (NCCN Guidelines®). Rectal Cancer. Version 1.2021—22 December. Available online: https://www.nccn.org/professionals/physician_gls/pdf/rectal.pdf (accessed on 15 April 2021).
19. Killeen, S.; Mannion, M.; Devaney, A.; Winter, D.C. Complete mesocolic resection and extended lymphadenectomy for colon cancer: A systematic review. *Colorectal Dis.* **2014**, *16*, 577–594. [CrossRef]
20. Moher, D.; Liberati, A.; Tetzlaff, J.; Altman, D.G. Preferred Reporting Items for Systematic Reviews and Meta-Analyses: The PRISMA Statement. *Ann. Intern. Med.* **2009**, *151*, 264–269. [CrossRef]
21. Wells, G.; Shea, B.; O'Connell, D.; Peterson, J.; Welch, V.; Losos, M.; Tugwell, P. The Newcastle-Ottawa Scale (NOS) for Assessing the Quality of Nonrandomised Studies in Meta-Analyses. 2013. Available online: http://www.ohri.ca/programs/clinical_epidemiology/oxford.asp (accessed on 15 April 2021).

22. Trastulli, S.; Desiderio, J.; Farinacci, F.; Ricci, F.; Listorti, C.; Cirocchi, R.; Boselli, C.; Noya, G.; Parisi, A. Robotic right colectomy for cancer with intracorporeal anastomosis: Short-term outcomes from a single institution. *Int. J. Colorectal Dis.* **2013**, *28*, 807–814. [CrossRef]
23. Petz, W.; Ribero, D.; Bertani, E.; Borin, S.; Formisano, G.; Esposito, S.; Spinoglio, G.; Bianchi, P. Suprapubic approach for robotic complete mesocolic excision in right colectomy: Oncologic safety and short-term outcomes of an original technique. *Eur. J. Surg. Oncol. (EJSO)* **2017**, *43*, 2060–2066. [CrossRef] [PubMed]
24. Spinoglio, G.; Bianchi, P.P.; Marano, A.; Priora, F.; Lenti, L.M.; Ravazzoni, F.; Petz, W.; Borin, S.; Ribero, D.; Formisano, G.; et al. Robotic Versus Laparoscopic Right Colectomy with Complete Mesocolic Excision for the Treatment of Colon Cancer: Perioperative Outcomes and 5-Year Survival in a Consecutive Series of 202 Patients. *Ann. Surg. Oncol.* **2018**, *25*, 3580–3586. [CrossRef] [PubMed]
25. Ngu, J.C.-Y.; Ng, Y.Y.-R. Robotics confers an advantage in right hemicolectomy with intracorporeal anastomosis when matched against conventional laparoscopy. *J. Robot. Surg.* **2018**, *12*, 647–653. [CrossRef] [PubMed]
26. Yozgatli, T.K.; Aytac, E.; Ozben, V.; Bayram, O.; Gurbuz, B.; Baca, B.; Balik, E.; Hamzaoglu, I.; Karahasanoglu, T.; Bugra, D. Robotic Complete Mesocolic Excision Versus Conventional Laparoscopic Hemicolectomy for Right-Sided Colon Cancer. *J. Laparoendosc. Adv. Surg. Tech.* **2019**, *29*, 671–676. [CrossRef]
27. Yang, Y.; Malakorn, S.; Zafar, S.N.; Nickerson, T.P.; Sandhu, L.; Chang, G.J. Superior Mesenteric Vein-First Approach to Robotic Complete Mesocolic Excision for Right Colectomy: Technique and Preliminary Outcomes. *Dis. Colon Rectum* **2019**, *62*, 894–897. [CrossRef] [PubMed]
28. Esch, J.S.A.; Iosivan, S.-I.; Steinfurth, F.; Mahdi, A.; Förster, C.; Wilkens, L.; Nasser, A.; Sarikaya, H.; Benhidjeb, T.; Krüger, M. A standardized suprapubic bottom-to-up approach in robotic right colectomy: Technical and oncological advances for complete mesocolic excision (CME). *BMC Surg.* **2019**, *19*, 72. [CrossRef]
29. Bae, S.U.; Yang, S.Y.; Min, B.S. Totally robotic modified complete mesocolic excision and central vascular ligation for right-sided colon cancer: Technical feasibility and mid-term oncologic outcomes. *Int. J. Colorectal Dis.* **2018**, *34*, 471–479. [CrossRef] [PubMed]
30. Ramachandra, C.; Sugoor, P.; Karjol, U.; Arjunan, R.; Altaf, S.; Patil, V.; Kumar, H.; Beesanna, G.; Abhishek, M. Robotic Complete Mesocolic Excision with Central Vascular Ligation for Right Colon Cancer: Surgical Technique and Short-term Outcomes. *Indian J. Surg. Oncol.* **2020**, *11*, 674–683. [CrossRef]
31. Petz, W.; Bertani, E.; Borin, S.; Fiori, G.; Ribero, D.; Spinoglio, G. Fluorescence-guided D3 lymphadenectomy in robotic right colectomy with complete mesocolic excision. *Int. J. Med. Robot. Comput. Assist. Surg.* **2021**, *17*, eRCS2217. [CrossRef]
32. Ceccarelli, G.; Costa, G.; Ferraro, V.; De Rosa, M.; Rondelli, F.; Bugiantella, W. Robotic or three-dimensional (3D) laparoscopy for right colectomy with complete mesocolic excision (CME) and intracorporeal anastomosis? A propensity score-matching study comparison. *Surg. Endosc.* **2021**, *35*, 2039–2048. [CrossRef]
33. Larach, J.T.; Rajkomar, A.K.S.; Narasimhan, V.; Kong, J.; Smart, P.J.; Heriot, A.G.; Warrier, S.K. Robotic complete mesocolic excision and central vascular ligation for right-sided colon cancer: Short-term outcomes from a case series. *ANZ J. Surg.* **2021**, *91*, 117–123. [CrossRef]
34. Siddiqi, N.; Stefan, S.; Jootun, R.; Mykoniatis, I.; Flashman, K.; Beable, R.; David, G.; Khan, J. Robotic Complete Mesocolic Excision (CME) is a safe and feasible option for right colonic cancers: Short and midterm results from a single-centre experience. *Surg. Endosc.* **2021**, 1–9. [CrossRef]
35. Bianchi, P.P.; Salaj, A.; Giuliani, G.; Ferraro, L.; Formisano, G. Feasibility of robotic right colectomy with complete mesocolic excision and intracorporeal anastomosis: Short-term outcomes of 161 consecutive patients. *Updates Surg.* **2021**, *73*, 1065–1072. [CrossRef]
36. Fleshman, J.; Sargent, D.J.; Green, E.; Anvari, M.; Stryker, S.J.; Beart, R.W.; Hellinger, M.; Flanagan, R.; Peters, W.; Nelson, H. Laparoscopic Colectomy for Cancer Is Not Inferior to Open Surgery Based on 5-Year Data From the COST Study Group Trial. *Ann. Surg.* **2007**, *246*, 655–664. [CrossRef]
37. Buunen, M.; Veldkamp, R.; Hop, W.C.J.; Kuhry, E.; Jeekel, J.; Haglind, E.; Pahlman, L.; Cuesta, M.A.; Msika, S.; Morino, M.; et al. Survival after laparoscopic surgery versus open surgery for colon cancer: Long-term outcome of a randomised clinical trial. *Lancet Oncol.* **2009**, *10*, 44–52. [CrossRef]
38. Green, B.L.; Marshall, H.; Collinson, F.; Quirke, P.; Guillou, P.; Jayne, D.G.; Brown, J.M. Long-term follow-up of the Medical Research Council CLASICC trial of conventional versus laparoscopically assisted resection in colorectal cancer. *BJS* **2012**, *100*, 75–82. [CrossRef]
39. Bae, S.U.; Saklani, A.P.; Lim, D.R.; Kim, D.W.; Hur, H.; Min, B.S.; Baik, S.H.; Lee, K.Y.; Kim, N.K. Laparoscopic-Assisted Versus Open Complete Mesocolic Excision and Central Vascular Ligation for Right-Sided Colon Cancer. *Ann. Surg. Oncol.* **2014**, *21*, 2288–2294. [CrossRef]
40. Storli, K.E.; Søndenaa, K.; Furnes, B.; Eide, G.E. Outcome after Introduction of Complete Mesocolic Excision for Colon Cancer Is Similar for Open and Laparoscopic Surgical Treatments. *Dig. Surg.* **2013**, *30*, 317–327. [CrossRef] [PubMed]
41. Athanasiou, C.; Markides, G.A.; Kotb, A.; Xia, X.; Gonsalves, S.; Miskovic, D. Open compared with laparoscopic complete mesocolic excision with central lymphadenectomy for colon cancer: A systematic review and meta-analysis. *Colorectal Dis.* **2016**, *18*. [CrossRef]
42. Chow, C.F.K.; Kim, S.H. Laparoscopic complete mesocolic excision: West meets East. *World J. Gastroenterol.* **2014**, *20*, 14301–14307. [CrossRef] [PubMed]

43. Spasojevic, M.; Stimec, B.V.; Dyrbekk, A.P.H.; Tepavcevic, Z.; Edwin, B.; Bakka, A.; Ignjatovic, D. Lymph Node Distribution in the D3 Area of the Right Mesocolon. *Dis. Colon Rectum* **2013**, *56*, 1381–1387. [CrossRef] [PubMed]
44. Bertelsen, C.A.; Neuenschwander, A.U.; Jansen, J.E.; Kirkegaard-Klitbo, A.; Tenma, J.R.; Wilhelmsen, M.; Rasmussen, L.A.; Jepsen, L.V.; Kristensen, B.; Gögenur, I.; et al. Short-term outcomes after complete mesocolic excision compared with 'conventional' colonic cancer surgery. *BJS* **2016**, *103*, 581–589. [CrossRef] [PubMed]
45. Xu, L.; Su, X.; He, Z.; Zhang, C.; Lu, J.; Zhang, G.; Sun, Y.; Du, X.; Chi, P.; Wang, Z.; et al. Short-term outcomes of complete mesocolic excision versus D2 dissection in patients undergoing laparoscopic colectomy for right colon cancer (RELARC): A randomised, controlled, phase 3, superiority trial. *Lancet Oncol.* **2021**, *22*, 391–401. [CrossRef]
46. Waters, P.S.; Cheung, F.P.; Peacock, O.; Heriot, A.G.; Warrier, S.K.; O'Riordain, D.S.; Pillinger, S.; Lynch, A.C.; Stevenson, A.R.L. Successful patient-oriented surgical outcomes in robotic vs. laparoscopic right hemicolectomy for cancer—A systematic review. *Colorectal Dis.* **2020**, *22*, 488–499. [CrossRef]
47. Sun, Z.; Kim, J.; Adam, M.A.; Nussbaum, D.P.; Speicher, P.J.; Mantyh, C.R.; Migaly, J. Minimally Invasive Versus Open Low Anterior Resection. *Ann. Surg.* **2016**, *263*, 1152–1158. [CrossRef]
48. Trastulli, S.; Coratti, A.; Guarino, S.; Piagnerelli, R.; Annecchiarico, M.; Coratti, F.; Di Marino, M.; Ricci, F.; Desiderio, J.; Cirocchi, R.; et al. Robotic right colectomy with intracorporeal anastomosis compared with laparoscopic right colectomy with extracorporeal and intracorporeal anastomosis: A retrospective multicentre study. *Surg. Endosc.* **2015**, *29*, 1512–1521. [CrossRef]
49. Morpurgo, E.; Contardo, T.; Molaro, R.; Zerbinati, A.; Orsini, C.; D'Annibale, A. Robotic-Assisted Intracorporeal Anastomosis Versus Extracorporeal Anastomosis in Laparoscopic Right Hemicolectomy for Cancer: A Case Control Study. *J. Laparoendosc. Adv. Surg. Tech.* **2013**, *23*, 414–417. [CrossRef] [PubMed]
50. Lujan, H.J.; Maciel, V.H.; Romero, R.; Plasencia, G. Laparoscopic versus robotic right colectomy: A single surgeon's experience. *J. Robot. Surg.* **2011**, *7*, 95–102. [CrossRef] [PubMed]
51. Park, J.S.; Choi, G.; Park, S.Y.; Kim, H.J.; Ryuk, J.P. Randomized clinical trial of robot-assisted versus standard laparoscopic right colectomy. *BJS* **2012**, *99*, 1219–1226. [CrossRef] [PubMed]
52. Chengwu, J.; Jin, C.; Hu, T.; Wei, M.; Wang, Z. Intracorporeal Versus Extracorporeal Anastomosis in Laparoscopic Right Colectomy: A Systematic Review and Meta-Analysis. *J. Laparoendosc. Adv. Surg. Tech.* **2017**, *27*, 348–357. [CrossRef]
53. Ricci, C.; Casadei, R.; Alagna, V.; Zani, E.; Taffurelli, G.; Pacilio, C.A.; Minni, F. A critical and comprehensive systematic review and meta-analysis of studies comparing intracorporeal and extracorporeal anastomosis in laparoscopic right hemicolectomy. *Langenbeck's Arch. Surg.* **2017**, *402*, 417–427. [CrossRef]
54. Emile, S.H.; Elfeki, H.; Shalaby, M.; Sakr, A.; Bassuni, M.; Christensen, P.; Wexner, S.D. Intracorporeal versus extracorporeal anastomosis in minimally invasive right colectomy: An updated systematic review and meta-analysis. *Tech. Coloproctol.* **2019**, *23*, 1023–1035. [CrossRef]
55. Benz, S.; Tannapfel, A.; Tam, Y.; Grünenwald, A.; Vollmer, S.; Stricker, I. Proposal of a new classification system for complete mesocolic excison in right-sided colon cancer. *Tech. Coloproctol.* **2019**, *23*, 251–257. [CrossRef] [PubMed]

MDPI
St. Alban-Anlage 66
4052 Basel
Switzerland
Tel. +41 61 683 77 34
Fax +41 61 302 89 18
www.mdpi.com

Journal of Personalized Medicine Editorial Office
E-mail: jpm@mdpi.com
www.mdpi.com/journal/jpm

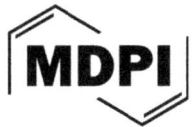